WITHDRAWN

PROVIDING
QUALITY
CARE

Also Available from the American College of Physicians

Bedside Diagnosis: An Annotated Bibliography of Recent Literature on
    Interviewing and Physical Examination
A Curriculum for Internal Medicine Residency: The University of Wisconsin
    Program
Clinical Efficacy Reports
    (evaluations of medical tests and procedures; in looseleaf form)
Common Diagnostic Tests: Use and Interpretation
Drug Prescribing in Renal Failure: Dosing Guidelines for Adults
Guide for Adult Immunization—Second Edition
Hospital Clinical Privileges: Guidelines for Procedures in Gastroenterology
    and Nephrology
Medical Ethics: An Annotated Bibliography
Women and Medicine
Zebra Cards: An Aid to Obscure Diagnoses

Ordering Information:
Subscriber Services
American College of Physicians
Independence Mall West
Sixth Street at Race
Philadelphia, PA 19106-1572
(215) 351-2600
(800) 523-1546

PROVIDING QUALITY CARE

The Challenge to Clinicians

NORBERT GOLDFIELD, MD
DAVID B. NASH, MD, MBA
Editors

Published by the American College of Physicians
Philadelphia, Pennsylvania

First Edition

Printed in the United States of America

Library of Congress Cataloging-in-Publication Data
Main entry under title:
Providing quality care: the challenge to clinicians/[edited by]
  Norbert Goldfield, David B. Nash.
     p.   cm.
  Includes bibliographies.
  ISBN 0-943126-11-8
  1. Medical care—Quality control.   2. Health services
administration.   3. Quality assurance.   I. Goldfield, Norbert.
II. Nash, David B.
  [DNLM: 1. Quality of Health Care—United States. W 84 P969]
RA399.A1P77   1989
362.1'068—dc19

Library of Congress Catalog Card No. 89-6453
ISBN 0-943126-11-8

Table of Contents

Contributors

Paul B. Batalden, MD
Vice President
Medical Care
Hospital Corporation of America
One Park Plaza
P.O. Box 550
Nashville, TN 37202-0550
(615) 320-2759

E. David Buchanan
Director
Quality Program Policy
Hospital Corporation of America
One Park Plaza
P.O. Box 550
Nashville, TN 37202-0550
(615) 320-2182

James B. Couch, MD, JD
Associate Executive Officer
Medical Systems
Metropolitan Hospital
Suite 303
Philadelphia, PA 19106
(215) 238-2068

Robert W. Dubois, MD, PhD
Vice President
Value Health Services
1448 15th Street
Suite 202
Santa Monica, CA 90404
(213) 394-2212

Norbert Goldfield, MD
President
Goldfield and Associates
72 Laurel Park
Northampton, MA 01060
(413) 586-5617

Sheldon Greenfield, MD
Senior Scientist
Institute for the Improvement of
    Medical Care and Health
New England Medical Center
750 Washington Street
Box 345
Boston, MA 02111
(617) 350-8080

Lisa I. Iezzoni, MD
Director of Health Services Research
Health Policy Institute
Boston University
53 Bay State Road
Boston, MA 02215
(617) 353-4520

Sherrie H. Kaplan, PhD
Research Scientist
Institute for the Improvement of
    Medical Care and Health
New England Medical Center
750 Washington Street
Box 345
Boston, MA 02111
(617) 350-8080

Orley H. Lindgren, PhD
Director
Institute for Medical Risk Studies
493 Bridgeway
Sausalito, CA 94965
(415) 332-3414

Don Harper Mills, MD, JD
Director
Institute for Medical Risk Studies
493 Bridgeway
Sausalito, CA 94965
(415) 332-3414

Laura Morlock, PhD
Associate Professor
Department of Health Policy and
    Management
The Johns Hopkins School of Hygiene
    and Public Health
624 North Broadway
Baltimore, MD 21205
(301) 955-6547

David B. Nash, MD, MBA
Assistant Professor of General Internal
    Medicine
Health Evaluation Center, 3 Ravdin
Hospital of the University of
    Pennsylvania
3400 Spruce Street
Philadelphia, PA 19104
(215) 662-2715

Sam Shaprio
Professor Emeritus
Health Services Research and Development Center
The Johns Hopkins University
624 North Broadway
Baltimore, MD 21205
(301) 955-6562

Donald M. Steinwachs, PhD
Professor and Director
Health Services Research and Development Center
The Johns Hopkins University
624 North Broadway
Baltimore, MD 21205
(301) 955-6562

John E. Ware, Jr., PhD
Senior Scientist
Institute for the Improvement of Medical Care and Health
New England Medical Center
750 Washington Street
Box 345
Boston, MA 02111
(617) 350-8080

Jonathan P. Weiner, Dr. PH
Associate Professor of Health Policy and of Medicine
The Johns Hopkins University
624 North Broadway
Room 605
Baltimore, MD 21205
(301) 955-5660

Foreword

America's relationship with its physicians, never a simple association to describe or define, is changing. The public, through its surrogates who largely pay the bill — government and private business — is demanding greater access to the physician's world. This activity, which moves in uncertain fits and starts, is not meant to stifle the clinical autonomy of the physician, but is an effort to better understand the processes and outcomes of medical care. Although medicine will remain largely a self-regulated profession, we have entered what Dr. Arnold S. Relman labeled not long ago "a new era of assessment and accountability... [that] is the third and latest—but probably not the last—phase of our efforts to achieve an equitable health care system, of satisfactory quality, at a price we can afford" (1).

The public and those who pay for medical care are far from alone in this new pursuit of greater accountability. The medical profession itself recognizes that because the care its practitioners render is imperfect, new approaches and applications must be continually sought. This search for greater efficacy and efficiency is in the best tradition of a profession. A learned profession is, after all, a keeper of a body of knowledge, a substantial portion of which derives from experience, as Dr. Samuel O. Thier, president of the National Academy of Sciences' Institute of Medicine, wrote not long ago (2). Moreover, a profession is responsible for advancing that knowledge and transmitting it to the next generation. Lastly, a profession sets and enforces its own standards, and values performance above financial reward. Although one may argue with society's uncertain methods, its challenge to physicians does not represent a central assault on our professionalism. Rather, society is searching for better answers to complex questions that relate to resource allocation, medical decision making, and the role of the patient. And it is asking the medical profession to meet this challenge.

It is appropriate that the American College of Physicians, which has for so long been at the cutting edge of constructive change in medicine, should take up this challenge through publication of this book. These chapters represent an essential summary of the work of leading researchers — physicians, economists, and individuals of other disciplines — who are dissatisfied with the status quo of medicine and are seeking to improve its future, not in isolation but in concert with persons who have a major stake in the outcome.

The title of the overview chapter is illuminating in this regard. The two physicians who edited this volume, David B. Nash and Norbert Goldfield, obviously recognize that without an exchange of information between the profession, payers, and patients, no meaningful dialogue will occur. They come at the question not with fear and trembling, but with enthusiasm that infuses a new generation in search of improving the clinical arsenal of physicians as the 21st century beckons. While physicians struggle with these new forms of scrutiny, they should remember that medical care remains the most highly valued service in our society, despite its imperfections.

One of the' common characteristics of the authors of this book is that although much of their work is published in the professional medical literature, they also are seeking to reach broader audiences — particularly the health policy community. In their search for better answers, they are demonstrating leadership. And the physicians among them are saying that it is inappropriate for medicine as a leadership profession to shrink from the self-examination necessary to propose better allocations of medical resources, grounded in clinical insight and practice, than has heretofore been the case.

John K. Iglehart
Editor, *Health Affairs*

References

1. Relman AS. Assessment and accountability: the third revolution in medical care. *N Engl J Med.* 1988; **319**:1220-2.
2. Thier SO. Reexamining the principles of medicine. *Health Aff (Millwood).* 1987; Winter:70-4.

Introduction

A dozen "Fortune 500" sized companies collaborate in Chicago (under the auspices of an employer-sponsored health care cost containment organization) to develop a system for monitoring the quality of health care. The companies, as a unit, join to negotiate lower rates and monitor provider performance. In Miami, a large trucking firm sends questionnaires to local physicians asking for detailed information about their training, fees, and malpractice history. In Philadelphia, a large teaching hospital distributes a special report each month detailing the cost to the hospital for every patient case, by Diagnosis Related Group, for individual physicians. Clinicians whose performance is more than two standard deviations from the mean of their colleagues are singled out for mandatory attendance at several continuing medical education programs. Lastly, outpatient office charts are coming under intense scrutiny and health maintenance organizations (HMOs) routinely send out patient-satisfaction survey questionnaires matching up chart notations with consumer reports about the quality of the medical intervention.

These are not draconian scenarios drawn from some future dominated by a mandatory national health insurance program. Rather, they are actual programs functioning as part of our multifaceted, pluralistic delivery system.

What common theme ties these scenarios together? In a phrase, *access to information*. Information about consumers, providers, hospitals, and HMOs. Information in vast new quantities. So much new information that researchers are just now sorting and cataloguing before the real analytical work can start.

We believe that physicians have been slow to appreciate the consequences of compiling this new database. Who will have access to information about the practice patterns of physicians? Will utilization data be tied to the delineation of clinical privileges? Can hospital mortality rates be used to rank hospitals with regard to quality, and, if so, how will these rankings be released?

These are just some of the pressing questions we seek to answer in this book. We have assembled a talented group of contributors from across the country, and each is an expert in his or her own right. We challenged them, successfully we believe, to focus their analytic talents for a clinical audience.

This is not a "how to" book with neat solutions to the knotty problems laid out above. Rather, we seek to provide clinicians with a working vocabulary of the terms and concepts involved in utilization review, mortality measures, severity-of-illness indices, and other quality of care research tools. Now, armed with this new vocabulary, physicians can sit at any hospital and medical staff negotiating table without an interpreter. They can act as co-equals with those controlling the resources — hospital administrators, insurance company executives, and others.

Each chapter has been subjected to a rigorous peer review process. This helped us sharpen our focus and provide you, the reader, with the most authoritative and reliable information available. Naturally, any errors of commission or omission are ours alone; that is the ultimate responsibility we bear as editors.

After each chapter, one of us offers a "commentary" meant in part to further elucidate complex points but, more importantly, to help weave the disparate chapters into a coherent whole volume. Our contributors have delivered on their promises, made almost 18 months ago, to bring us absolutely the most current critical thinking on the issues. Our "commentaries" are shaped by our bias that clinicians are woefully unprepared for the information overload about to influence their practice patterns.

Who should read this book? We believe it has a wide audience among *all* clinicians concerned about quality. Physicians in all fields are the primary audience. Nurses, medical records technicians, medical staff administrators, and attorneys concerned with health-related issues would also find much useful information. Certainly, physicians in training and their program directors would benefit from an early reading of this book. No clinician will be immune from the fallout generated by the explosive concepts so clearly articulated by our contributing authors.

We are indebted to Edward J. Huth, Editor, *Annals of Internal Medicine* and head of the Publication Division, American College of Physicians — for his willingness to publish our book. Kathleen Case, Director of the Department of Scientific Publishing, Diane McCabe, Publishing Projects Coordinator, and Laini Berlin, Production Editor, were helpful from the conception of this book through a prolonged gestation.

We owe a special thanks to John Iglehart, an accomplished fellow editor (of *Health Affairs*) and special health policy correspondent to *The New England Journal of Medicine*, for writing an insightful foreward.

Lastly, our wives, Sandra and Esther, and all of our children, bore a good part of our burden while the book began to take its present final form. They tolerated our late night calls between Philadelphia and Hartford with mostly good humor and a shrug that conveyed the message, "Oh well, what can we do about them anyway?" The truth is, without Sandra and Esther, the entire project would never have been undertaken, as they are our beacons to new horizons and our anchors to the realities of family life. We owe the Goldfield and Nash households a big collective thanks for a supportive job well done.

Norbert Goldfield, MD
Northhampton, Massachusetts

David B. Nash, MD, MBA
Philadelphia, Pennsylvania

Winter 1988

Chapter 1

Information Needs of Purchasers

DAVID B. NASH, MD, MBA
NORBERT GOLDFIELD, MD

INTRODUCTION

Leaders of American business and government are tired of paying the increasing costs of health care for their employees. In the past 5 years payers in both the public and private sector have attempted to hold down health care costs in many ways. What are the financial results of these efforts? Have these efforts resulted in questions about the quality of care delivered in this country? Although the measurement of quality of health care has always had merit, the current push to measure quality of care arises out of the realizations that efforts at reducing costs have resulted in poorer care for certain segments of the population, and that improvements in quality will result in decreased costs.

Since the early 1960s health care costs have quadrupled and now consume 11% of the gross national product, with estimates of 15% by the year 2000 (Simmons HE. Speech given to the National Leadership Commission on Health Care, Washington, DC, April 14, 1988). In 1986 increases in hospital charges outstripped the rate of inflation by 10 to 1 (1). Wide differences were seen in the daily costs of inpatient care; a hospital patient in California pays an average of $1,109 a day whereas a patient in New York pays $512 a day (1). In 31 states, a hospital bed was empty as often as it was occupied; in 35 states, beds were vacant an average of 150 days a year.

Faced with rising costs in all segments of the health care system, experts have proposed various interventions in the physician-patient relationship. The Canadian and European models limit total outlay for various health care sectors. However, the American model, a mixed private and public model, encourages smaller interventions that inevitably affect the physician-patient relationship. It is this effect on the relationship between the physician and patient that has raised concern regarding the deterioration of quality of care.

Three 'types of interventions have emerged. Health maintenance organizations (HMOs) have received the greatest attention. Although HMOs decrease health costs compared with traditional indemnity, they also attempt for financial reasons to enroll healthier patients, leaving the sicker patients in traditional indemnity plans. Enrollment in HMOs has skyrocketed from 10 million in 1980 to nearly 30 million in 1988 (Simmons HE. Speech given to the National Leadership Commission on Health Care, Washington, DC, April 14, 1988).

A second intervention occurred, in part, as a consequence of this increase in HMO enrollment. Health insurers responded to the perceived attempt by HMOs to enroll healthier patients (as well as to the onset of Diagnosis Related Groups and other government efforts to cut costs) by mitigating their risk and carefully monitoring efforts of health care institutions to shift costs or increase charges for paying patients. This action has occurred in the face of increasing numbers of uninsured or low-paying HMO contract patients. In the past 10 years, the number of uninsured persons in this country has risen dramatically to nearly 30 million in 1988. Access to care is as important a measure of quality as is the prescription of appropriate medication.

Third, health insurers have attempted to cut costs through interventions such as preadmission certification, second surgical opinions, and concurrent review. These efforts are a result of research by John Wennberg that highlights the variations in practice patterns for medical conditions throughout the United States. Variations in practice patterns have caused concern about the appropriateness of care for many illnesses. For example, determining the appropriate conditions under which coronary arteriography is done has both quality and cost implications. Physicians and payers alike realize that although cost considerations have increased concern about quality, quality measurements, whether in the areas of appropriateness, severity, or patient satisfaction, can themselves affect the cost of medical care.

Henry Simmons, MD, president of the National Leadership Commission on Health Care, listed the critical questions on quality of care for those who purchase health care at the Commission's April 1988 meeting. What are the medical practice standards guiding the care your employees receive? How are these standards being set? Are they based on solid science? Are there adequate systems that continually monitor adherence and, when necessary, cause timely corrective action? How effectively are these medical resources being used and how are they affecting the health of your employees and their families?

Physicians must understand these issues if they are to participate in the debate on controlling costs and assuring quality. There is no question that quality of care measuring can be considerably improved. However, quality of care is multifaceted, and although our quality control mechanisms are at a rudimentary stage, many measurement tools are available. The challenge for physicians is to adopt these tools when appropriate to highlight quality deficiencies and achieve cost savings. Although physicians are less than one half of 1% of the population, they determine how nearly 11% of the gross national product will be spent (2).

DEFINING QUALITY OF CARE

Physicians have traditionally been reluctant to define quality, claiming that it is an elusive concept. In part, the traditional physician-patient relationship was unequal; the physician held sway, making all decisions regarding care. Each physician had his or her own definition of quality directed to a particular patient. Caper (3) defined the three components of quality as efficacy, appropriateness, and the caring function of medicine. *Efficacy* is the concern that a diagnostic or therapeutic procedure accomplishes its goal. Although a particular diagnostic or therapeutic course of action may be *appropriate* in some circumstances, the costs, risks, and benefits must be assessed in each case. *The caring function of medicine* involves the interpersonal, supportive, and psychological aspects of the physician-patient relationship.

More recently, researchers and practitioners have been refining their definitions of quality, searching for a paradigm that all concerned parties would accept. Quality could be defined as the *capacity* of patient care to achieve a goal (4). Accordingly, this definition shifts the focus of quality from the property of the treatment to its capacity to achieve a goal, and makes the goal the factor that determines quality. Therefore, quality can be measured only with reference to a goal.

The American Medical Association (5) considered eight elements as essential to good quality care. In brief, quality care should produce optimal improvement in the patient's health; emphasize health promotion and disease prevention; be provided in a timely fashion; include informed consent; be based on accepted medical principles; be provided with empathy; use technology efficiently; and be documented in such a way to allow for peer review (5). However, as Steffen (4) has pointed out, this definition does not state how all of these elements are connected; quality must include an assessment of patient goals and values.

The federal government has several definitions of quality care. One recent definition states, "the quality of medical care is the degree to which the process of care increases the probability of outcomes desired by patients and decreases the probability of undesired outcomes, given the state of medical knowledge" (6).

Avedis Donabedian has established a framework for assessing quality — the triad of structure, process, and outcome (7-9). Structural measures of quality include tangible and quantifiable items such as the ratio of physicians to patient beds and the composition of certain hospital committees. Measures of process include utilization review functions such as the average length of stay for certain procedures, adherence to established standards, and a general sense of proficiency based on volume and conditions treated (10). Outcome measures go beyond simple morbidity and mortality measures to include rates of iatrogenic complications, nosocomial infections, and unexpected returns to the operating room.

Lastly, quality care can be viewed as having two principal dimensions, the "technical" and "interpersonal" aspects of care (11). Technical quality depends on how well the science and technology of medicine are applied to diagnosing and treating the patient's problems. Interpersonal quality depends on how well the patient's personal needs are met.

Some critics may argue that these definitions are not helpful and, in fact, are dated. As early as 1910, Dr. Ernest A. Codman (12), a surgeon at the Massachusetts General Hospital in Boston, was promulgating his quality assurance idea known as the "end result system." Codman claimed that "to effect improvement, the first step is to admit and record the lack of perfection" (12). He did a case-by-case review of surgical outcomes and kept a file card system for reviewing his own performance. Although Codman was a strong proponent of peer review, his ideas were considered radical, and he was eventually forced to leave his position. Eventually, his work was influential in the organization of the American College of Surgeons in 1913, and the Hospital Standardization Program that the College carried on until it evolved into the Joint Commission on Accreditation of Hospitals in 1952.

By 1952 other physicians were linking hospital statistics with quality care. Paul Lembcke (13) showed wide variations in appendectomy rates in New York State, foreshadowing the seminal work in small-area analysis by John Wennberg over 20 years later.

PUBLIC AND PROFESSIONAL PERCEPTIONS

Before answering the question "Can purchasers make the right decisions, given good information?" one needs to examine what purchasers think about health care today. Are the public's perceptions about health care markedly different from the physicians' viewpoints? Purchasers of care, whether large organizations or individual consumers, *assume* a high quality of care — they do not consciously think they may be purchasing inadequate care. The public may feel that the implicit threat of malpractice serves as a guardian of quality.

Joseph Califano, Jr., (now a Washington, DC, lawyer after serving as Secretary of Health, Education, and Welfare from 1977 to 1979 under President Carter) has written that medicine is too important to be left to physicians and politicians (14). Citing his experience as chairman of the health care committee at Chrysler Corporation, Califano shows that 5% of the claims submitted by employees generated 40% of the costs, and that employees holding the same job took different periods of leave for the same medical conditions and diagnoses. Based on a new program of establishing medical guidelines for physicians treating Chrysler workers, the company has saved more than $3 million in 6 months, not to mention 52,000 days of work.

Believing that government policymaking in health care often mirrors public opinion polls, some researchers have discovered surprising trends among the public. Blendon (15) reported six major public opinion trends most likely to influence the quality of health care: Americans appear to be happier with the status quo of their personal health care than is commonly recognized. Americans want *more* health spending, not less. The continuation of public support for increased health spending will depend on there not being an economic crisis in the 1990s. The public does not see the staggering federal deficit as a problem requiring major cuts in health care spending. In the event of a serious economic crisis the public would reduce health spending by freezing fees, regionalizing expensive technologies, reducing inefficiencies, and limiting care to the poor. The commercialization of care may lead to a decline in the public's trust in health professionals.

Contrary to expert forecasts, the public is not inclined to participate in newer forms of practice such as HMOs, preferring their current arrangements — especially the freedom to choose a personal physician or hospital. These polls point to a national contradiction: the concern regarding quality as well as a desire to maintain the status quo (16). Some observers note that the progressive medicalization of daily life has brought unrealistic expectations of cure; these expectations have created a climate of apprehension, insecurity, and alarm among the public (17).

Other public opinion polls support Blendon's findings. Harvard Community Health Plan, a large HMO in Boston, commissioned a firm to conduct a national opinion survey about making difficult health care decisions (18). Contradictory opinions between the public and physicians were evident. By a margin of 91% to 8% the public believes that people should have the right to get the best possible health care. By a margin of 71% to 26% the public believes that health insurance should pay for any treatment that will save lives, regardless of the cost to save one life. Physicians, on the other hand, disagree with this statement by a margin of three to one. Lastly, although less than one third of the public believes they get good-to-excellent value for their health care dollar, more than three quarters of physicians believe we get *excellent* value.

The various definitions of quality care and the results of national opinion polls make formulating a policy difficult. If purchasers agree on the definitions, can they make appropriate decisions about where to spend their health care dollars? The core questions for purchasers are "What kind of information do I need about the supplier or provider of care to help me make a rational, best-buy decision for my employees? Who should get this information, how should it be structured, and how should it be used by corporate decision makers?

THE INFORMATION FLOW

Because the federal government is the largest single purchaser of medical care, it is worthwhile to examine quality guidelines for consumers developed for a recent Office of Technology Assessment (OTA) report (6). The OTA describes 10 possible indicators for quality care that consumers should use when purchasing health services (Table 1). However, it is unrealistic to assume

TABLE 1. Summary of Quality of Care Indicators Evaluated by the Office of Technology Assessment

Hospital mortality rates
Adverse events, including nosocomial (hospital-acquired) infections
Formal disciplinary actions by state medical boards against physicians
PRO/HHS sanctions
Malpractice compensation
Evaluation of physicians' performance for a specific condition, such as hypertension, by process or outcome measures
Volume of services in hospitals or performed by physicians
External standards and guidelines for scope of hospital services, including emergency rooms, cancer care, and neonatal intensive care units
Physician specialization as measured by specialty board certification or by practicing in one's area of training
Patients' assessment of their care

From U.S. Congress, Office of Technology Assessment. *The Quality of Medical Care: Information for Consumers.* Washington, DC: U.S. Government Printing Office, June 1988 (OTA-H-386).

that most of these data would be available to any one provider. But this is a beginning that helps establish a clearinghouse to maintain the critical flow of information.

The OTA (19) cautions purchasers that current techniques are not adjusted adequately for patients and that environmental factors may influence their health and satisfaction independently of the quality of care. There are no uniform methods to record, collect, and report data. For outpatients, this is particularly true as there is never a discharge abstract available to review each patient encountered. In addition, although some information, like hospital mortality rates, is becoming available to the public, some relevant quality information, such as the results of hospital accreditation, is regularly compiled but not publicly available.

Finally, how individuals and organizations use quality-of-care information, and how information can most effectively be communicated remain largely unexplored. The OTA recommends that consumers combine information from more than one quality indicator and draw information from more than 1 year.

The OTA recognizes that consumers may not have "perfect market access." That is, "consumers' choices occur in an environment that is partly restricted by physician referral and limitations imposed by employers, third-party payers, geographic location, and lack of health insurance" (6).

The OTA speculated as to how to make more and better quality information available to consumers. The recent release of hospital mortality information by the Health Care Financing Administration (HCFA) was cited as a case in point. Although the HCFA statistics were cited in the print media, radio, and television, the OTA reported (6) that another step might be

> . . . to make quality-related information continuously available to consumers in hard copy and through computer terminals in libraries, senior citizen centers, adult education centers, community centers, and other facilities. Hard copy information could be provided to physicians, particularly referral physicians;

this would assist them to make wise referral choices and to help patients who want the information interpreted. Cable television exposures could be considered as "hot lines" that could provide a source of continuous information.

The report (6) contends that

The acceptance of information on the quality of a provider's care is increased when it is accessible in familiar settings, such as libraries and senior citizen centers, where needed social support is present. Studies of consumers' reasons for choosing health services indicate that consumers often rely on the recommendations of friends and relatives; lay opinions and social networks play an important role in the evaluation and decision processes regarding choice of physicians and hospitals. Consumers need social support from peers, family, and friends in making choices of health providers. Expert-based information may seem less foreign if it is presented in familiar settings.

In essence, the OTA suggests integrating information on quality care into available sources.

The OTA concludes that only a few indicators have the most validity for consumers: formal disciplinary actions by state medical boards against poor-quality physicians; physicians practicing in the area of their training; and patients' ratings of the interpersonal aspects of their care.

Many researchers have studied the issue of patients' ratings and concluded that consumers can accurately and reproducibly judge certain aspects of the quality of medical care services. The process of care can be thought of as having two basic components: the scientific or technical, and the interpersonal (20). Research using patient questionnaires and a review of the literature has shown some surprising results (21) that are summarized here:

- Bias from personal characteristics is not so strong as to invalidate consumers' ratings of the interpersonal or technical quality of their care.

- Consumers' ratings of technical quality do reflect, at least in part, how many services they received.

- For common problems, consumers can distinguish between the technical aspects of care judged good and less-than-good by physicians.

- Interpersonal features of care do not obscure consumers' abilities to distinguish levels of the technical process for common outpatient problems.

- Whatever "quality" means to consumers, their perceptions of quality affect their choices among health care alternatives.

- Consumers' reports (as distinct from ratings) hold considerable promise as a data source for quality assessment and assurance activities.

- The costs of obtaining data from consumers are not higher, and are probably lower, than those for obtaining data from more traditional sources such as record audits.

- Consumers are the best source of data on the interpersonal aspects of care; moreover, consumers can provide some of the data on technical quality of outpatient care not available from such traditional data sources as claims and records.

This research seems to confirm what all good clinicians already intuitively know: Listen to your patients; they can make the diagnosis for you. To which can be added: They can also tell the clinician how good a job he or she is doing!

CORPORATE "BUY RIGHT" PROGRAMS

As the manager of employee benefits for Aluminum Company of America (ALCOA), Richard Wardrop told his employees, "When we buy a car or a household appliance, we bore in like lions. When we buy health care, we act like lambs. We do exactly what we're told to do, because we simply don't have enough information to make good decisions" (22).

This firm and other members of the Pennsylvania Business Roundtable have joined the Buy Right Project. Buy Right, developed by Walter McClure, from the Center for Policy Studies in Minneapolis, helps employees and their beneficiaries choose among providers with good quality and efficiency (23,24). McClure has said, "The individual patient can no more determine the quality and efficiency of his providers from one or two medical episodes than he can tell the quality of a hitter after watching one or two ball games . . . . Who sees the whole season for the providers? The Purchasers" (25).

Buy Right rewards the efficient high-quality provider with patients, not artificial bonuses. Buy Right requires that purchasers be able to assess the quality and efficiency of providers, and then provide their employees with the means and incentives to choose the most efficient quality providers. These principles raise two technical problems: How do you measure quality and efficiency, and how can the purchaser help beneficiaries shift to the "better" provider?

McClure (25) believes that quality has three components: patient satisfaction, effectiveness, and innovation. These components are best measured by comparing provider performance using available expert quality assessment systems such as the Horn Severity Index and the MedisGroups Staging System. If purchasers demand this type of information, providers will install these expert systems to remain competitive. (However, physicians must help corporations and other big purchasers see the distinction between severity and quality).

In terms of shifting to the better provider, McClure's plan changes the incentives that are currently based solely on price. Companies score providers on quality and efficiency and then give beneficiaries incentives to choose good providers over those who are inefficient or of poor quality. McClure calls this solution "incentive technology." Although Buy Right programs recognize the limitations in state-of-the-art quality assessment tools, companies who join are getting useful information rather than basing all purchase decisions on cost alone. One must also remember that access to care is part of the decision-making process.

Buy Right programs are a kind of disclosure tool, forcing hospitals to release information on cost and quality. Other, less widespread information disclosure systems are also being used. Some companies, like Ryder Systems, Inc., of Miami, have developed their own clearinghouse for quality information called Medfacts (26). Ryder sent a questionnaire to 1400 physicians in the Miami area asking for detailed information about their training, fees, and local hospital privileges. Although only a first step toward ranking physicians by quality performance, Medfacts has computerized its database, and an employee can search for specific kinds of information. For example, the system can easily find "a board-certified female gynecologist between the ages of 35 and 55 practicing in southern Dade County who provides second opinions."

Although these information assembly techniques are still being developed, Pennsylvania and Colorado have recently enacted legislation that requires hospitals to furnish data on medical outcomes and severity of illness, and to make the data available through appropriate state agencies (27). These state agencies will issue public reports on "hospital quality" not later than 1990. However, both states have adopted different systems. Which one is the best and most accurate? New Jersey will soon adopt another system measuring severity. Hospitals may one day face the problem of reclassifying a patient's level if the patient transfers from one state to another, despite the fact that the patient is clinically unchanged.

Although comparisons of severity of illness are relevant, they are not the same as quality. However, it appears that the desire to obtain any kind of relevant information becomes an overriding force. These information systems have spawned a new industry where academicians have set up for-profit companies to sell their wares across the country. Physicians now must cope with this evaluation of their daily activities (28).

NEW WAYS TO PURCHASE BENEFITS (AND QUALITY)

Although some companies join Buy Right programs in their local areas, others have taken broader action on their own. In 1987 Allied-Signal saw its health care bill jump 39% to $355 million (29). Allied recently created a single, national health care plan by making their 67,000 employees the customers of one insurer, CIGNA Corporation. According to Allied's chairman (30), " . . . by offering volume business to CIGNA, we've secured a three-year fixed rate of increase in costs for comprehensive medical and dental care for our U.S. employees. CIGNA is able to share the risk with us because it in turn has contracted with a network of physicians, hospitals, and other health care providers to deliver services." By using one insurer, there is the potential opportunity for stricter quality control measures, uniform data reporting, and better assessment of outcomes all geared toward improved quality at a lower cost.

Other companies have taken Allied's lead. Southwestern Bell Corporation, based in St. Louis, entered its 57,300 employees and retirees in 18 cities in five Midwestern and Southern states into a network of HMOs operated by the Prudential Insurance Company of America (the nation's largest group health insurer) (31). The company has increased the burden on employees who do not use the network by making them pay higher deductibles and out-of-pocket costs for physician visits. Although the company admits that there have been some "growing pains," medical costs have been reduced by at least 10% from the rate under the old indemnity plan.

United HealthCare, the second largest publicly held HMO company in the country, has teamed up with Honeywell by agreeing to tailor a special health care plan to Honeywell's specifications. According to Dr. John M. Burns, Honeywell's health and resources vice president, "We said, 'Here is the product we intend to buy. We want certain benefits and we have certain requirements. If you want to supply us, you have to provide them' " (32). The plan includes strict financial monitoring of physicians, allowing benefits managers to examine claims that are several standard deviations from the norm and to force physicians to practice differently.

Ultimately, a purchaser, whether a corporation or the government, can adopt different options when negotiating with a health care provider. Each option has implications for quality of care measurement. Allied and other corporations have chosen to work with one health care provider. There are administrative advantages to this approach. When uniform data exist, the purchaser can demand both financial and quality of care data in summary form. Medicare, Xerox, and General Electric have adopted a different approach. These organizations have concluded that the Allied approach represents a fundamental misunderstanding of the way health care is delivered in this country. General Electric has adopted the position that health care is a local phenomenon and not a fundamentally uniform commodity, and therefore cannot be organized in an efficient manner on a national basis. Medicare, for example, is currently adopting the strategy of negotiating with either local or regional preferred provider organizations. It becomes readily apparent that the approach to quality of care measurement is different in these two purchasing strategies.

The beneficial effects on quality under these various options are arguable, but the message is clear: Big purchasers can wield clout. Companies are moving aggressively from passive payers to savvy shoppers for health care.

BEYOND UTILIZATION REVIEW

There are few topics as irksome to clinicians as utilization review (33): Many believe that utilization review is simply a euphemism for "physician interference." Now, researchers have begun to look at the relationship between utilization review and quality. Major companies are hiring outside consulting firms to conduct independent reviews of clinician decision making — moving beyond the simple preadmission certification programs of the early 1980s. There are new corporate programs that focus on the two arms of utilization review: appropriateness (quality) and efficiency (scheduling, length-of-stay, evaluations, prescribing habits, among others).

Individual companies that lack market clout may not be able to force hospitals to renegotiate rates or disclose mortality information. Smaller companies can now turn to private utilization review companies to analyze their insurance claims. In one recent study (35), researchers found that utilization review reduced admissions by 12.3%, inpatient days by 8.0%, hospital expenditures by 11.9%, and total medical expenditures by 8.3%. When the same authors analyzed only groups that had relatively high admission rates before adopting utilization review, it was found that they had a 34% reduction in inpatient days and a 30% reduction in hospital expenditures. The savings-to-cost ratio of utilization review overall was about 8 to 1.

Utilization review is the assessment of the appropriateness and efficiency of hospital care through review of the medical record (35). Implicit review criteria usually means that physicians review the entire record and make summary judgments. Explicit review criteria are predetermined. Generally, nonphysicians review the medical records to ascertain whether the care rendered met review criteria. There are four generally accepted dimensions to utilization review (35):

- What care was provided? Did it meet the patient's medical needs?

- When was the care provided? Did the admission occur an appropriate length of time before the surgery, or were there unneeded preoperative days of care?

- How much care was provided in terms of the duration and frequency of care? Was the hospital stay the appropriate length? Was the number of laboratory tests appropriate?

- Where was the care provided? Did the patient require hospital-level care, or could he or she have been treated in an alternative site such as an outpatient clinic, an ambulatory surgery center, or a nursing home?

Utilization management goes beyond these traditional definitions to include the deliberate action by payers to influence providers to increase the efficiency and effectiveness with which services are provided (35). Now, companies are turning to case-management firms to help them bring down costs and bolster quality through utilization management.

For example, with 12,000 employees nationally, Sheraton Corporation spent $12.2 million on health care in 1986. The birth of three premature infants accounted for 10% of the total cost (36). Sheraton retained a case-management company to work with physicians, patients, and family members to minimize hospital stays and find alternative treatments such as home outpatient care or the use of specialized facilities. Case managers know what local resources are available and can blunt the effects from catastrophic cases. No controlled trials have been done that show a positive impact on quality from these programs, but corporations will not wait for these trials. The bottom-line savings appear to be sufficient evidence for them to move ahead. One utilization management company helps firms analyze competing HMOs by doing comparative audits of quality of care. This company claims that although costs are in the center of controversy today, employee relations, union relations, and *liability* costs of poor quality care will be critical in the future (37).

Clinicians should not regard these maneuvers as attempts by companies to encroach on traditional professional concerns. Some companies have abandoned second opinion surgical programs and preadmission certification due to a lack of proven cost savings and, more importantly, employee complaints about the unwieldy nature of the bureaucracy these programs have spawned. Limited evidence suggests that preadmission screening has few deleterious effects on patient care outcomes (38).

PAYING FOR QUALITY

With the advent of computerized indices of severity of illness, hospitals can now compare their patients' status with competitive institutions. It seems only natural that hospitals could use these new tools and work together to set clinical performance standards. If hospitals met these explicit utilization standards, which were bolstered by measures of patient severity, their success could be rewarded and their shortfalls could be penalized.

Four hospitals in Rochester, New York, have signed an agreement with the state and Blue Cross that apparently would make them the nation's first hospitals to receive bigger payments if they achieve better clinical outcomes (39). The hospitals have set aside 1% of their pooled revenues from all non-Medicare sources in 1988, rising to 2% in 1989. From the pool these hospitals will allocate *extra* per diem payments to facilities that meet morbidity and mortality goals they establish for themselves. One state official estimated their combined revenues to be $340 million.

The 3-year experiment, because it takes severity of illness into account, would not penalize member hospitals if patients had complications as long as the complications were "anticipated or explained" (40). Rochester is the only city in the nation where hospitals have a financial incentive to do a better job. No doubt this is the most sophisticated step in a national movement toward the use of severity of illness systems to evaluate, and perhaps control, medical quality and utilization. The Hospital Experimental Program Phase III, as the project is called, will also allow the hospitals to be compared with a "norm" calculated from the proprietary software system used to measure severity of illness (41). Purchasers of care will have powerful market information on the cooperating hospitals rivaling the programs set up by Allied, CIGNA, and others previously discussed.

Individual physician quality ratings will get a real boost if the HCFA, which controls the Medicare plan, pushes through its proposal. The HCFA hopes to begin funding a study that would rate physicians by name with results eventually being made public (42). There are many factors to be considered in rating physicians, including mortality rates, speed of recovery, and complexity and severity of illness — basically the same criteria now used by HCFA to rate hospitals with regard to their treatment of Medicare beneficiaries (43).

Hospitals may soon get computer software that would enable them to track physician performance precisely and provide some quality indicators, however crude. The Medical Group Management Association in Denver developed the program at its Center for Research in Ambulatory Health Care Administration under a 42-month, $625,000 grant from the W.K. Kellogg Foundation of Battle Creek, Michigan (44). The software uses a relative value scale to measure the differences in physicians' productivity. The potential of this system to identify nonproductive physicians in a large group is impressive. There is an intellectual leap of faith when one has to relate mundane procedure reports, without variation between physicians, to differences in perceived quality among practitioners.

The trend toward ranking individual physician performance is the result of ranking hospital performance. The business community and consumers, together with consumer advocacy groups concerned about the impact of cost containment on health, demand criteria, standards, and data — information flow — with which to measure physician performance.

A Boston research group points out (45) that physician performance rating still is dominated by subjective assessment, and hampered by poor information and a lack of quantifiable criteria. This group believes that computerized claims data, audits of office practices, and patient satisfaction surveys will allow composite ratings of individual physicians over time. Some of the important criteria that will be used to establish these profiles include tracer conditions to assess how primary care clinicians treat hypertension, diabetes mellitus, and the like. Table 2 shows the entire proposed composite profile, an inevitable consequence of medical information flow.

Perhaps one way to prepare for these inevitable changes in the evaluation of clinicians is to incorporate a quality management program into residency training. Faculty at the University of Vermont College of Medicine (46) have emphasized the importance of the problem-oriented medical record and its relation to quality assurance activities. The program stresses thoroughness, reliability, analytic sense, and efficiency — all critical skills for the future practitioner. The researchers claim that it *is* possible to define explicit standards against which to judge analytic capabilities. The residency directors are striving to teach the complex interrelationship between cost and quality.

HMO QUALITY

No section on information flow as it relates to quality could conclude without a brief discussion of HMO quality. Luft (47) has shown that the large, traditional, group and staff model HMOs were eager to participate

TABLE 2. Developing a Composite Profile of the Primary Care Physician

Component	Examples
Institute of Medicine criteria score	
Accessibility	Arrangements for on-call coverage
Comprehensiveness	Range of services provided in office
Coordination	Review mechanisms for collecting information from other providers
Continuity	Review medical record for quality of documentation
Accountability	Peer review mechanisms in practice; liability coverage
Process tracer score	Review of explicit and implicit process tracers for: Illnesses common in primary care practice (hypertension, urinary tract infections, congestive heart failure) Screening and preventive health care (compliance with Canadian Task Force guidelines for mammography, breast examination, Papanicolaou smears, stool guaiac/rectal examination)
Outcome tracer score	Rates of hypertensives with controlled blood pressure Rates of smoking cessation, weight loss, lowering of cholesterol levels
Physician credentials	Residency completed in accredited program Board certification
Education and teaching profile	Recertification in specialty Active in teaching program
Patient satisfaction score	Access to office Physician behavior Continuity of care
Psychosocial and bioethical profile	Evidence of health promotion and health education activity Discussion and management of critically ill or dying patient's wishes

Reproduced with permission. Daley J, German PM, Delbanco TL. Looking for quality in primary care physicians. *Health Aff (Millwood)*. 1988; 7:107-13.

in studies comparing HMO quality. Kaiser and Group Health Cooperative of Puget Sound were the mainstays of the now famous, but severely outdated, RAND Health Insurance Study. That study showed that HMOs saved money but delivered care equal to, *if not better than*, care available in the fee-for-service sector. Proponents of HMOs saw the group practice setting "as encouraging consultation and the shared medical record as an informal method of ongoing peer review" (47). With the advent of increased competition and the corporatization of care, these findings may now be called into question.

For example, the Midwest Business Group on Health (MBGH), a consortium of businesses interested in health policy issues, recently polled HMOs in the Chicago area as to their quality of staff, facilities, care, and reporting capabilities. Twelve of twenty-four HMOs competing for purchasers' business in the Chicago area responded to the survey. James Mortimer, the president of MBGH, explained that "wide variation in HMO responses was noted. Their ability to answer specific questions and the comprehensiveness of the documentation differed rather dramatically" (10). There was particularly wide variation in the policies of criteria for patient referral to specialists, performance evaluation of nonphysician providers, and monitoring of hospitals' readmission rates, patient severity of illness on admission, and mortality rates — all key to the maintenance of quality.

The issue of HMO quality has become particularly important in the independent practice association form of an HMO. The possibility of underutilization exists if physicians fear they will lose money if they refer their patients elsewhere. However, several financial arrangements provide bonus payments on the basis of referred (to either hospitals or specialists) expenses. The financial issue can be addressed in two ways: First, no physician can receive a bonus on the basis of utilization until quality screens are first met. Quality screens may include patient satisfaction, medical records, and audits of primary care physician offices. Once the quality concerns are met, costs can be measured. Second, physicians can recommend a year-end evaluation with integration of quality of care, quality of service, and cost effectiveness. Alternatively, the quality process can be undertaken either quarterly or semiannually, thus allowing the measures of cost effectiveness to proceed on an ongoing basis.

One HMO has begun to take the MBGH survey to heart. U.S. HealthCare (USHC), a for-profit, multistate, open panel HMO in Pennsylvania and New Jersey, will pay their physicians bonuses based partly on their performance on quality measurement scales (48). The HMO company will rely on patient satisfaction surveys and medical care evaluations based on semiannual sample chart audits.

At the Harvard Community Health Plan (HCHP), the largest HMO in New England with 310,000 members, 1% of their budget is allocated for quality assurance activity (49). Dr. Donald Berwick at HCHP has been a leader in the field of HMO quality and heads the Department of Quality-of-Care Measurement. This department is charged with developing methods to measure and track quality, implementing those methods, and reporting continually on how the plan is doing in taking care of patients.

The Quality-of-Care Measurement program contains the classic triad of performance, including structure, process, and outcome. But the program goes beyond these dimensions to look at access (in terms of waiting time for appointments), telephone response rate, interpersonal sensitivity, staff morale, and reliability.

As a financially successful operation, HCHP can take advantage of available resources to examine quality. Large organized group practices have the staff to administer a quality assurance program and physicians can be allotted time to participate. By spreading the fixed costs of quality assurance programs over more patients and providers, the cost of each audit decreases with the volume of activity (50).

Yet, as Berwick (49) argues:

> If HCHP displays for its consumers that it complies with certain screening practices 82% of the time, how will that act upon the decisions of purchasers who know nothing comparable about our local HMOs because they themselves know nothing comparable? Unfortunately, HCHP performance data create

a problem for potential users such as employers because of the absence of normative standards with which companies can compare HCHP with other plans.

The paradox here is that those who measure quality first will be the first to know their flaws. They will also be the first to act on the basis of this new information with the possibility of lowering costs and improving services.

APPROPRIATENESS AND OUTCOME MEASURES

Berwick (49) emphasized the lack of normative standards in many aspects of quality care measurement. How can we enforce what we cannot define or standardize? Those interested in quality care have shifted their attention to explore basic questions relating to the appropriateness of certain procedures and the ability to track the outcomes from physician-patient encounters. The central issues are what procedures are inappropriate, can they be eliminated, can money be saved, and will quality of care automatically improve?

Researchers at RAND contend that we can measure clinical appropriateness for a wide range of procedures using expert panels of physicians and explicit chart review criteria (51). The limitations of this method notwithstanding (52), RAND investigators reviewed the "appropriateness" of performing coronary artery bypass surgery in almost 4,900 cases. They found 56% of the surgeries were done for appropriate reasons, 30% for equivocal reasons, and 14% for inappropriate reasons (53). The percentage of appropriate surgeries varied by hospital, from 37% to 78%. The investigators conclude that "if society wishes not to pay for procedures in the equivocal or inappropriate categories, then one could almost double the number of appropriate coronary bypass surgeries without raising health care expenditures. Thus it may be possible to control costs while maintaining quality" (53). Similar evaluations by RAND have been done for carotid endarterectomies (54) and upper gastrointestinal endoscopies (55) with similar conclusions.

The impact of these studies will be great. Standards of care and guidelines for procedures are developed by evaluating appropriateness indications. Willis Goldbeck, president of the Washington Business Group on Health, favors establishment of these standards and the eventual publication of a national database that would name physicians following the standards as a guide for insurers (56). Dr. Paul Ellwood (57) has taken us one step beyond the appropriateness argument laid out above to ponder "our inability to measure and understand the effect of the choices of patients, payers, and physicians on the patient's aspirations for a better quality of life." This statement harks back to one of the first definitions of quality offered earlier; it encompasses the medical and nonmedical goals of care.

Outcomes management is a "technology of patient experience designed to help patients, payers, and providers make rational medical care-related choices based on better insight into the effect of these choices on the patient's life" (57). Outcomes management has four main components: It places greater reliance on standards and guidelines that physicians can use in selecting interventions; it routinely and systematically measures the functioning and well-being of patients; it pools clinical and outcome data on a massive scale; and it attempts to analyze and disseminate results from the segment of the database most appropriate to the concerns of each decision maker. Ellwood envisions a shift in emphasis within the "chaotic" health system (58). He believes that payers are making purchasing decisions with inadequate information about the impact of those decisions on patients' quality of life. Currently, the acceptability of care, access to care, and the quality of the physician-patient relationship are not part of the standard record from a medical encounter.

However, merely looking at outcomes such as mortality data may skew our assessment of institutions (59). More information is needed on the *patient's* evaluation of the actual encounter, as outlined by Ellwood, to draw accurate conclusions about the quality of care rendered.

CONCLUSIONS AND PROSPECTS

Despite the quantity and type of new and powerful information available to purchasers of medical care — from Buy Right coalitions to HMO self-assessments — one could argue that purchasers still will not be able to answer the basic questions posed earlier. The bulk purchaser of medical care has entered an area formerly reserved solely for the clinician and patient. Clinicians must now deal with the bulk purchaser with the same concern and attention once reserved for individual patients. Yet, how can purchasers pay for procedures when providers cannot agree on a basic premise such as its appropriateness for a presenting medical condition or the patient's eventual clinical outcome? This question leads us back to the development of standards of care—not rigid laws to be blindly followed "but data elements and recommendations that respond continually to what is learned from application and subsequent research" (57).

How are standards derived? Major quality care research efforts are underway at diverse organizations (60) such as the Joint Commission on Accreditation of Healthcare Organizations, the Institute of Medicine (IOM), and the National Leadership Commission on Health Care.

The federal government, through the Consensus Development Conferences held on the campus of the National Institutes of Health (NIH), has tried to tackle knotty clinical problems (61). By publishing their recommendations, it is hoped that the NIH can influence individual physician practice patterns and thus directly improve quality of care. The results, after more than a decade, are decidedly mixed (62).

Private organizations such as the American Medical Association (AMA) and the American College of Physicians (ACP) have mustered their resources to help measure quality. The AMA is conducting an evaluation of severity adjustment and quality assurance systems. The ACP, through its Clinical

Efficacy Assessment Project, has been evaluating the performance and cost effectiveness of various technologies to determine where they can be used more effectively. The ACP has also begun to wrestle with individual physician quality issues by developing guidelines for granting hospital privileges to physicians (63) under the Clinical Privileges Project.

The diversity of groups at work in this area is impressive. To catalogue it all, the IOM recently published a directory that is "... intended to facilitate the search for information on the safety, efficacy, and cost effectiveness of medical technology" (64).

Public and private agencies, business coalitions, and academic researchers will no doubt continue to provide information on the state of medical care. In the final analysis, however, clinicians must be at the forefront, interpreting severity measures, validating quality research programs, and helping purchasers find the best quality care at a reasonable cost to everyone.

References

1. Bean E. Latest survey shows hospital charges increasing far more quickly than CPI. *Wall Street Journal.* April 4, 1988.
2. Eisenberg JM. Physician utilization: the state of research about physician's practice patterns. *Med Care.* 1985;**23**:461-83.
3. Caper P. Defining quality in medical care. *Health Aff (Millwood).* 1988;**7**:49-61.
4. Steffen GE. Quality medical care: a definition. *JAMA.* 1988;**260**:56-61.
5. Quality of care: AMA Council on Medical Service. *Conn Med.* 1986;**50**:832-4.
6. U.S. Congress, Office of Technology Assessment. *The Quality of Medical Care: Information for Consumers.* Washington, DC: U.S. Government Printing Office, June 1988 (OTA-H-386).
7. Donabedian A. Evaluating the quality of medical care. *Milbank Mem Fund Q.* 1966;**44**(Suppl):166-206.
8. Donabedian A. The epidemiology of quality. *Inquiry.* 1985;**22**:282-92.
9. Donabedian A. Quality assessment and assurance: unity of purpose, diversity of means. *Inquiry.* 1988;**25**:173-92.
10. The Hospital Research and Educational Trust. *Focus on Measuring the Value of Health Services.* Chicago: American Hospital Association; 1986.
11. Ginsburg PB, Hammons GT. Competition and the qualilty of care: the importance of information. *Inquiry.* 1988;**25**:108-15.
12. Codman EA. A study in hospital efficiency. *Surg Gyn Obstet.* 1914; January: 491-6.
13. Lembcke PA. Measuring the quality of medical care through vital statistics based on hospital service areas: I. Comparative study of appendectomy rates. *Am J Public Health.* 1952;**42**.
14. Califano JA. The health-care chaos. *New York Times Mag.* March 20, 1988.
15. Blendon RJ. The public's view of the future of health care. *JAMA.* 1988;**259**:3587-93.
16. Blendon RJ, Altman DE. Public attitudes about health care costs: a lesson in national schizophrenia. *N Engl J Med.* 1984;**311**:613-6.
17. Barsky AJ. The paradox of health. *N Engl J Med.* 1988;**318**:414-8.
18. Louis Harris and Associates. *Making Difficult Health Care Decisions.* Boston, Massachusetts: Harvard Community Health Plan; 1987.
19. Carveth WB (ed). The quality of medical care: information for consumers. In: *Medical Benefits: The Medical-Economic Digest.* Charlottesville, Virginia: Kelly Communications; 1988.
20. Cleary PD, McNeil BJ. Patient satisfaction as an indicator of quality care. *Inquiry.* 1988;**25**:25-36.
21. Davies AR, Ware JE Jr. Involving consumers in quality of care assessment. *Health Aff (Millwood).* 1988;**7**:33-48.
22. Koenig R. Comparison shopping: companies seek new data on health-care costs to gain leverage in bargaining for services. *Wall Street Journal.* April 22, 1988.

23. McClure W. Buying right: how to do it. *Bus Health.* 1985;2(10):41-4.
24. McClure W. Buying right: the consequences of glut. *Bus Health.* 1985;2(9);43-6.
25. McClure W. Competition and the pursuit of quality: a conversation with Walter McClure [interview by John K. Iglehart]. *Health Aff (Millwood).* 1988;7:79-90.
26. Ricks TE. New corporate program lets employees compare local doctors fees and training. *Wall Street Journal.* August 4, 1987.
27. Tresnowski BR. The current interest in quality is nothing new [Editorial]. *Inquiry.* 1988;25:3-5.
28. Couch JB, Nash DB. Severity-of-illness measures: opportunities for clinicians [Editorial]. *Ann Intern Med.* 1988; 109:3-5.
29. Rundle RL. Insurers step up efforts to reduce use of free-choice health plans. *Wall Street Journal.* May 11, 1988.
30. Hennessy EL. A completely new way to purchase medical benefits. *Wall Street Journal.* July 18, 1988.
31. Kramon G. A company tests H.M.O. approach. *New York Times.* July 12, 1988.
32. Gannes S. Strong medicine for health bills. *Fortune.* April 13, 1987.
33. Ruffenach G. Painful medicine; how one bid to trim Medicare expenses has doctor battling doctor. *Wall Street Journal.* October 31, 1988.
34. Feldstein PJ, Wickizer TM, Wheeler JR. Private cost containment: the effects of utilization review programs on health care use and expenditures. *N Engl J Med.* 1988;318:1310-4.
35. Payne SM. Identifying and managing inappropriate hospital utilization: a policy synthesis. *Hlth Serv Res.* 1987;22:709-69.
36. Ricklefs R. Firms turn to "case management" to bring down health-care costs. *Wall Street Journal.* December 30, 1987.
37. Milstein A, Nash D, Sands J. Auditing quality of care: an employer based approach. *Bus Health.* 1986;3(8):10-2.
38. Imperiale T, Siegal A, Crede WB, Kamens EA. Preadmission screening of Medicare patients: the clinical impact of reimbursement disapproval. *JAMA.* 1988; 259:3418-21.
39. Meyer H. NY hospitals to have payment adjusted by clinical outcome. *AM News.* December 4, 1987.
40. Anonymous. Four Rochester hospitals tie costs to quality of care. *New York Times.* November 15, 1987.
41. Wagner M. Pilot payment program yields quality results. *Modern Hlthc.* 1988; 18(30):46.
42. Tolchin M. U.S. plans to rate doctors treating Medicare patients. *New York Times.* June 12, 1988.
43. Tolchin M. U.S. challenged on data on hospital death rates. *NY Times.* July 11, 1988.
44. Mindell B. Measuring MD productivity. *AM News.* June 10, 1988.
45. Daley J, Gertman PM, Delbanco TL. Looking for quality in primary care physicians. *Health Aff (Millbank).* 1988;7:107-13.
46. Bouchard RE, Tufo HM, Beaty HN. The impact of a quality assurance program on postgraduate training in internal medicine. *JAMA.* 1985;253:1146-50.
47. Luft HS. HMOs and the quality of care. *Inquiry.* 1988;25:147-56.
48. Meyer H. Two HMOs offer MD bonuses for high quality marks. *AM News.* March 11, 1988.
49. Berwick DM. Monitoring quality in HMOs. *Bus Health.* 1987;5(1):9-12.
50. Eisenberg JM, Kabcenell A. Organized practice and the quality of medical care. *Inquiry.* 1988;25:78-89.
51. Kahn KL, Kosecoff J, Chassin MR, et al. Measuring the clinical appropriateness of a procedure: can we do it? *Med Care.* 1988;26:415-22.
52. Knauss W, Nash DB. Predicting and evaluating patient outcomes [Editorial]. *Ann Intern Med.* 1988;109:521-2.
53. Winslow CM, Kosecoff JB, Chassin M, Kanouse DE, Brook RH. The appropriateness of performing coronary artery bypass surgery. *JAMA.* 1988;260:505-9.
54. Winslow C, Solomon DH, Chassin MR, Kosecoff J, Merrick NJ, Brook RH. The appropriateness of carotid endarterectomy. *N Engl J Med.* 1988;318:721-7.
55. Morrissey JF. The problem of the inappropriate endoscopy [Editorial]. *Ann Intern Med.* 1988;109:605-6.
56. Freudenheim M. Costly procedures under scrutiny. *New York Times.* July 26, 1988.
57. Ellwood PM. Shattuck lecture — outcomes management: a technology of patient experience. *N Engl J Med.* 1988; 318:1549-56.
58. Meyer H. National healthcare outcome data base proposed. *AM News.* July 22, 1988.
59. Luft HS, Hunt SS. Evaluating individual hospital quality through outcome statistics. *JAMA.* 1986;255:2780-4.

60. Heinen L, Gorski JA, Roe W. Quality of care research and projects in progress. *Health Aff (Millbank).* 1988;7:145-50.

61. Perry S. The NIH consensus development program. *N Engl J Med.* 1987;**317**:485-8.

62. Kosecoff J, Kanouse DE, Rogers WH, McCloskey L, Winslow CM, Brook RH. Effects of the National Institutes of Health Consensus Development Pro-gram on physician practice. *JAMA.* 1987;**258**:2708-13.

63. Roberts JS, Radany MH, Nash DB. Privilege delineation in a demanding new environment. *Ann Intern Med.* 1988;**180**:880-6.

64. Kramon G. Guide assesses new technology. *New York Times.* May 17, 1988.

Chapter 2

The Patient's Role in Health Care and Quality Assessment

SHERRIE H. KAPLAN, PhD
JOHN E. WARE, JR., PhD

INTRODUCTION

One of the thornier issues currently facing practitioners, medical educators and health policy makers is the definition of a reasonable and appropriate role for patients in the medical care process. The crux of the problem is the need to balance the increasing sophistication of patients and the values they bring to health and health care, with the need to maintain a sensible level of autonomy for physicians in practice. The most rational integration of patients in medical care would be to bring them into the medical decision-making process so that their preferences and values are systematically incorporated in diagnosis and treatment, and to make their evaluations of the care they receive part of routine quality assessment.

This chapter is to provide an overview of the research and practical issues surrounding two distinct roles for patients — as evaluators of care, both directly and indirectly, supplying information used by others in evaluating care, and as active participants in care, shaping the nature of the care they receive.

There is no question that these are two completely separable roles. Patients can be part of medical decisions without being asked to evaluate the quality of those decisions, and, conversely, patients can and have been asked to evaluate the care they receive without helping to shape its course. Information from patients about their health and health care is now used by and is of benefit to physicians and administrators in the delivery of patient care. There is emerging evidence (1-4) that including patients in their care can positively affect its quality, measured even in clinical terms. Both thrusts are consistent with an overall change in the patients' role in medical care. It follows that if patients better understand their care — the rationale behind medical decisions, the goals of treatment, and the side effects, risks, and consequences of treatment — they will be better evaluators of that care.

All fine rhetoric, but what is the evidence that involving patients in health care and the evaluation of its quality is practical and is beneficial both to the patient and to the physician? After all, although patient participation in care has generally been limited to membership on the governing boards of hospitals, comprehensive health planning agencies, government agencies, and medical quality review organizations (5,6), such participation has not had a smooth history (7-9). At best, such involvement has been ineffective, and, at worst, it has lead to conflicts between patients and providers. Systematic involvement of patients in care and the assessment of its quality will require serious reconsideration of ethical issues such as redefinition of the boundaries of responsibility for care between physicians and patients, wholesale revisions in quality assessment data collection methods, revisions in existing and development of new training programs for physicians and patients, and a potentially profound reformulation of the physician-patient relationship (10,11).

Why bother and why now? Especially at a time when physicians are being required to respond to cost-containment pressures, to the changes in health care delivery in response to increasing costs, to runaway technologic advances, and to heightened visibility via media access to medical research and to consumers, involving patients in medical care and its assessment seems too overwhelming a task.

First, particularly with respect to access to care and the physician-patient relationship, patients' evaluations of the quality of care they receive are the most practical source of information. No other data source currently part of the traditional quality assessment machinery incorporates patients' values or preferences in the same way as directly as surveys of patients' opinions. Over 10 years of empirical research has produced valid, reliable, and feasible measures of patient satisfaction with care that can now be used in practice settings (12-28).

Second, patients' assessments of, or "patient satisfaction" with care have been shown to affect both the physician-patient relationship and patients' health status (29-38). Dissatisfied patients physician-shop (29-32), change health plans (33,34), sue (35), do not follow-through on treatment recommendations (36-38), and avoid physician visits (39). Further, patients are already making decisions about their health care. A recent survey (40) has shown that one third of Americans choose the hospital in which they receive care themselves, one third decide with their physicians, and one third have the physician decide for them. Patients usually choose their own physicians (41,42). A recent national survey (41) of consumers showed that 79% knew that hospitals differ in the quality of care they deliver. Further, information about the quality of care provided by institutions as well as individual providers is increasingly available to consumers (43,44). State medical boards supply information to consumers on formal disciplinary actions taken against individual physicians, and state medical societies make information on board certification available. It is not known from the literature whether, how, and to what extent people access the information available or whether patients use available quality of care information when making decisions about care. It is estimated that as many as one third of patients will change physicians in any given year (45). It is also known that patients do not follow a large number of treatment recommendations made by their providers (46,47).

Third, research has shown a link between clinical measures of health and patient-reported health outcomes. Better control of blood sugar and blood pressure, as well as higher levels of forced expiratory volume in 1 second (FEV$_1$) have been associated with fewer disease-related restrictions on patients' functioning (48,49). To the extent that patients' *reports* of their health (for example, abilities to perform usual daily activities) or their ratings of their health status (for example, as overall "excellent, very good, good, fair, or poor") augment clinical data and have relevance for disease management, the integration of such information into routine clinical practice may substantially improve the outcomes of care.

Fourth, there is evidence (50-55) that patients want a more expanded role in their medical care and more information from their physicians. Empirical research using both clinical and patient-reported outcome measures suggests that expanding the role of patients in their care may augment the medical care process to produce better health outcomes. (1-4,56,57). Interventions designed to include patients in decision making by incorporating their values in discrete decisions (57) and by training them to obtain information and to negotiate effectively on their own behalf during office visits (1-4) have been shown to change patients' behavior in ways that positively influence their health and enhance disease management.

Fifth, if not satisfied with the care they receive or if not permitted to participate in their care, some patients may turn to self-care. Self-care is viewed negatively by physicians (58). Some forms of self-care are increasingly fraught with hazards to patients' health and may prevent them from receiving benefits they might have derived from traditional medical care.

Finally, three recent developments underscore the importance of providing a role for patients in health care and its assessment. First, the American Board of Internal Medicine has completed a study designed to determine the feasibility of using patients' evaluations of the interpersonal skills of residents as a potential element of the certification process (59-62). If such measures are to become part of future recertification processes it is necessary to ensure that the science of measurement of patients' assessments of quality (patient satisfaction with care) has been adequate for this purpose, and moreover to understand the relationships between patient satisfaction with care and physicians' behavior.

Second, large-scale data collection efforts to gather patients' evaluations of the quality of care they receive have recently been undertaken by at least two major organized systems of health care delivery (63,64). Integration of data from patients is being planned for system-wide quality assurance programs.

Third, a national data collection effort (65) is underway that uses patients' reports of their functional status and health perceptions as the discriminating measures to distinguish health care delivery systems by the quality of care they provide. In the context of this study, profiling individual providers by outcome measures, including patient functioning, patient satisfaction, and technical and interpersonal styles of care, is being studied.

For these reasons, it is an appropriate time to address several issues regarding patients' involvement in the medical care process and the assessment of its quality. Specifically, what can patients tell about the quality of care provided to them? Which aspects of care are appropriate for patients to evaluate? What do patients' subjective evaluations or reports add to objective clinical assessments of the quality of care? Does what the patient tell us have any bearing on health outcomes? How can patient evaluations of their care and reports about their health outcomes be integrated into organized quality assessment programs? Can a reasonable role for patients in medical decision making be defined — one that enhances the outcomes of their care and does not interfere with physicians' judgment or ability to provide high-quality technical care?

This chapter is not intended to provide a thorough discussion of the important policy and ethical considerations surrounding each of these issues. Rather, we will discuss the research and practical implications of three different ways to integrate patients into their care — in the evaluation of the process of care; in the evaluation of the outcomes of care; and in the care itself, by participating in medical decision making. Our discussion will focus on a review of research evidence and questions remaining in these areas, along with practical considerations, such as the integration of patient information into organized quality assessment programs with patients and providers as consumers of information.

In the context of this discussion, we make the subtle, but important distinction between patient *reports* and patient *ratings* of both their *health* and the *health care they receive*. These distinctions tap an issue central to the definition of the patient's role in care — whether they will be asked to *evaluate* (through ratings) or whether the information they provide (through reports) will be used by others to evaluate health and health care. Figure 1 shows how ratings of health, defined narrowly for this example as physical functioning, and of health care are distinguished from reports of each.

Patients' ratings and reports of their health provide information about the outcomes of care; ratings and reports of health care provide information about the process of care. Both ratings and reports provide valuable and non-overlapping information. As noted elsewhere (69), if asked only whether they are able to participate in sports or move heavy objects, two individuals may give the same response. However, each may give very different answers when asked to rate the level of effort required to do so. Similarly, when asked whether or not information regarding medication side effects was discussed during an office visit, two patients of the same physician might both respond positively, yet rate the quality of that information differently. Thus, both ratings and reports are needed to obtain the most comprehensive and interpretable information from patients about their health and health

	RATINGS	REPORTS
HEALTH	Rating of Physical shape or condition[66] (Excellent -- Poor)	Able to participate in sports, strenuous activities[67] (Yes/No)
HEALTH CARE	Rating of quality of doctors' explanations[60] (Excellent -- Poor)	Side effects of medications discussed?[68] (Yes/No)

Figure 1. Differences between ratings and reports of health and health care.

care. These distinctions and their implications for the role of patients in the assessment of health and health care are important to keep in mind through the remainder of this discussion.

PATIENTS' ASSESSMENTS OF THE HEALTH CARE PROCESS

Determining the quality of medical care involves judgment. That judgment is based on the values, standards, and expectations of the evaluator. Judgments of the quality of health care are traditionally made by providers of that care, based on conformance with accepted standards of technical performance. These standards generally do not include patients' values or preferences, nor do they refer to aspects of care other than technical quality (such as interpersonal care). Thus, patients' assessments of care provide information not available elsewhere.

Before incorporating patients' assessments of health care into the routine evaluation of quality of care, it is reasonable to ask whether the currently available measures of patients' opinions about the care they receive are suitable for this purpose, whether patients' assessments of care have any meaningful consequences, and whether patients' assessments of care are subject to change as a function of anything physicians do or do not do.

Is the Science of Measurement up to the Task?

Extensive research in the area of obtaining patients' ratings and reports of the health care they receive has produced sensitive and specific measures that can be used to target those aspects of care that need improvement to meet patients' standards (70). There is a clearer relationship between patients' assessments of health care (or patient satisfaction with care) and what physicians, nurses, receptionists, and administrators can do "Monday morning" to change those assessments, than there is between patients' assessments of their health and how care can be modified to change health outcomes.

Several measures of patient satisfaction with care are now available (12-28). In an extensive review published by the Office of Technology Assessment (70), the reliability, validity, and feasibility of various patient rating methods were summarized. Other studies have compared the relative strengths of two or more of these measures in assessing patient satisfaction in the same patient sample (26). There is substantial evidence that the short answer to the question above is yes. However, a more considered response would be: It depends on the purposes for which patient assessments of their care are being used. Just as diagnostic tests are designed to be as specific as possible, so patient assessments of their care cannot diagnose all aspects of poor quality in all situations.

Reliability of Patients' Assessments of Care. The goal of obtaining a reliable measure of patients' assessments of care is consistency of scores. This consistency can be determined over time (test-retest reliability), across raters (inter-rater reliability), across two or more forms of the same measure (alternate forms), or across several items measuring the same thing (internal consistency reliability). Reliability does not address the "correctness" of a measure, but rather the extent to which a measure is able to distinguish real differences in scores (between people, groups, points in time) from differences in scores caused by random fluctuations (measurement error). Reliability scores range from 0.0 to 1.0; a reliability score of 0.65 is considered acceptable for comparisons between groups (for example, physicians or hospitals). Most multiple-item patient satisfaction scales have good internal consistency reliability. Scores on patient satisfaction scales related to the technical and interpersonal care provided by physicians range from 0.63 to 0.94 with most scoring roughly 0.80 (70), a level that allows for comparisons of groups.

The issues of concern when considering the reliability of patients' assessments of health care are *whose* care is being evaluated and which care (physicians, hospitals, delivery systems) is being evaluated? The "unit of analysis" or the group whose care is to be evaluated shapes the reliability question. If the concern, for example, is whether patients evaluate care provided in one delivery system (Health Maintenance Organization [HMO] compared with fee-for-service) as better or worse than that provided in another, as has been done in some studies of patient satisfaction with care (34,71,72), then the reliability questions are "is the measure of patients' assessments of (satisfaction with) care precise enough to distinguish real differences in patients' assessments of these systems from those due to errors in measurement (for example, patient's mood at the time)" and "how many patients per system of care are needed to obtain a reliable score for that system?"

The latter is rarely discussed in the patient satisfaction literature or addressed in the quality of care literature. However, because a prominent goal of traditional quality assessment is the estimation of a score for the individual physician, the question "how many patients per physician are needed to obtain a reliable score" is important. Gauging performance based on fewer observations may lead to incorrect conclusions regarding physicians' performance.

Empirical evidence from studies of patient satisfaction begins to address this question, although the evidence is less prevalent for this type of reliability than for internal consistency reliability. Two studies (73,74) indicate that the ratings of 10 patients per physician are needed to obtain reliable scores; one study (59) suggests that the number may range from 20 to 40 depending on the level of reliability desired. These data should be interpreted in the context of reliability for other quality assessment measures. Traditional quality assessment measures rely on the correspondence between data obtained from the medical record and standards set by an expert panel. There is only very recent evidence indicating the number of scores for each physician that would be needed to obtain a reliable score for that physician using these traditional quality of care measures. This evidence suggests that roughly 40 patients per physician are needed to obtain quality of care scores using chart audits that are sufficiently reliable to compare one physician's care with another's (75). Thus, it appears that the 10 to 40 patients per physician indicated as needed to obtain a reliable score for measures of patient satisfaction with care may be comparable with other methods of assessing the quality of physician performance.

It should be noted that the reliability of scores per physician was determined in all three of the patient satisfaction studies cited for the entire range of scores. Although it may be desirable for medical educators to discriminate between superlative and "only excellent" physicians to identify role models for patient care, usual quality assurance activities are focused on physicians and hospitals scoring below some cutoff point. With this intent, many fewer patients per physician may be needed to obtain a reliable profile of patient dissatisfaction for each physician.

The second reliability question raised above involves which care, rendered by physician, hospital, or system, is being evaluated, and how that care should be sampled. Does the care provided by a physician or hospital for one disease condition represent all care provided by that physician or hospital? If not, as has been suggested (76), how many disease conditions are needed to obtain a reliable score for the individual physician or hospital? Moreover, within a disease condition, should a single visit represent all care for that condition, or should several visits be sampled to obtain a reliable assessment of care?

These questions are not unique to patients' assessments of health care but are true for quality of care assessment in general. They raise sampling issues that press the state of the art of measurement in this area. We are only beginning to see these issues addressed in the literature. Ongoing work in this area (59,75,76) and other research will need to address these sampling issues if we are to use measures of patients' assessments of care to make judgments about the care of individual physicians, hospitals, or delivery systems.

Validity of Patients' Assessments of Care.   The question of validity in evaluating assessments of patient care asks "to what extent are the realities of health care represented by patient ratings and reports?" The kind of evidence brought to bear on this question depends on the purposes to which patients' assessments of care are to be put. If, for example, patients' assessments of care are being sought to maintain a stable patient population in an individual physician's practice, then patients' tenure with the practice (continuity of care) is the outcome measure against which patients' assessments should be compared to determine their validity. If patients' assessments of care are to be used to improve the quality of care provided to them, then some other measure of the quality of care they receive, such as health outcomes, should be used to "validate" their assessments of care. There will never be a perfect correspondence between patients' assessments of care and any other measure of that care. Patients' evaluations are in part a reflection of their own values and preferences. There should, however, be an association between patients' assessments of the care they receive and other measures of the quality of that care that demonstrates some credible interrelationship.

Another important issue involves the capacity of measures of patients' assessments of care to discriminate different *levels* of care, from the highest to lowest quality. Empirical evidence has shown that patients generally give high ratings to the care they receive. On a scale from 0 to 100, for example, patients will typically give their care scores of 82 or above (27). If all patients are so happy, why bother to measure patients' satisfaction or evaluations of care? Research (29-38) has shown that small differences even at the upper end of the scale (those that distinguish patients who are very satisfied with care from those who are satisfied, but slightly less so) have important implications for patients' subsequent behavior with respect to health and health care. In another study (30), roughly an 8-point difference in patients' satisfaction with care at the upper end of a scale ranging from 1 to 100 was associated with a 10-fold increase in the probability of patients' disenrollment from a health care plan.

Using the example of a thermometer to measure patients' temperature, although it is theoretically possible to make distinctions in temperature at all levels of the scale, all the "action," or the critical values that indicate the presence of some disease process, occurs in a very narrow range. Similarly, although it is possible to measure patients' assesments of care over the entire continuum of scores, all the action apparently happens at the ceiling. If the goal of measuring patients' assessments of care is to intercede at some level below which negative events (bad health outcomes, ruptures of physician-patient relationships, disenrollment from health plans) will occur, then current research should be targeted at identifying those "critical values." If, however, the goal of measuring patients' assessments of care is to promote high-quality health care, then the goal of current research should be to determine the characteristics of care that receive the highest patient ratings.

Given a specific purpose, the validity of patients' assessments of care can and has been determined in several different ways. The validity of new clinical measures, such as glycosylated hemoglobin, is determined by their correspondence with the former "gold standard," in this case fasting blood glucose. However, for quality of care there is no criterion with known properties and relationships to variations in levels of illness against which to compare patients' assessments of quality. Under such circumstances, this type of validity, called "criterion validity," is sometimes determined by the correspondence of a measure with the judgments of an expert. Several studies have shown that, although patients' assessments of care tend to be consistently higher than the ratings of that same care by physicians and nurses, care judged as excellent or good by physicians or nurses is also judged as excellent or good by patients (28,60,77-80)

In two separate sets of experiments, staged videotaped visits in which professional actors portrayed a physician and a patient with varying levels of quality of interpersonal and technical care, were shown to patients and physicians. Patients were able to match the judgments of the physicians who viewed the tapes for both aspects of care (28,79). Using a similar format, Kaplan and associates (60) have shown that patients' evaluations of certain aspects of interpersonal care match the judgments of experts. To evaluate whether the level of correspondence between expert and patient raters of care observed in these studies (roughly 75%) is high or low, they can be compared with the extent of agreement between other, more traditional measures of quality. In a study using four data sources — physician interview, patient interview, chart audit, and a videotape of the encounter — Gerbert and colleagues (81) found that the conclusions about care drawn using any two of these methods were in agreement roughly 78% of the time.

The validity of a quality assessment measure can also be determined by its correspondence with other known measures of the same aspects of quality (for example, satisfaction with interpersonal care and another measure of the quality of interpersonal care) and its lack of or weak correspondence with other aspects of quality (for example, satisfaction with technical care when interpersonal care has been experimentally manipulated). Substantial research has demonstrated a relationship between interpersonal care, specifically, certain elements of physician-patient communication and patients' satisfaction with interpersonal care (31,45,82-98). Most studies of the ways physicians and patients communicate during office visits have applied standardized coding schemes to audiotapes or videotapes of office visits. Using this approach, it is possible to identify the specific elements of the conversation of physicians and patients that are most closely related to patients' ratings of care. The amount of information provided by the physician during the visit has shown the most consistent relationship to patient satisfaction (Table 1).

TABLE 1. Behaviors of Physicians During Office Visits Associated with Patient Satisfaction with Care.

Satisfaction Correlated with:	Additional Modifiers*	Type of Ratings†	Reference
Amount of information given	. . .	I	82
	. . .	NS	83
	. . .	G	84
	. . . and retained by the patient	I/T	85
	. . . at the end of the visit only	Inf	86
	. . . of an explanatory nature (what was done and why)		87
	. . . about the expected outcome	G	99
Attentiveness, listening, answering questions	. . .	G	88
	. . .	I	86
	. . . at the conclusion of the visit	I	84
Emotional warmth	. . .	G	89,90
	. . .	G	91
	. . .	G	92
	. . .	G	93
	. . .	I	84
Attention to psychological issues	. . .	Inf	94
	. . .	I	82
	. . .	I	95
	. . .	I	96
Courtesy, empathy, reassurance	. . .	I	82
Less controlling	. . .	G	89
	. . .	G	97
	. . .	G	98
	. . .	G	93
	. . .	G	45
	. . .	G	94
	. . .	I	84
More time spent communicating	. . .	NS	83
	. . .	G	89
	. . .	G	31
	. . .	I	95

*Elaboration to category presented in the studies cited.
†Type of satisfaction associated with individual behaviors: I=interpersonal; G=general satisfaction; T=technical; Inf=informativeness; NS=not significant.

The science of physician-patient communication analysis is not developed enough to distinguish the way in which information is delivered from its content, nor do existing studies provide much information about the nature of information that "produces" patient satisfaction. There is some evidence (87) that patients rate their interpersonal care more favorably when physicians provide explanations about what is being done and why, and can distinguish information that is irrelevant, although highly technical, from information presented in lay language that is meaningful to their care. Another consistent finding has been that when during the visit the information is provided is important. Stiles and associates (86,100) have shown that patients' ratings of satisfaction with the visit were only associated with information provided at the conclusion of the visit as summary comment.

Other aspects of interpersonal care as measured by physician-patient communication have also shown an association with patients' ratings of interpersonal care. Patients' ratings were more favorable when physicians: were attentive, spending more time listening and answering patients' questions (84,86,88); showed more emotional warmth (84,89-93); paid more attention to patients' social or psychological concerns (82,94-96); were courteous and reassuring (82); were less controlling (made suggestions instead of giving directions) (45,84,89,93,94,97,98); and spent more time communicating (compared with performing the physical examination, recording in the chart, and so forth) (31,83,89,95,98). Although less well studied, there is similar evidence for inpatients' ratings of interpersonal care while hospitalized (101, 102).

As evidence of validity, these findings indicate that patients are rating something real, and that their ratings reflect the way they are treated by physicians during office visits and are not simply a reflection of some internal cognitive process. Does better interpersonal care have any clinical relevance beyond patients' ratings? Do these differences in physicians' communication, for example, affect patients' health outcomes? Although this relationship has not been widely studied, recent research suggests that the quality of physician-patient conversation improves the resolution of patients health problems (103-106), blood pressure control (2,107), and blood glucose control (3) (Table 2).

How patients' ratings of their care are related to their health outcomes is not yet known. More research is needed to determine whether the recognition and delivery of higher quality interpersonal care by physicians motivates patients to cooperate in their treatment more effectively, producing better health outcomes. Longitudinal studies currently underway will help to sort out these relationships (65).

TABLE 2. Studies Relating Physician-Patient Conversation to Patients' Health Outcomes.

Data Source	Health Outcome	Effect	Reference
Audio tapes	Blood pressure control	Observed	107
Questionnaire	Problem resolution	Observed	103
Questionnaire	Perceived recovery	Observed	104
Questionnaire	Problem resolution	Observed	105
Questionnaire	Problem resolution	Observed	106
Questionnaire	Functional status	Not observed	99
Questionnaire	Blood sugar control	Nob observed	68
Audio tapes	Blood pressure control; blood sugar control	Observed	2,3

Reprinted with permission. Kaplan SH, Greenfield S, Ware JE Jr. Assessing the effects of physician-patient interactions on the outcomes of chronic disease. *Med Care.* 1989; In press.

Patient Reports of the Process of Care

That patients can evaluate the interpersonal aspects of care, and that their ratings of and reports about the quality of interpersonal care are valid is not as controversial as whether and in what areas they can provide valid information about the quality of technical care. Patients do not have the same technical knowledge as physicians. Evaluations of physicians by their peers has much greater intuitive appeal as a superior way to assess the quality of technical care. What can patients tell us about technical care? Are there aspects of the process of care for which patients can provide reliable and valid information? Further, if not on technical knowledge, on what do they base their evaluations? Opponents to the use of patients' assessments of technical care argue that patients cannot distinguish highly competent technical care from nice or warm or humane care (28), that is, their ratings of technical care are not valid.

The limited evidence available suggests that patients may be able to supply some types of information, such as whether certain tests were ordered, whether treatments were recommended, or whether medications were prescribed, at least as accurately as other sources of information traditionally used in quality of care assessment, such as the medical record or reports from physicians (81,108). Whether and to what extent patients can or should add to data available from other sources and how such data should be evaluated remains to be determined.

Patients may also augment traditional data sources for assessing the quality of the medical care process. In a series of studies (81,108), patients have been shown to provide valid information on tests that were ordered, treatments recommended, and whether or not patient education occurred during an office visit, compared with information obtained from videotapes, medical records, and physicians' reports.

As discussed above, there is also some empirical evidence (28,79) that when asked to rate the technical quality of care that has been experimentally manipulated, patients' ratings correspond with the ratings of physicians and nurses. Further, these studies showed that patients could distinguish higher quality interpersonal care from better technical care. There is other evidence gathered in clinical settings that patients' evaluations of care match experts' judgments. In a study of 1,418 patients in 20 emergency rooms, Linn (78) found that patients' ratings of the burn care delivered in the emergency room were significantly lower when the technical process of care was poorer, as judged against a clinical algorithm.

Some research findings (34,109) suggest, however, that patients' evaluations of their care are influenced by red herrings — that they confuse quantity with quality. Appropriateness of care is not reflected in patients' ratings. The technically perfect but unnecessary operation or procedure would probably not be judged as poor quality by the average patient. Conversely, if the findings of Sox and associates (109) are found to be generalizable, patients may incorrectly view the appropriate nonperformance of diagnostic tests or procedures as evidence of poor quality.

The appropriate role of the patient in the assessment of the quality of technical care has been debated more than studied. We are now seeing noteworthy differences in evaluations of the technical care provided by different health care delivery systems by some groups of patients (34). If not due to real differences in the technical quality of care rendered in these systems, to what are these differences attributable? Much more scientific attention must be focused on this issue if we are to understand the meaning of patients' assessments of the quality of technical care.

It is reasonable to assume that improving patients' understanding of the details of the medical care process, at least as it pertains to the management of any illness they may have, will provide them with a better foundation from which to make assessments about the quality of that process. Improvements in patients' understanding of the care process could also help to assure that they get good care. Fledgling efforts to engage patients in medical care decision making have shown that it is possible to change the way they behave during office visits, and that these changes have salutory effects on disease management and health outcomes (1-3, 57). Whether and to what extent patients can understand enough about their care to serve as proxies for expert judgments about quality of technical care remains an important research and policy issue.

Bias in Patients' Assessments of Care.   The term bias in measurement terms means systematic error — differences in a measure that are caused by something other than real differences in the object being measured. In the measurement of patients' assessments of care, the question of bias is, "are we measuring the care or some attribute of the patient?" Bias, or systematic error, in estimating the quality of care rendered by individual physicians, clinics, or systems of care, can occur in two ways: First, as a function of some inherent bias in the way certain patients assess care (for example, some groups of patients may be prone to rate physicians or medical care in general less favorably than others, based on factors other than the way they are treated); and second, in analysis, as a function of the disproportionate representation of a group of patients who give higher or lower ratings of care, based on real differences in the way they are treated (for example, patients who are new to a physician or practice setting are prone to give lower ratings than continuing patients).

Several patient characteristics, as well as physician and health care delivery system characteristics, have been associated with patients' ratings of the care they receive. The characteristics of patients associated with less favorable ratings of physicians' care are listed in Table 3. If these patients (for example, younger, better educated, sicker) gave less favorable ratings because of some internal factor (such as general skepticism or disaffection) (113) then these patients' ratings would be considered to be biased. If, as is more likely, these patients gave less favorable ratings because of real differences in the way they are treated by physicians, then their ratings are not biased, but simply a reflection of real world differences in the care they receive.

There is little empirical evidence on this issue. Two studies (114,115) have shown that primary care physicians refer some patients more frequently

TABLE 3. Characteristics of Patients Associated with Dissatisfaction with Care.

Characteristic	Reference
Younger patients	110
Better educated patients	111
Higher income patients	12
White patients (compared with any other ethnicity)	15,19,79
Sicker patients	23
Psychologically distressed*	112

*These patients were dissatisfied only with the humaneness of their care, not the competence of their physicians or with the overall quality of care they received.

than others. Another study (116) has shown that physicians' interviewing behavior varied with the sex, age, appearance, and ethnicity of the patient. Some recent experimental research (60) may begin to untangle the issue of bias in ratings from actual care differences. It is important to understand whether any patient characteristics should be adjusted for when comparing patients' ratings of one physician (system of care, specialty group) with another, or when declaring physicians' care as substandard.

There have also been studies (84,117) showing that certain characteristics of physicians, such as age, sex, ethnicity, specialty, and socioeconomic background, influence patients' ratings of care. Other investigators (25,71,118) have shown that ratings of care in different health care delivery systems (for example, fee-for-service compard with HMOs) are systematically different, although this finding is less consistent (72,117). Whether these differences are due to bias, that is, some systematic prejudice in the way patients view younger, female physicians in primary care compared with older, male specialists, or whether there are real differences in the care provided by these groups of physicians remains an issue when comparing patients' ratings of one group of physicians with another.

Bias in ratings can result from the tendency of people responding to surveys to agree with every item. Called "acquiescence response set," this behavior results in answers that the respondent did not mean, and therefore in inaccurate ratings of care. This type of bias has been studied with respect to patient satisfaction ratings, and has been shown to influence the ratings of patients of low socioeconomic status (14). To counter the effects of this form of bias, items in the best patient satisfaction questionnaires are balanced to include a roughly equal number of favorably and unfavorably worded items.

Another form of bias, referred to as "social desirability response set," or the tendency of people to represent themselves in the best possible light, has also been studied (24) with respect to patient satisfaction. This form of bias would produce artificially higher ratings of physicians for patients most interested in presenting themselves positively (for example, patients of lower socioeconomic status). This form of bias has been shown to inflate the ratings of poorer patients, although not substantially (24). Nevertheless, if a large number of upper socioeconomic status patients were included in the sample used to give ratings for the care of an individual physician, it may be reasonable to adjust for patients' socioeconomic status before that physician's care was compared with the care of other physicians.

In summary, if patients' ratings of individual physicians are to be used to judge the quality of care provided by that physician, or to compare one physician's care with another's, the issues of bias, in both patients' ratings and in analysis, must be considered. Just as case mix should be used to adjust health outcomes to make fair comparisons between individual physicians, groups of physicians, hospitals, or groups of health care delivery systems, so the patient characteristics that may cause misinterpretation of patients' ratings for those comparisons — such as access to care, length of office waits, proportion of new patients — must be considered if the care provided by physicians, clinics, or hospitals is to be evaluated fairly.

Other Methodologic Issues.   There has been some concern among those who have studied patient satisfaction with care that patients' ratings of their care are almost too high to be believable, particularly because patients also seem to view medical care as in crisis (119). This paradox may in part be explained by patients' tendency to view their own care in a more favorable light than the care received by others (24). It may also be an accurate reflection of the quality of care received — that most patients get very good to excellent care. However, when patients who say they are very satisfied with the care they receive are asked whether their care could be improved, a substantial proportion say yes. Although these patients profess to be satisfied, they view their care as nonoptimal.

High patient ratings should not be used as evidence that care need not be improved. Small differences among patients who generally rate the care they receive from physicians as excellent have been shown to produce substantial differences in whether or not patients will continue to see that physician (27). It is important, therefore, to make finer discriminations where the variability is — at the upper end of the scale. This is particularly true if the goal in obtaining patients' assessments of care is to target those "threshhold" values below which patients will take some undesirable action (for example, change physicians or health plans, sue, experience negative health outcomes).

Recent refinements have been made in the way patients' ratings of the care they receive are measured that have improved the variability at the upper end of the scales (27,61-63). These refinements include asking patients to rate specific behaviors of providers thought by experts to represent high-quality care and using a rating scale that ranges from "excellent to poor." This type of rating scale produces a more even distribution of quality of care scores, and is a more direct evaluation of care by the patient (27,61). The content of items in newly developed patient evaluation questionnaires was designed to be useful in giving specific feedback to physicians, medical educators, or administrators regarding what behaviors to change to improve patients' ratings of care (60-62). These refinements should produce a more interpretable quality of care score for individual physicians, groups, or systems of care.

Another important issue involved in obtaining patients' evaluations of the quality of care is the multidimensional nature of care. Substantial research

(12,17,18,21) has shown that when rating the care they receive, patients are able to distinguish the elements of physician care (interpersonal and technical) from access to care, availability of care, continuity of care (that is, whether they see the same physician from visit to visit), cost of care, and services provided by health care staff other than physicians. As discussed above, with respect to the care provided by physicians, patients may or may not be able to distinguish high-quality interpersonal from competent technical care (28,79). Whether within each of these broad areas — interpersonal and technical care — patients can distinguish among specific behaviors that contribute uniquely to a physician's overall score for interpersonal or technical care is only beginning to be studied (61). It is important to identify specific elements of care that lead to positive and negative evaluations of care if these evaluations are to provide useful information for training and feedback regarding physicians' performance.

Do Patients' Assessment Have Consequences for Health and Health Care?

Asking for patients' assessments of health care would have merit if only for token enfranchisement of the patient in the medical care process in an era where consumerism is socially valued (113). However, cost-containment in health care requires that such data collection efforts meet cost-benefit standards, especially in view of the expense of traditional quality assessment activities (28). It is therefore important to ask not only what can be done to change patients' assessments of the care they receive, but what is likely to happen if patients view their care as nonoptimal.

There is considerable evidence that patients' assessments of care have important consequences for their health and for the health care they receive. Patients who are dissatisfied with their health care are more likely to engage in activities that disrupt their medical care and could compromise their health outcomes (Table 4). Patients who give less favorable ratings to their technical and interpersonal care have been shown (29-32,120) to physician-shop and to be more likely to disenroll from their health care plan in the subsequent year (33,34). Further, disgruntled patients initiate frivolous malpractice claims more frequently (35). Although the empirical evidence is somewhat mixed (99,121), patients who rate the interpersonal aspects of their care more favorably are more likely to follow through on treatment recommendations (36-38). At least one study (39) has shown that patients who rate their care more favorably are more likely to make visits to the physician.

The relationship between patient satisfaction and transitions in health is not well studied. Research evidence from two cross-sectional studies is contradictory. Linn and Greenfield (110) reported that sicker patients are more dissatisfied with care, while Patrick and colleagues (122) reported that healthier patients are more dissatisfied with care. Neither study explored the causal relationship between satisfaction and health outcomes. The National Study

TABLE 4. Consequences of Dissatisfaction with Care.

Dissatisfaction Associated with:	Findings	Reference
Physician shopping	Patients who rate their technical and interpersonal care more favorably are significantly less likely to change physicians in the subsequent year	29-32, 120
Disenrollment from health plan	Plans with the lowest patient satisfaction ratings had disenrollment rates 10 times higher than those with higher ratings	33, 34
Malpractice suits	Poor relationship with the physician is the most important contributing factor to filing of frivolous claims	35
Noncompliance*	Patients who rate their interpersonal care favorably are more compliant with treatment recommendations	36-38

*The association between dissatisfaction and noncompliance is not consistent across all studies (121,99).

of Medical Outcomes will provide longitudinal data to explore the nature of the relationship between patients' evaluations of the care they received and their health outcomes (65).

The relationship between patients' assessments of health care and their health outcomes should not be expected to be more substantial than the previously observed relationships between medical care process and outcomes using traditional quality of care assessment methods (123). The magnitude of this relationship is one of the "cutting edge" research questions in the area of patient assessments of health and health care.

What Produces Favorable Patient Assessments of Care?

The most useful feedback to medical educators or physicians in practice regarding patients' assessments of care would include the identification of behaviors that need to be changed to improve patients' ratings. Some recent questionnaires contain items with this kind of behavioral content — for example, "how would you rate the physician's ability to give information about treatment side effects in nonmedical language (excellent to poor)?" Even without knowing the content of patients' evaluations, at least one study (80) has shown that feedback of overall scores from patients' assessments of care to individual physicians leads to improvements in their scores. Such research has not been conducted among physicians in practice.

Some research conducted in practice settings identifies specific behaviors of physicians that lead to better and worse ratings of care from patients. This research has been done primarily by those interested in physician-patient communication, and therefore focuses on the specific conversational behaviors of physicians that are associated with positive and negative assessments of care by patients (Table 1). Patients' ratings are more favorable, for example, when physicians explain what is being done and why (87); give information in lay language (60); summarize their findings and plans at the conclusion of the visit (86,100); show emotion during the visit (84,89,93); pay more attention to patients' social or psychological concerns (82,94,96); are less controlling during the visit (45,84,89,93,97,98); and spend more time giving patients information (31,83,89,95,98).

If the purpose in obtaining patients' assessments of care is to improve patient care in the areas that patients find important, then understanding the relationship between the specific behaviors of physicians that influence those assessments becomes critical. Research in this area provides empirical evidence that specific behaviors of physicians *are* related to better and worse ratings by patients — that patients "are not just saying" that their care is good or bad based on things that have nothing to do with the ways they are treated by physicians.

However, studies in this area have explored a relatively narrow range of physicians' and patients' behaviors using a limited number of observational techniques. The complex and rich fabric of the individual physician-patient relationship and the dynamic elements of that relationship that are gratifying for both physician and patient may not be captured in a microanalysis of any given office visit. Therefore, although some generalizations regarding the behaviors of physicians that may result in more and less favorable ratings from patients can be made from the existing literature, it would be inappropriate to suggest that high-quality care is a series of unrelated, automatically performed gestures and bits of conversation. Rather, what is important to conclude from this literature is that the behavior of physicians during office visits has an important influence on patients' evaluations of the care they receive, that patients are not evaluating some abstract concept of "doctoring," and that changes in behavior during office visits can produce changes in patients' ratings.

SUMMARY

This section began with the question "is the science of obtaining patients' assessments of care up to it" (that is, up to the purpose of evaluating the performance of individual physicians, groups of physicians, or health care institutions)? The answer is a qualified yes. Some key facts warrant underscoring. First, since 1970, substantial research has produced some questionnaires that with a relatively small number of items can provide valid, reliable scores for obtaining patients' assessments of the care provided by groups of physicians or health care delivery systems. Most technical problems in obtaining accurate and consistent assessments from patients have been solved with good measurement.

Second, although most patients rate the care they receive very favorably, small differences have been shown to have notable consequences for patients' behavior with respect to health and health care.

Third, patients assess different aspects of care — access, office waiting time, facilities, physicians' interpersonal and technical skills, nurses' interpersonal and technical skills, receptionists' manner — differently. These different dimensions of care should be, and are in many available measures of patients' assessments of care, measured separately. Recent research (60,61) in this area suggests that the most difficult distinctions to make may be between the interpersonal and technical care provided by physicians. If patients' assessments of care are to serve any meaningful purpose in quality assurance, via feedback to physicians, for example (80), more measurement work must be done to understand and to sharpen the distinctions patients make between the quality of interpersonal and technical care.

Fourth, patients' assessments of care have only recently been used to evaluate the performance of individual physicians or health care institutions (59,63,64). Evidence from these studies indicates that, if the care by the individual physician, clinic, or hospital is the object of measurement, it is more important to have fewer questionnaire items from a larger sample of patients, than more information from fewer patients.

Recent studies have made considerable progress toward making patients' assessments of care feasible to obtain and useful in quality assurance activities. Questions remain that need to be resolved when patients' assessments of care are used to compare the care provided by one physician or one health care institution, with a group of physicians or health care institutions with another. How many patients, for example, are needed to obtain a reliable score for an individual physician? How should an individual physician's or health care institutions' patient assessments of care be adjusted for patient characteristics, such as age, sex, health status, or expectations of care, if at all? What scores from patients' assessments of physicians' care are within the "normal range," below which other negative outcomes (ruptures of the physician-patient relationship, disenrollment from health plans, failures to adhere to treatment recommendations, poor health outcomes) will ensue? For which aspects of care? Integrating patients' assessments of care into existing quality assurance mechanisms will require that on-going research be directed at providing answers to these questions.

PATIENTS' ASSESSMENTS OF HEALTH OUTCOMES

The previous section explored the issues surrounding the patient as the direct evaluator of the health care process. A less direct, but equally important role for patients in the comprehensive assessment of the quality of health care is that of information source about health outcomes. Patients may be the only source of certain kinds of health outcome information central to quality assessment. With respect to *reports* of health (Figure 1), patients' functional status, for example, the ability to perform usual daily activities, is not gathered routinely or in a standardized fashion in any of the sources of information used in traditional data collection for quality of care assessment (for example, medical records, claims data, and so forth).

For information regarding how illness affects the quality of patients' lives, or patients' subjective evaluations or *ratings* of their health, patients are the only reasonable data source. On the negative side, only the patient can tell how bad a symptom feels or how much an illness extracts in human terms — suffering, pain, level of effort, worry, or concern about health. On the positive side, only the patient can evaluate his or her sense of well-being, energy level, vitality, quality of life, and outlook for future health. Further, only the patient knows his or her own internal referent for gauging what constitutes "excellent" or "poor" health. Again, it is important to make fine distinctions among those who give very favorable ratings. For example, variations in patients' use of health services and 5-year survival rates have been noted (124) even among those who rate their health as "excellent."

How should patients' ratings and reports of health be used in the continuous improvement of patient care and are they suitable for this purpose? As with patients' assessments of the *process* of health care, patients' ratings and reports of health as evidence of the *outcomes* of that care must be carefully scrutinized to ensure that they meet the standards of measurement for this purpose. Further, it is reasonable to ask whether and to what extent patients' assessments of their health have any recognizable and important consequences and whether patients' assessments of health are influenced by medical care. Finally, and perhaps of greatest consequence for the improvement of patient care, how can information from patients about their health be used most effectively by physicians and administrators?

Progress in the Science of Measuring Patients' Ratings and Reports of Health

Compared with patients' assessments of *health care*, the link between patients' assessments of their own *health*, and the process of health care is not as well understood. Interest in this area has grown as the search for ways to contain health care costs without compromising quality intensifies. That interest, coupled with the increasing need to understand the efficacy of clinical treatment modalities in other than strictly physiologic terms (125), has refocused attention on the meaningful integration of "quality of life" or health status measures and patient care. At least two studies (125,126) have shown that, for the same gain in clinical terms, physicians may be able to choose drugs, for example, that have fewer undesirable consequences for specific aspects of patients' health in terms of daily functioning and well-being.

Several well-tested measures of patients' assessments of their health and limitations imposed on their health by disease are available (49,65,67,126-131). The behavioral measures (reports) of patients' health, often referred to as "functional status" measures, provide information on the extent to which patients are or are not limited, as a consequence of illness, in the performance of activities that make up their daily routine. The subjective or evaluative measures (ratings) of patients' health provide information on the extent to which patients *feel* that their health is optimal or compromised.

The most comprehensive measures of patients' self-assessed health tap at least five distinct health concepts: physical health, mental health, social functioning, role functioning, and general well-being. Because each of these dimensions makes a unique contribution to the total picture of patients' overall health status, each must be measured and interpreted separately to understand patients' health status over time. Table 5 shows selected examples of health survey questions designed to represent each of these dimensions.

It should be noted that items in Table 5 represent both ratings and reports of patients' health. Being unable to participate in strenuous sports, for example, may affect the state of health of an athlete differently than a person who does not exercise. Thus, the evaluation or rating of health status by the patient adds to the conceptual understanding and measurement precision with which health is assessed.

How reliable are the available measures of patients' self-assessed health status (49,65,67,126-131,145)? How sensitive and specific are these measures to differences in levels of health? What methodologic issues should be addressed before they can be used with confidence to improve patient care? Some of these questions are addressed more completely in other chapters. The following discussion highlights the progress made and research needed to further the use of patients' assessments of health in clinical settings.

Reliability of Patients' Assessments of Health.   The issues of reliability in measuring patients' self-assessed health status parallel those discussed above with respect to patients' assessments of health care. The internal consistency reliability scores of most multidimensional measures of patients' functional status, for example, exceed the 0.65 accepted standard for group comparisons.

There are two concerns regarding the reliability of patients' assessments of their health status that are particularly important in improving patient care. To assess changes in patients' health status over time, as a product of good medical care, for example, the *measure* of health must be sufficiently precise to distinguish real differences in health status from those due to the random fluctuations (measurement error). For a patient with a given disease or health problem, how much change should be expected in a specified period? If health in the time frame being considered is relatively stable, that is, if expected changes are small but meaningful, then identifying those differences becomes particularly important. The precise measurement of health transitions is especially relevant when the impact of medical care on patients' health is being evaluated. Work in progress in the National Study of Medical Care Outcomes (147) will begin to address this issue. Other research is needed for a wide representation of disease conditions and patient populations to improve our understanding of "expected" transitions in health.

A second reliability issue of concern when considering patients' assessments of health in the context of improving the quality of care involves sampling. If the care provided by individual physicians, hospitals, or health care delivery

TABLE 5. Selected Items Measuring Generic Health Concepts.

Concepts	Definition
Physical	
Physical limitations	Limitations in performance of self-care, mobility, and physical activities.
Physical abilities	Ability to perform everyday activities.
Days in bed	Confinement to bed due to health problems
Physical well-being	Personal evaluation of physicl condition
Mental	
Anxiety and depression	Feelings of anxiety, nervousness tenseness, depression, moodiness, downheartedness.
Psychological well-being	Frequency and intensity of general positive affect.
Behavioral and emotional control	Control of behavior, thoughts and feelings during specified period.
Cognitive functioning	Orientation to time and place, memory, attention span, and alertness.
Social	
Interpersonal contacts	Frequency of visits with friends and relatives. Frequency of telephone contacts with close friends or relations during specified period.
Social resources	Quantity and quality of social ties, network.
Role	
Role functioning	Freedom from limitations in performance of usual role activities (for example, work, housework, school) due to poor health.
General health perceptions	
Current health	Self-rating of health at present
Health outlook	Expectations regarding health in the future.
Pain	Ratings of the intensity, duration and frequency of pain as well as limitations in usual activities due to pain.

Ware JE Jr. Standards for validating health measures: definitions and content. *J Chron Dis.* 1987; **40**:473-80.

systems is to be evaluated based on a summary score, for example, the average self-assessed health status of their patients, then the number of patients needed per physician, hospital, or system, the number of disease conditions, and the number of visits (to the physician, hospital, or system) that will make up the sample must be carefully considered to estimate those scores reliably and interpret them correctly.

Validity of Patients' Assessments of Health. The question of validity with respect to patients' assessments of health asks "to what extent is the patients' *real* health status reflected in their ratings and reports?" Because we lack a gold standard against which to evaluate patients' assessments of their health, the validity of their ratings and reports must be judged using other strategies.

What other health measures should serve as the appropriate comparison? It depends on the purpose for measuring patients' self-assessed health status. If the purpose is to compare the health of two or more groups of patients, for example, those with health insurance and those without health insurance (148), then the measures used should capture important differences between those groups. The validity of many of the comprehensive, "generic" measures of patients' health status for this purpose has been widely studied and discussed extensively in the literature (67,130,134,149-151).

If the purpose is to evaluate the effectiveness of various treatment modalities or to explore the effects of certain diseases on patients' assessments of their health status, then "disease-specific" measures of health may be useful

Table 5 continued

Abbreviated Items	References
Needs help with bathing, dressing; in bed, chair, couch, for most of day; does not walk at all.	132-136
Able to walk uphill, upstairs; able to participate in sports; strenuous activities.	
During past 30 days, number of days health keeps one in bed all day or most of day.	136
Rating of physical shape or condition.	66, 137
Depressed or very unhappy; bothered by nervousness or nerves.	66, 138
Happy, pleased, satisfied with life. Wake up expecting an interesting day; feel cheerful, lighthearted.	26, 27, 137, 139-141
Feel emotionally stable; lose control of behavior, thoughts, feelings; laugh or cry suddenly.	134, 137, 139, 141
Feel confused, forget a lot, make more mistakes than usual.	134
Number of friends visited; going out less often to visit people.	134, 142
How often on telephone with close friends or relatives, past month.	142
Number of close friends, people to talk with.	142
Limited in kind or amount of major role activity; health causes problem at work; unable to work because of health.	7, 67, 136, 143
In general, is health excellent, good, fair, or poor?; health is excellent; energy, pep, vitality; been feeling bad lately.	1, 139, 144
I expect to have a very healthy life.	145
During the past three months, how much pain have you had?	136
How much pain interfered with things?	146

in addition to the information provided by the more generic health status measures. Used in this way, disease-specific measures improve the sensitivity and specificity of patients' assessments of health and can help to improve patient care. For example, if information were available regarding the extent to which certain drugs improved the dexterity and decreased the pain of an arthritic patient, but produced side effects (for example, gastropathy) that compromised patients' overall functioning, physicians could weigh the trade-offs between these two health states, incorporate patient preferences, and come to a more comprehensively considered treatment strategy. Well-tested disease-specific measures have been developed for arthritis (126) and prostatism (152).

Using patients' assessments of health in the continuous improvement of patient care requires that some practical measures be available for routine use in medical practice. Several measures have been shown to be practical for data gathering in office practice (131,143,153,154). Now that we have more practical measurement instruments, their routine use in medical practice settings will provide the experience needed to address important issues remaining in the integration of patients' health status assessments in direct patient care and in the evaluation of the quality of that care. For example, how should case mix be used to adjust patients' health status scores for individual or groups of physicians, hospitals, or health care systems? How are generic and disease-specific measures of patients' self-assessed health related to recognized clinical endpoints? How do changes in patients' assessments of health correspond with changes in clinical markers of disease progression or improvement? Some studies have linked patients' self-assessed health status with clinical outcomes, such as levels of FEV$_1$ (49), glycosylated hemoglobin (48), and diastolic blood pressure (125). How much overlap between clinical endpoints and patients' assessments of health should be expected? To the extent that this overlap identifies the area in which medical care has its maximum effect, research on a wide spectrum of diseases in which several measures of patients' health, clinical and self-assessed, are gathered simultaneously will begin to clarify our understanding of the relationship between medical care and health.

What Causes Changes in Measures of Patients' Health?

How much change should be expected in measures of patients' health status over time? What is the appropriate time window for observing these changes for a given disease, a specific group of patients, and so forth? How much can medical care affect these changes? This last question is particularly of concern when evaluating the performance of an individual physician using patients' functional status. Two patients at the same level of functioning at any given point may have very different probabilities for remaining at that level. For example, a patient in bed for a broken leg has a very different likelihood for remaining in bed 3 months later than a patient in bed because of severe chronic obstructive pulmonary disease. Medical care may also have a limited relationship to patients' functioning. Individual patients may limit their activities for reasons unrelated to medical care. Research (48,156-158) shows there is considerable variability in individuals' response to physical signs and symptoms, causing more patients to limit usual activities in the face of minor health problems and others to function well with serious disease.

The impact of the best medical care may also be modified by the values patients place on certain levels of functioning (159,160). If a patient chooses not to function at the maximum level possible given restrictions reasonably imposed by disease severity and comorbidity, how much and in what way should the assessment of the quality of care provided by the individual physician be affected? On which aspects of patients' self-assessed health can physicians, through technically competent medical care or "effectively persuasive" interpersonal care, have influence? What is the effect of "prescribed dysfunction"; that is, do some physicians advise bed rest or reduced activity beyond what is needed for maximum recovery of health for a given disease or group of patients? Which aspects of care are immutable or beyond the scope of reasonable medical intervention?

The accumulated experience in the area of patients' assessments of health demonstrates their great potential for evaluating health outcomes for groups of individual patients. Further experience is necessary to assure the correct interpretation of scores on measures of patients' self-assessed health and to forecast changes in health, particularly those that are subject to change through medical care. While this experience is being gained, these measures should be used only with caution in evaluating the medical care provided by individual physicians or groups of physicians.

What are the Consequences of Poor Patient Assessments of Health?

Both conceptually and empirically, we know relatively little about the consequences of patients' views of their health status. Does impaired physical functioning, for example, impede health behaviors, such as exercise, that ultimately change physiology (48)? If so, for which diseases, for which aspects of patients' health, for which groups of patients? Imposing a causal order on the iterative nature of health and medical care may be an entertaining but fruitless academic exercise. For the improvement of routine patient care, however, it may be important to understand the interrelationships between patients' assessments of their health and the degree to which those assessments are related to engagement in or avoidance of the behaviors that will augment or compromise the effectiveness of medical treatment.

Using Measures of Patients' Health to Improve Patient Care

Pilot programs designed to integrate patients' assessments of their health into organized quality of care assessment and assurance programs have begun in some large health care delivery systems (63,64). These systems are using data collected from patients to make decisions regarding the quality of care provided by physicians, nurses, clinics, and hospitals. Users of these data must confront all of the problems and limitations noted above. The measurement and interpretation issues surrounding patients' assessments remain to be addressed. Nonetheless, measures that meet the standards demanded for quality of care assessment are available; their use in the context of these quality assessment and assurance programs will provide information needed by researchers to continue their refinement.

To maximize the impact of these measures on quality of care, it is necessary to close the loop — to provide feedback to physicians and patients. Some research has been done in which patients' functional status scores were provided to individual physicians to improve those scores (161). Although the feedback was not shown to be effective in changing patients' scores, similar studies are now in progress to assess the impact of other forms of feedback regarding patients' functional status. Whether or not these studies identify the optimal form of feedback to maximize change in patients' functional status scores for the individual physician, users of quality assessment information must consider the form and content of such feedback.

Providing feedback to physicians, hospitals, and systems of health care delivery regarding the quality of care they provide becomes even more critical when quality of care information is made available to patients (162-164). Recent evidence from a survey (165) conducted in the top 20 U.S. metropolitan areas showed that 35% of respondents actively sought out quality of care information before seeking health care services. If one third of patients will use quality of care data in the face of present difficulties in obtaining such data, and if the data available to such patients may mislead them about the quality of care provided (166), it is timely to develop strategies for providing quality assessment information to patients, and to address the ethical and policy issues surrounding the dissemination of such information, including the role of the media and government agencies, and the rights of physicians and patients to privacy.

PATIENT PARTICIPATION IN MEDICAL CARE

The most direct role for patients in the continuous improvement of health care is as active participants in both the formulation and implementation of diagnostic and treatment decisions. There are at least three current approaches to expanding patient participation in care: informed consent; the application of decision-analysis to evoke patient preferences for treatment alternatives; and techniques for increasing patients' involvement in medical decision making during office visits. Each of these approaches has its own conceptual and research history and will be discussed separately below.

The underlying assumption linking each of these approaches to expanding the patient's role in care is that beyond being ethically correct, some measurable benefit in patients' health and well-being can be derived from including them in the medical decision-making process. How valid is this assumption? How much and in what ways does involving patients in the details of their care influence the benefit they derive from that care? What are the implications of an expanded role for patients for the physician-patient relationship? What are the elements of the most effective, most promising programs for involving patients in care?

These questions are addressed to varying degrees in empirical studies of informed consent, eliciting patient preferences, and involving patients in medical decision making during office visits. They raise other important questions, such as, which are the "correct" outcomes (for example, generic health status, information transfer, patients' assessments of care) against which to evaluate the effectiveness of programs to involve patients in care? The following discussion provides an overview of the research evidence and questions that remain as patients are increasingly brought into the medical care process.

Informed Consent and Informed Choice

It is beyond the scope of this chapter to cover the 30 years of accumulated ethical, policy, and empirical literature addressing the intent and effectiveness of informed consent. Extensive reviews of this literature, from medical, legal, and social science perspectives, can be found elsewhere (167-169). Rather, we will focus on where the informed consent process, as a form of participation in care, occurs in the span of an individual's health care, what elements of the informed consent process maximize and minimize the likelihood that patients will make intelligent choices among diagnostic and treatment alternatives, and what are the observed benefits to patients of participating in care through informed consent.

The Location of Informed Consent in the Span of Health Care. In the context of a patient's health care, the informed consent process usually occurs in the hospital when the patient is at minimum, distressed, and at maximum, very sick. In either case, by the time the patient is in the hospital, he or she has already committed to a course of treatment, or a diagnostic or surgical procedure (170). At this point in their history of contact with the health care system, most patients have not had any formal training in how to make good health-related decisions under optimal, much less stressful circumstances. Stress impedes effective decision making (171,172). The lack of prior preparation for decision making, coupled with a stressful situation, minimizes the likelihood that most patients will be able to make a well-reasoned, intelligent choice among alternatives presented to them.

To make an informed choice among health care alternatives, patients must pay attention to information they obtain or are presented with, understand that information, remember it, objectively evaluate it, weigh it according to their values and preferences, and reach a decision about the course of action most appropriate for them (167). How can patients be better prepared for this kind of role in the medical care process so that, should hospitalization become necessary, they have experience with health-related decision making? Including patients in the medical decision-making process at some point before hospitalization would increase their familiarity with decision-making skills in the health care context. Training programs for adults that are designed to sharpen patients' decision-making skills during routine office visits (1,3), and during offices visits focusing on a specific treatment decision (57) have been developed.

Although these training programs have been shown to be effective in changing patients' outcomes, they are implemented well into the course of patients' health care, when most patients have had several contacts with a health care system that does not support an active role for patients in care (11,173-175). A more successful approach to ensure adequate preparation for health-related decision making might be to begin training programs well before the individual becomes sick and needs health care. Training programs aimed at improving health-related decision-making skills among children have been shown to be successful, both in teaching decision-making skills and in changing the health and illness behaviors of those children (176-181). Recent evidence (181) suggests that the changes these programs effect, including greater competency in decisions to use health care services, persist into the adult years. Informed consent among patients prepared from childhood to participate in health care decisions might have a different character and different consequences than the current informed consent process.

As a mechanism for increasing patients' participation in their care, the informed consent process, even as currently practiced, can have a positive effect on the benefits that patients derive from care. Research and practical experience point to specific elements of the informed consent process that can enhance or compromise its success in helping patients reach informed health care decisions.

Barriers and Aids to Providing Informed Choices.   There is substantial evidence that involving patients in their care through the informed consent process can be more or less effective, depending on the character and manner in which information about health care options is delivered. The type of information usually considered essential to making voluntary, informed choices among treatment alternatives is the nature of and rationale behind the treatment or procedure that the patient is endorsing, the risks and benefits involved, the probability of occurrence of those risks and benefits after a treatment or procedure, and the risks and benefits of alternatives to that treatment or procedure, along with their probabilities of occurrence. Observational studies have shown that physicians selectively omit information about risks, benefits, and alternatives when explaining diagnostic and therapeutic procedures to obtain patient consent (182,183). When asked why, physicians cite patients' inabilities to comprehend and cope with information, the seriousness of patients' illnesses, and disinterest of patients in the information as reasons for withholding or selectively imparting information (184). Regarding comprehension, at least one study has shown that most patients do not understand written and oral information provided during the informed consent process, nor do they understand the intent of the process (185). In addition, even the more assertive patients do not ask a lot of questions (1-3,89,186), and sicker patients ask even fewer questions; patients who ask fewer questions get less information (1-3).

Sicker, more distressed patients are also more prone to errors in decision making, particularly those involving probabilistic thinking (171,187). The distress caused by hospitalization may be enough to compromise effective decision making. Further, insufficient time to process information and come to a decision impairs decision making. Individuals under pressure have been noted to give systematically greater weight to negative information and to exaggerate the implications and seriousness of relatively insignificant consequences (187).

Finally, patients may be unfamiliar with their own values and preferences with respect to treatment alternatives and the implications for their health. If, as has been noted, "people are most likely to have clear preferences regarding issues that are familiar, simple, and directly experienced," (188) then patients who have less experience with the illness, hospital, or clinic, or who are faced with a complex decision, are likely to be unclear about their values and preferences for specific health care alternatives and health outcomes.

TABLE 6. Barriers and Aids to Effective Communication of Information Related to Health Care Decisions.

Barriers	Aids
Complexity of treatment, procedure and alternatives	Use of lay language
Severity of patients' illness: distress	Feedback from patient regarding what they understood
Poor information-seeking skills of patients	Use of multiple media (written forms, personal communication, video-tape)
Time pressures	Repetition of information
Biases in interpreting probabilities	Personalizing risk/benefit information
Patients' ignorance of their own values	Consistency of presentation method across all alternatives Grouping information by type Time to ponder; take home information

Given these barriers to effective transmission of complex information to distressed patients, does anything work? Table 6 summarizes the techniques that are likely to maximize the effectiveness of the informed consent process. The avoidance of medical jargon has been consistently associated with more effective physician-patient communication (68,85,89-91,100). Querying patients regarding what they understood from the informed consent process has been proposed as an effective way to ensure that the information was received and to clarify any misconceptions patients may have (167-169).

Repetition of information also helps patients remember and process relevant details. Such repetition may be most effective when several media (written materials, verbal communication with physicians, videotapes) are used to impart decision-relevant information (189). For patients to make the best decision about the desirability of a treatment or procedure, they must understand how the risks and benefits of that treatment or procedure and its alternatives apply to them. Although risk or benefit information may not always be known, helping patients to personalize the information and arrive at some estimation of their individual risk or benefit will reduce errors in judgment based on biases in interpreting probabilities (190,191).

Other elements of an effective strategy for helping patients make optional health-related decisions and avoid common biases in judgment include grouping information so that the patient is presented with all information of a similar type at once. That is, the description of the treatment or procedure and the array of alternatives, risk information for each alternative, benefit information, and so forth should be grouped together to facilitate reasoned decision making (190). In addition, patients should be given probability information consistently across all treatment alternatives to minimize interpretation errors (192). For example, ratios or percentages should not be used to describe risk for death from one treatment or procedure if qualitative statements such as "insignificant" or "trivial" are used to describe risk for death from an alternative treatment.

TABLE 7. Positive Health Effects of Information before Treatment.

Health Effect	Patients Sampled	Reference
Decreased postoperative anxiety	Surgical patients	171
Decreased pain medication	Endoscopic patients	194
	Surgical patients	195
	Burn patients	196
Decreased discomfort	Blood donors	197
Decreased recovery time	Surgical patients	198
Decreased length of hospital stay	Surgical patients	171,195,199,200

Finally, as noted above, time pressures impair decision-making abilities. In nonemergency situations, patients are most likely to make well-reasoned decisions if given some time to consider and reflect on the information they have obtained. In a study of breast cancer patients, patients who took consent forms home showed better understanding of proposed treatment and its alternatives compared with a control group who signed forms immediately after the usual informed consent procedure (193).

Impact of Providing Informed Choices. Given the difficulties, can meaningful benefit be gained from informing patients about their health care alternatives and the consequences they can expect? Considerable empirical evidence has accumulated that suggests that for various indicators of patients' health, patients who receive information about what to expect from care fare better than those who do not (Table 7). Other experimental research has shown that patients who are offered choices have more positive health outcomes than those who are not (201,202). Providing patients with alternatives and enough information to make intelligent choices appears to be well worth the effort.

Eliciting Patient Preferences

Weighing treatment alternatives against personal values and preferences is a key element of effective health-related decision making. As noted above, patients are often poorly prepared to think about their values and preferences in specific health care situations. For example, patients facing cholecystectomy who have never considered whether they would prefer the risks and benefits of lithotripsy or medication as alternative therapies might not be able to give credible or consistent weights to each alternative.

Techniques derived from utility theory have been developed to elicit patient values for specific treatment decisions (203-205). Although such techniques might not be practical for use in routine health care delivery, when decisions have important consequences for patients' health status, and are nonemergency in nature, using modifications of these techniques might provide clinicians with useful information about patient preferences for various health care alternatives.

Designing techniques that can be used by physicians in routine office practice is therefore an important avenue for further research in this area. Other important research issues must also be addressed for physicians to be able to interpret information from patients regarding their values and preferences for specific treatment alternatives correctly. Because patients are subject to the biases in judgment involving probabilities noted above (190,192), because patients are unfamiliar with the thinking processes involved in making trade-offs, especially when choices have negative consequences (206,207), and because patients are often in some distress in medical settings, the validity and reliability of assessments of patient preferences must be studied.

How should the validity of measures of patients' values and preferences be determined? How stable are patients' values (different from measures of those values) over time? Do patients' reference points, used to assess their values, shift as their life circumstances change? What is valid on one day for a patient who is apparently free from disease may change the next day when breast cancer is diagnosed. How do variations in the setting in which patients' values are measured (home compared with physician's office compared with hospital) affect the reliability of these measures? How much are measures of patients' values affected by other threats to reliability such as random variation in patients' mood? Research must begin to address these questions before measures of patients' values can be incorporated in clinical practice.

Involving Patients in Care during Office Visits

As noted by Greenfield in Chapter 7, many important decisions that shape the course of patients' care occur during the office visit. Although including patients in their care at any point of contact with the health care system (physician's office, clinic, hospital) has the dual disadvantages of patients' anxiety and lack of preparation that impede effective decision making as noted above (171,172,187), from a behavioral perspective the office visit may represent a highly desirable opportunity to effect change aimed at enhancing the patient's role in medical decision making.

First, the patient is less sick or less distressed during the office visit than when in the hospital. Second, the physician and patient are more likely to know each other in the office than hospital setting. Third, the physician can often take advantage of a series of sequential office visits to present decisions, review alternatives, and elicit and verify patient values. Between visits, patients return to family, friends, and advisors with whom they can review decision-related information and reflect on their values and preferences in a less time-pressured and anxiety-producing environment. Patients can then modify, negotiate, or discuss original decisions with the physician on subsequent visits.

Are Office-Based Training Programs Available? Training programs developed specifically for use in office practice to improve patients' decision-making skills are now available. Two examples of existing programs illustrate the spectrum of approaches to orienting patients to the process of medical care and involving them in medical decisions.

One approach focuses on providing patients access to the logic of the medical care process for the outpatient management of a specific chronic disease (1-3). Using modified treatment algorithms displayed in branching logic format, this approach orients patients to the entire decision-making framework for the management of their disease. Mapping the process the physician follows in arriving at a treatment decision, the branching nature of the algorithm individualizes the decisions relevant for specific patients, in the context of the care provided for most patients with their disease.

In the context of this framework, patients focus on decisions that are relevant for a specific office visit. For example, if a patient with rheumatoid arthritis is symptomatic, in the face of a trial of a nonsteroidal anti-inflammatory agent on a given visit, the algorithm is constructed to identify various options for care at that visit, including changing to another nonsteroidal agent, adding steroids, changing the dose of the current drug, adding an analgesic, or maintaining current therapy for an additional period. Although the specific decisions that are relevant may vary from office visit to office visit, patients can understand the context of and rationale for a specific decision, and gain predictability from the decision-making framework provided in the algorithm regarding what to expect next. Over the course of a year or two, the patient with rheumatoid arthritis may face various decisions, such as initiation of remittive therapy or surgery. The focus of this approach is therefore the entire framework for effective disease management.

This approach was designed to be conducted during the waiting time immediately preceding office visits to maximize the potential for changing patients' behavior during that visit. In 20-minute sessions conducted during this period, assistants use the information in the patient's medical record to focus the patient's attention on the decisions identified in the algorithm as pertinent to their current visit. Any diagnostic or treatment alternatives relevant to the patient's current disease management are reviewed with the patient as candidates for discussion and negotiation with his or her physician.

These options are reviewed with the patient before each visit, along with specific negotiation and information skills designed to reduce the likelihood that the patient will forget, or become embarassed or intimidated and impede the successful negotiation of decisions. Patients thus "coached" to participate in care, are then seen by their physicians for their usual office visits. Physicians, specifically trained to present decisions and to encourage patients to participate in care, provide behavioral reinforcement for patients' negotiating and decision-making attempts in the context of routine care. Between visits, patients are sent home with copies of the treatment algorithm and their medical records to review. "Coaching" sessions are repeated over the course of consecutive visits.

This approach is therefore characterized by its emphasis on *multiple decisions* that happen in long-term course of care for a specific disease; on the transmission of *individualized information* about the decisions relevant

**TABLE 8. Effects of the Interventions on Patients' Functional Limitations.*

Variable	Functional Limitations		tValue†
	Experimental	**Control**	
Diabetes, $n = 59$			
Before	2.69	3.57	
	(2.14)	(2.98)	
			3.19
After	1.31	3.30	
	(1.91)	(3.09)	
Hypertension, $n = 102$			
Before	2.91	3.11	
	(2.04)	(3.01)	
			4.04
After	1.71	3.40	
	(1.67)	(2.79)	
Ulcers, $n = 44$‡			
Before	3.11	3.45	
	(2.34)	(3.68)	
			2.89
After	1.17	3.71	
	(2.58)	(3.07)	

*Data presented are means with standard deviations in parentheses.
†Based on differences between groups adjusted for baseline scores in separate analyses of variance.
‡Baseline data reflect aggregated health status measure obtained by taking best linear combination of four health status measures from principal components analysis (41).
Reproduced with permission. Kaplan SH, Greenfield S, Ware JE Jr. Impact of the doctor-patient relationship on the outcomes of chronic disease. In: Stewart M. Roter D, eds. *Communicating with Patients in Medical Practice.* Newbury Park, California: Sage Publications, Inc.; In press.

to a patients' care, in the context of a framework outlined by the *algorithm* for understanding those decisions; on the training of *specific behaviors* (negotiating, information seeking, decision making) rather than the transmission of information about the disease and its management; on the need for including *both patients and their physicians* in training for greater patient involvement in care; on the use of *multiple media*, including written materials and personal contact with assistants or physicians; and on *repetition* over sequential visits to ensure that patients become accustomed to participating in decision making during office visits.

Another approach to including patients in care during office visits emphasizes a specific decision with noteworthy consequences for patients' health outcomes, such as surgery (57). This approach focuses intensively on that specific decision, enumerating specific treatment alternatives and their implications for patients' subsequent health outcomes, and eliciting patients' values and preferences for each treatment alternative. Patients are asked to view videotapes in which other patients who have experienced the outcomes of each treatment alternative discuss their values and preferences and their rationale for selecting that alternative. These tapes are also designed to address patients' expectations of each treatment alternative.

TABLE 9. Effects of the Interventions on Physiologic Health Outcomes.*

Variable	Experimental	Control	*t* Value[†]
Blood sugar (HbA1), $n = 59$			
Before	10.6	10.3	0.55
	(2.1)	(2.0)	
After	9.1	10.6	2.81[‡]
	(1.9)	(2.2)	
Diastolic blood pressure, $n = 102$			
Before	95	93	0.80
	(11)	(14)	
After	83	91	-5.0[‡]
	(8)	(8)	

*Data presented are means with standard deviations in parentheses.
[†]Based on comparison of group means with pooled variance.
[‡]$P < 0.05$
Reproduced with permission. Kaplan SH, Greenfield S, Ware JE Jr. Impact of the doctor-patient relationship on the outcomes of chronic disease. In: Stewart M. Roter D, eds. *Communicating with Patients in Medical Practice.* Newbury Park, California: Sage Publications, Inc.; In press.

Do Such Approaches Affect Health Outcomes?   Randomized controlled trials (208) on approaches such as those described above show that patients who are encouraged to participate in their care fare better, both in self-assessments and in clinical measures of their health status, than those exposed to traditional patient education programs. Tables 8 and 9 present data from randomized trials among patients with chronic diseases, of the approach by Greenfield and colleagues, described above (1-3). In these studies, patients in the experimental groups, although similar at baseline to patients in the control groups in reports of functional limitations due to illness, reported fewer functional limitations at 18-month follow-up after participating in the program (Table 8). Similarly, experimental patients with diabetes were shown to have significantly lower post-intervention levels of glycosylated hemoglobin compared with controls, and experimental hypertensive patients had significantly lower diastolic blood pressure at follow-up than patients in the control group (Table 9).

These findings are provocative and suggest that beyond being a health care "amenity," programs designed to involve patients in their care may influence both the process of care and the health outcomes that patients experience as a product of that care. Research currently underway to expand these approaches to other disease conditions, treatment settings, and patient populations will address the generalizability of these findings. Further research combining several approaches must be done to identify where, when, and in what manner patients are most effectively involved in the course of their health care.

CONCLUSIONS

This chapter has reviewed the research and practical issues involved in three distinct aspects of the patient's role in health care — in the evaluation of the *process* of care; in the evaluation of the *outcomes* of care; and in the shaping of the health care process itself, as *participants* in medical decision making. It is important to underscore progress made in each of these areas and to identify research issues remaining that will further the definition of a reasonable role for patients in routine patient care and the assessments of its quality.

With respect to the evaluation of the process of care, research since 1970 has solved many of the technical problems in obtaining patients' assessments of care with good measurement. Well-tested standardized measures of patients' ratings and reports of the technical and interpersonal care they receive are now available. Such measures consistently point to the need to distinguish among the various dimensions of patients' assessments of care including access to care (waiting time, transportation, financial access), facilities (for example, parking), office staff, as well as the technical and interpersonal care provided by physicians. If patients' assessments of care are to be used to evaluate the performance of individual physicians, it is important that physicians are not held accountable for aspects of care beyond their control.

Extremely important and least well understood is the distinction between patients' assessments of interpersonal and technical care they receive. This distinction is particularly important in an era of cost-containment where changes in the manner in which health care services are delivered place both at risk. Further, if patients' assessments of care are to be used to improve the care provided by physicians, these aspects of care must be distinguished.

Recent research underscores the importance of having a large sample of patients (compared with more information from fewer patients) to represent the care provided by individual physicians fairly. Research in this area has also shown that small differences in patients' assessments of care have important consequences for patients' health and health care behaviors over time. Such differences have been linked to physician-shopping, avoidance of physicians, propensity to sue, and noncompliance with medical advice.

To *use* patients' assessments of care in the continuous improvement of health care quality, continuing research must be aimed at specific issues. First, existing measures must be refined and improved to fashion the "Snellen Eye Chart" equivalent. Second, such measures must be built into a routine data collection system. Third, such a system must be included in a mechanism for using the data generated, providing feedback to individual physicians, and supporting changes necessary to improve the care they provide.

To *understand* patients' assessments of care, the links between what patients say about care and the actual process of care must be explored. Studies of the relationship between patients' assessments of care and physicians' assessments of care will address the effects of interpersonal dynamics on the quality of care provided. Such studies will also help evaluate the effects of changes made in health care delivery systems on both physicians and patients.

With respect to the evaluation of the outcomes of care, well-tested measures of patients' assessments of their health status are now available. Such measures are being used to understand the relationship between clinical evidence of a change in health status and changes in patients' perceptions of their health. If such measures are to be used in the evaluation of health care, especially at the level of individual physician performance, research must be done to determine whether more in-depth information is needed from fewer patients, or whether a fairer estimate is gained from less information gathered from a larger sample of patients.

If such measures are to be used in the improvement of quality of care, research must be done to identify and understand the meaning of "abnormal" functioning. As with abnormal laboratory values, identifying when a patient is outside the normal range is the first step in understanding what to do about it. To further this understanding, practical measures that can be used in routine office practice must be developed and refined. The use of such measures in routine data collection systems will forward their interpretation, for both patient care and quality assessment purposes.

There is evidence that levels of disease severity and comorbidity do not correspond perfectly with patients' assessments of their health. For situations and patient groups in which there is the least overlap, further research must be done to understand why. What produces these disparities? What causes can physicians control? How much should individual physicians be held accountable for patients' "dysfunctioning"?

With respect to the role of the patient in medical decision making, a few promising approaches have been developed that provide training for a reasoned expansion of patients into the medical care process. Evidence from randomized controlled trials of one approach suggest that such programs have positive effects on patients' health. To understand where and when such approaches are most and least effective in improving patients' health and the quality of patient care, they must be tested in various health care settings; among patients with different diseases, demographic characteristics, and attitudes about health care; among physicians of different specialties; and among physicians and patients with different lengths of association and different types of relationships.

The most rational approach for including patients in care links elements from existing programs. Ideally, preparation for making responsible health care decisions should begin in childhood with curricula for teaching general decision-making skills (176-181). Preparation for decision making for a specific disease could then build on such skills (1-3). Patients, prepared for decision making in the context of a specific disease, would then be more effectively prepared for, and benefit more from, intensive training programs aimed at highly specific, very consequential decisions (57). Such patients stand the best chance of shaping the quality of health care they receive.

If medical care is the "negotiated achievement" (209) of an optimal resolution of patients' health problems, methods must be sought that use patients' assessments of their health and health care, and involve them in medical decision making. These methods must enhance the technical and interpersonal quality of care from both patients' and physicians' perspective.

References

1. Greenfield S, Kaplan SH, Ware JE Jr. Expanding patient involvement in medical care: effects on patient outcomes. *Ann Intern Med.* 1985;**102**:520-8.
2. Kaplan SH, Greenfield S, Ware JE Jr. Expanded patient involvement in medical care: effects on blood pressure. National Conference on High Blood Pressure Control, Chicago, Illinois, April 1985.
3. Greenfield S, Kaplan SH, Ware JE Jr, Yano EM, Frank HJ. Patient participation in medical care: effects on blood sugar control and quality of life in diabetes. *J Gen Intern Med.* 1988;**3**:448-57.
4. Schulman BA. Active patient orientation and outcomes in hypertensive treatment: application of a socio-organizational perspective. *Med Care.* 1979;**17**:267-80.
5. Kelman HR. Evaluation of health care quality by consumers. In: Elinson J, Siegmann AE, eds. *Sociomedical Health Indicators.* Farmingdale, New York: Baywood Publishing Co.; 1979.
6. Anderson DM, Kerr M. Citizen influence in health service programs. *Am J Public Health.* 1971;**6**:1518-23.
7. Glassner M. Consumer expectation of health services. In: Corey L, ed. *Medicine in a Changing Society.* St. Louis, Missouri; CV Mosby; 1972.
8. Huntly RR. Improving the health services system through research and development. *Inquiry.* 1970;**1**:15-21.
9. Sheps CM. The influence of consumer sponsorship on medical services. *Milbank Mem Fund Q.* 1972;**50**:41-73.
10. Thomasma DC. Beyond medical paternalism and patient autonomy: a model of physician conscience for the physician-patient relationship. *Ann Intern Med.* 1983;**98**:243-8.
11. Brody DS. The patient's role in clinical decision making. *Ann Intern Med.* 1980;**93**:718-22.
12. Ware JE Jr, Snyder MK, Wright WR. *Development and Validation of Scales to Measure Patient Satisfaction with Health Care Services. Volume I, Part B: Results Regarding Scales Constructed from the Patient Satisfaction Questionnaire and Measures of Other Health Perceptions.* Springfield, Virginia: National Technical Information Service; 1976.
13. Doyle BJ, Ware JE Jr. Physician conduct and other factors that affect consumer satisfaction with medical care. *J Med Educ.* 1977;**52**:793-801.
14. Ware JE Jr. Effects of acquiescent response set on patient satisfaction ratings. *Med Care.* 1978;**16**:327-36.
15. Hulka BS, Kupper LL, Daly MD, Cassel JC, Schoen F. Correlates of satisfaction and dissatisfaction with medical care: a community perspective. *Med Care.* 1975;**13**:648-58.
16. Lebow JL. Consumer assessments of the quality of medical care. *Med Care.* 1974;**12**:328-37.
17. Zyzanski SJ, Hulka BS, Cassel JC. Scale for the measurement of satisfaction with medical care: modifications in content, format, and scoring. *Med Care.* 1974;**12**:611-20.
18. Ware JE Jr, Davies-Avery A, Stewart AL. The measurement and meaning of patient satisfaction. *Health Med Care Ser Rev.* 1978;**1**:13-15.
19. Linn LS. Factors associated with patient evaluation of health care. *Milbank Mem Fund Q Health Soc.* 1975;**53**:531-48.
20. Wolf MH, Putnam SM, James SA, et al. The medical interview satisfaction scale: development of a scale to measure patient perceptions of physician behavior. *J Behav Med.* 1978;**1**:391-402.
21. Linder-Pelz S, Struening EL. The multi-dimensionality of patient satisfaction with a clinic visit. *J Community Health.* 1985;**10**:42-54.
22. DiMatteo MR, Hays R. The significance of patients' perceptions of physician conduct: a study of patient satisfaction in a family practice center. *J Community Health.* 1980;**6**:18-34.
23. Linn LS, DiMatteo MR, Chang BL, Code DW. Consumer values and subsequent satisfaction ratings of physician behavior. *Med Care.* 1984;**22**:804-12.
24. Hays RD, Ware JE Jr. "My medical care is better than yours: social desirability and patient satisfaction ratings. *Med Care.* 1986;**24**:519-24.
25. Gray LC. Consumer satisfaction with physician provided services: a panel study. *Soc Sci Med.* 1980;**14A**:65-73.
26. Roberts JG, Tugwell P. Comparison of questionnaires determining patient satisfaction with medical care. *Health Serv Res.* 1987;**22**:637-54.
27. Ware JE Jr, Hays RD. Methods for measuring patient satisfaction with specific medical encounters. *Med Care.* 1988;**26**:393-402.
28. Davies AR, Ware JE Jr. Involving consumers in quality of care assessment. *Health Aff (Millwood).* 1988;**7**:34-48.

29. Kasteler J, Kane RL, Olsen DM, Thetford C. Issues underlying the prevalence of 'doctor-shopping' behavior. *J Health Soc Behav.* 1976;**17**:328-39.

30. Ware JE Jr, Davies AR. Behavioral consequences of consumer dissatisfaction with medical care. *Eval Prog Planning.* 1983;**6**:291-7.

31. Louis Harris and Associates. *Americans and Their Doctors.* Publication No. 28. New York: January, 1985.

32. Wolinsky FD, Steiber SR. Salient issues in choosing a new doctor. *Soc Sci Med.* 1982;**16**:759-67.

33. Ware JE Jr, Curbow B, Davies AR, Robins B. *Medicaid Satisfaction Surveys, 1977-1980: A Report of the Prepaid Health Research, Evaluation and Development Project.* Sacramento, California: California State Dept of Health Services; 1981.

34. Davies AR, Ware JE Jr, Brook RH, Peterson JR, Newhouse JP. Consumer acceptance of prepaid and fee-for-service medical care: results from a randomized controlled trial. *Health Serv Res.* 1986;**21**:429-52.

35. Vaccarino JM. Malpractice: the problem in perspective. *JAMA.* 1977;**238**:861-3.

36. Davis MS. Variation in patients' compliance with doctors' orders: medical practice and doctor-patient interaction. *Psychiatry Med.* 1971;**2**:31-54.

37. Francis V, Korsch BM, Morris MJ. Gaps in doctor-patient communication: patients' response to medical advice. *New Engl J. Med.* 1969;**280**:535-40.

38. Kallen DJ, Stephenson JJ. Perceived physician humaneness, patient attitude, and satisfaction with the pill as a contraceptive. *J Health Soc Behav.* 1981;**22**:256-67.

39. Mirowsky J, Ross CE. Patient satisfaction and visiting the doctor: a self-regulating system. *Soc Sci Med.* 1983;**17**:1353-61.

40. Jensen J. Choosing a hospital. *Amer Demographics.* 1987;**9**:45-7.

41. Inguanzo JM, Harju M. What makes consumers select a hospital. *Hospitals.* 1985;**59**:90-4.

42. Hickson GB, Stewart DW, Altemeier WA, Perrin JM. First step in obtaining child health care: selecting a physician. *Pediatrics.* 1988;**81**:333-8.

43. Komaroff AL. Quality assurance in 1984. *Med Care.* 1985;**23**:723-34.

44. Mosteller F. Assessing quality of institutional care [Editorial]. *Am J Public Health.* 1987;**77**:1155-6.

45. Lavin JH. Why 3 out of 5 patients switch. *Med Econ.* 1983;**60**:11-7.

46. Haynes RB, Sackett DL, Taylor DW. *Compliance in Health Care.* Baltimore: John Hopkins University Press; 1979.

47. Hayes-Bautista DE. Modifying the treatment: patient compliance, patient control and medical care. *Soc Sci Med.* 1976;**10**:233-8.

48. Kaplan SH. Patient reports of health status as predictors of physiologic health measures in chronic disease. *J Chronic Disease.* 1987;**40**:(Suppl 1):27S-40S.

49. Kaplan RM, Atkins CJ, Timms R. Validity of a quality of well-being scale as an outcome measure in chronic obstructive pulmonary disease. *J. Chronic Dis.* 1984;**37**:85-95.

50. Vertinsky IB, Thompson WA, Uyeno D. Measuring consumer desire for participation in clinical decision-making. *Health Serv Res.* 1974;**9**:121-34.

51. Faden RR, Becker C, Lewis C, Freeman J, Faden AI. Disclosure of information to patients in medical care. *Med Care.* 1981;**19**:718-33.

52. McIntosh J. Processes of communication, information seeking and control associated with cancer: a selective review of the literature. *Soc Sci Med.* 1974;**8**:167-87.

53. Haug MR, Lavin B. Public challenge of physician authority. *Med Care.* 1979;**17**:844-58.

54. Cassileth BR, Zupkis RV, Sutton-Smith K, March V. Information and participation preferences among cancer patients. *Ann Intern Med.* 1980;**101**:832-6.

55. Waitzkin H. Information giving in medical care. *J Health Soc Behav.* 1985;**26**:81-101.

56. Quill TE. Partnerships in patient care: a contractual approach. *Ann Intern Med.* 1983;**98**:228-34.

57. Wennberg JE, Mulley AG Jr, Hanley D, et al. An assessment of prostatectomy for benign urinary tract obstruction: geographic variations and the evaluation of medical care outcomes. *JAMA.* 1988;**259**:3027-30.

58. Linn LS, Lewis CE. Attitudes toward self-care among practicing physicians. *Med Care.* 1979;**17**:183-90.

59. Swanson D, Webster G, Norcini J. Precision of patient ratings of residents' humanistic qualities: how many patients are enough? Presented at the Annual Meeting of the American Public Health Association, Boston, Massachusetts, November 13-17, 1988.

60. Kaplan SH, Greenfield S, Linn LS, Cope D. Are patients just saying that? Relation of patient ratings to known differences

in physicians' humanistic behaviors. Presented at the Annual Meeting of the American Public Health Association, Boston, Massachusetts, November 13-17, 1988.

61. Ware JE Jr, Hays R. Validity of different patient rating methods in detecting differences in physicians' humanistic skills. Presented at the Annual Meeting of the American Public Health Association, Boston, Massachusetts, November 13-17, 1988.

62. Carter WB, Inui T. How patients judge humanistic skills of their physicians. Presented at the Annual Meeting of the American Public Health Association, Boston, Massachusetts, November 13-17, 1988.

63. Berwick D, Ware JE Jr, Nelson E, et al. *Patient Judgments of Hospital Quality: Report of a Pilot Study.* Cambridge, Massachusetts: Harvard Community Health Plan; In print.

64. Grossman J, Chairman and Chief Executive Officer, New England Medical Center, Inc, February 1, 1989, personal communication.

65. Stewart AL, Hays RD, Ware JE Jr. The MOS short-form general health survey: reliability and validity in a patient population. *Med Care.* 1988;**26**:724-35.

66. Chambers LW, Macdonald LA, Tugwell P, Buchanan WW, Kraag G. The McMaster Health Index Questionnaire as a measure of quality of life for patients with rheumatoid disease. *J Rheumatol.* 1982;**9**:780-4.

67. Stewart AL, Ware JE Jr, Brook RH. *Construction and Scoring of Aggregate Functional Status Measures Vol. I.* Santa Monica, California: The RAND Corporation (R-2551-HHS); 1982.

68. Hulka BS, Kupper LL, Cassel JC, Mayo F. Doctor-patient communication and outcomes among diabetic patients. *J Community Health.* 1975;**1**:15-27.

69. Ware JE Jr. Standards for validating health measures: definition and content. *J Chronic Dis.* 1987;**40**:473-80.

70. Ware JE Jr, Davies AR, Rubin HR. Patients' assessments of their care. In: U.S. Congress, Office of Technology Assessment. *The Quality of Medical Care: Information for Consumers.* Washington, DC: U.S. Government Printing Office, June 1988 (OTA-H-386).

71. Tessler R, Mechanic D. Consumer satisfaction with prepaid group practice: a comparative study. *J Health Soc Behav.* 1975;**16**:95-113.

72. Shortell SM, Richardson WC, LoGerfo LP, Diehr P, Weaver B, Green KE. The relationship among dimensions of health services in two provider systems: a causal model approach. *J Health Soc Behav.* 1977;**18**:139-59.

73. DiMatteo MR, Hays RD, Prince LM. Relationship of physicians' nonverbal communication skill to patient satisfaction, appointment noncompliance, and physician workload. *Health Psychol.* 1986;**5**:581-94.

74. DiMatteo MR, Taranta A, Friedman HS, Prince LM. Predicting patient satisfaction from physicians' nonverbal communication skills. *Med Care.* 1980;**18**:376-87.

75. Davis JE, Meyer DL, Murray JR. Obtaining stable estimates of performance for quality of care measures. Presented at the 16th Annual Meeting of the American Public Health Association, Boston, Massachusetts, November 1988.

76. Sanazaro PJ, Worth RM. Measuring clinical performance of individual internists in office and hospital practice. *Med Care.* 1985;**23**:1097-114.

77. Ehrlich J, Morehead MA, Trussell RE. *The Quantity, Quality and Costs of Medical and Hospital Care Secured by A Sample of Teamster Families in the New York Area.* New York: Columbia University School of Public Health and Administrative Medicine; 1961.

78. Linn BS. Burn patients' evaluations of emergency department care. *Ann Emerg Med.* 1982;**11**:255-9.

79. Chang BL, Uman GC, Linn LS, Ware JE Jr, Kane RL. The effect of systematically varying components of nursing care on satisfaction in elderly ambulatory women. *West J Nurs Res.* 1984;**6**:367-86.

80. Cope DW, Linn LS, Leake BD, Barrett PA. Modification of residents' behavior by preceptor feedback of patient satisfaction. *J Gen Intern Med.* 1986;**1**:394-8.

81. Gerbert B, Stone G, Stulbarg M, Gullion DS, Greenfield S. Agreement among physician assessment methods: searching for the truth among fallible methods. *Med Care.* 1988;**26**:519-35.

82. Comstock LM, Hooper EM, Goodwin JM, Goodwin JS. Physician behaviors that correlate with patient satisfaction. *J Med Educ.* 1982;**57**:105-12.

83. Smith CK, Polis E, Hadac RR. Characteristics of the initial medical interview associated with patient satisfaction and understanding. *J Fam Pract.* 1981;**12**:283-8.

84. Buller MK, Buller DB. Physicians' communication style and patient satisfaction. *J Health Soc Behav.* 1987;**28**:375-88.

85. Bertakis KD. The communication of information from physician to patient: a method for increasing patients' retention and satisfaction. *J Fam Pract.* 1977;**5**:217-22.

86. Stiles WB, Putnam SM, James SA, Wolf MH. Dimensions of patient and physician roles in medical screening interviews. *Soc Sci Med.* 1979;**13A**:335-41.

87. Carter WB, Inui TS, Kukull WA, Haigh VH. Outcome-based doctor-patient interaction analysis. II. Identifying effective provider and patient behavior. *Med Care.* 1982;**20**;550-66.

88. Korsch BM, Gozzi EK, Francis V. Gaps in doctor-patient communication. I. Doctor-patient interaction and patient satisfaction, *Pediatrics.* 1968;**42**:855-71.

89. Korsch BM, Negrete VF. Doctor-patient communication. *Sci Am.* 1972;**227**:66-74.

90. Korsch BM. Doctor-patient communication. In: Henderson G, ed. *Physician-Patient Communication: Readings and Recommendations.* Springfield, Illinois: Thomas; 1981.

91. Freemon B, Negrete VF, Davis M, et al. Gaps in doctor-patient communication: doctor-patient interaction analysis. *Ped Res.* 1971;**5**:298-311.

92. Pantell RH, Stewart TJ, Dias JK, Wells P, Ross AW. Physician communication with children and parents. *Pediatrics.* 1982;**70**:396-402.

93. Street RL Jr, Wiemann JM. Patients' satisfaction with physicians' interpersonal involvement, expressiveness and dominance. In McLaughlin M, ed. *Communication Yearbook.* Volume 10. Beverly Hills, California: Sage Publications; 1987.

94. Weinberger M, Greene JY, Mamlin JJ. The impact of clinical encounter events on patient and physician satisfaction. *Soc Sci Med* [*E*]. 1981;**15**:239-44.

95. DiMatteo MR, Prince LM, Taranta A. Patients' perceptions of physician behavior: determinants of patient commitment to the therapeutic relationship. *J Community Health.* 1979;**4**:280-90.

96. Friedman HS, DiMatteo MR, Taranta A. A study of the relationship between individual differences in nonverbal expressiveness and factors of personality and social interactions. *J Res Pers.* 1980;**14**:351-64.

97. Hall JA, Roter DL, Rand CS. Communication of affect between patient and physician. *J Health Soc Behav.* 1981;**22**:18-30.

98. Lane SD. Compliance, satisfaction and physician-patient communication. In: Bostrom R, ed. *Communication Yearbook.* Beverly Hills, California: Sage Publications; 1983.

99. Woolley FR, Kane RL, Hughes CC, Wright DD. The effects of doctor-patient communication on satisfaction and outcome of care. *Soc Sci Med.* 1978;**12**:123-8.

100. Stiles WB, Putnam SM, Wolf MH, James SA. Interaction exchange structure and patient satisfaction with medical interviews. *Med Care.* 1979;**17**:667-81.

101. Ley P, Bradshaw PW, Kincey JA, Atherton ST. Increasing patients' satisfaction with communication. *BR J Soc Clin Psychol.* 1976;**15**:403-13.

102. Kane RL, Klein SJ, Bernstein L, Rothenberg R, Wales J. Hospice role in alleviating the emotional stress of terminal patients and their families. *Med Care.* 1985;**23**:189-97.

103. Starfield B, Wray C, Hess K, Gross R, Birk PS, D'Lugoff BC. The influence of patient-practitioner agreement on outcome of care. *Am J Public Health.* 1981;**71**:127-31.

104. Stewart MA, McWhinney IR, Buck CW. The doctor-patient relationship and its effect upon outcome. *J R Coll Gen Pract.* 1979;**9**:77-81.

105. Bass MJ, Buck C, Turner L, Dickie G, Pratt G, Robinson HC. The physicians' actions and the outcome of illness in family practice. *J Fam Pract.* 1986;**23**:43-7.

106. The Headache Study Group of the University of Western Ontario. Predictors of outcome in headache patients presenting to family physicians — a one year prospective study. *Headache.* 1986;**26**:285-94.

107. Orth JE, Stiles WB, Scherwitz Hennrikus D, Vallbona C. Patient exposition and provider explanation in routine interviews and hypertensive patients' blood pressure control. *Health Psychol.* 1987;**6**:29-42.

108. Gerbert B, Hargreaves WA. Measuring physician behavior. *Med Care.* 1986;**24**:838-47.

109. Sox HC Jr, Margulies I, Sox CH. Psychologically mediated effects of diagnostic tests. *Ann Intern Med.* 1981;**95**:680-5.

110. Linn LS, Greenfield S. Patient suffering and patient satisfaction among the chronically ill. *Med Care.* 1982;**20**:425-31.

111. Linder Pelz S. Social psychological determinants of patient satisfaction: a test of five hypotheses. *Soc Sci Med.* 1982;**15**:583-9.

112. Greenley JR, Young TB, Schoenherr RA. Psychological distress and patient satisfaction. *Med Care.* 1982;**20**:373-85.

113. Hibbard JH, Weeks EC. Consumerism in health care: prevalence and predictors. *Med Care.* 1987;**25**:1019-32.

114. Penchansky R, Fox D. Frequency of referral and patient characteristics in group practice. *Med Care.* 1980;**8**:368.

115. Greenfield S, Linn LS, Purtill NA, Young RT. Reverse consultations: profiles of patients referred from subspecialists to generalists. *J Chronic Dis.* 1983;**36**:883-9.

116. Hooper EM, Comstock LM, Goodwin JM, Goodwin JS. Patient characteristics that influence physician behavior. *Med Care.* 1982;**20**:630-8.

117. Ross CE, Wheaton B, Duff RS. Client satisfaction and the organization of medical practice: why time counts. *J Health Soc Behav.* 1981;**22**:243-55.

118. Dutton DB. Patterns of ambulatory health care in five different delivery systems. *Med Care.* 1979;**17**:221-43.

119. Andersen RM, Fleming GV, Champney TF. Exploring a paradox: belief in a crisis and general satisfaction with medical care. *Milbank Mem Fund Q Health Soc.* 1982;**60**:329-54.

120. Marquis MS, Davies AR, Ware JE Jr. Patient satisfaction and change in medical care provider: a longitudinal study. *Med Care.* 1983;**21**:821-9.

121. Wartman, SA, Morlock LL, Maltiz FE, Palm EA. Patient understanding and satisfaction as predictors of compliance. *Med Care.* 1983;**21**:886-91.

122. Patrick DL, Scrivens E, Charlton JR. Disability and patient satisfaction with medical care. *Med Care.* 1983;**21**:1062-75.

123. McAuliffe WE. Studies of process-outcome correlations in medical care evaluations: a critique. *Med Care.* 1978;**16**:907-30.

124. Ware JE Jr, Brook RH, Rogers WH, et al. *Health Outcomes for Adults in Prepaid and Fee-for-Service Systems of Care: Results from the Health Insurance Experiment.* Santa Monica, California: The RAND Corporation (R-3459-HHS), 1987.

125. Croog SH, Levine S, Testa MA, et al. The effects of antihypertensive therapy on the quality of life. *N Engl J Med.* 1986; **314**:1657-64.

126. Meenan RF, Anderson JJ, Kazis LE, et al. Outcome assessment in clinical trials: evidence for the sensitivity of a health status measure. *Arthritis Rheum.* 1984; **27**:1344-52.

127. Bergner M, Bobbitt RA, Carter WB, Gilson BS. The sickness impact profile: development and final revision of a health status measure. *Med Care.* 1981;**19**:787-805.

128. Jette AM. Functional capacity evaluation: an empirical approach. *Arch Phys Med Rehabil.* 1980;**61**:85-9.

129. Patrick DL, Bush JW, Chen MM. Methods for measuring levels of well-being for a health status index. *Health Serv Res.* 1973;**8**:228-45.

130. Reynolds WJ, Rushing WA, Miles DL. The validation of a functional status index. *J Health Soc Behav.* 1974;**15**:271-88.

131. Nelson E, Conger B, Douglass R, et al. Functional health status levels of primary care patients. *JAMA* 1983;**249**:3331-8.

132. Katz S, Ford AB, Moskowitz RW, et al. Studies of illness in the aged. *JAMA.* 1963;**185**:94-9.

133. Kaplan RM, Bush JW, Berry CC. Healthy status: types of validity and the index of well-being. *Health Serv Res.* 1976;**11**:478-507.

134. Berner M, Bobbitt RA, Pollard WE, Martin DP, Gilson BS. The sickness impact profile: validation of a health status measure. *Med Care.* 1976;**14**:57-67.

135. Hulka BS, Cassel JC. The AAFP-UNC study of the organization, utilization, and assessment of primary medical care. *Am J Public Health.* 1973;**63**:494-501.

136. NCHS: *Health* United States. Washington DC: U.S. Department of Health and Human Services; 1981.

137. Dupuy HJ. The psychological section of the current Health and Nutrition Examination Survey. In: *Proc Public Health Conf on Records and Statistics Meeting Jointly with the National Conference on Health Statistics.* Washington, DC: National Conf on Health Statistics; 1972.

138. Bradburn NM. *The Structure of Psychological Well-Being.* Chicago: Aldine Publishing Co.; 1969.

139. Dupuy, HJ. The Psychological General Well-being (PGWB) Index. In: Wenger NK, ed. *Assessment of Quality of Life in Clinical Trials of Cardiovascular Therapies.* New York: Le Jacq Publishing Co.; 1984:170-83.

140. Costello CG, Comrey AL. Scales for measuring depression and anxiety. *J Psychol.* 1967;**66**:303-13.

141. Veit CT, Ware JE Jr. The structure of psychological distress and well-being in general populations. *J Consult Clin Psychol.* 1983;**51**:730-42.

142. Donald CA, Ware JE Jr. The measurement of social support, In: Greenley JR, ed. *Research in Community Mental Health.* Greenwich, Connecticut: JAI Press, Inc.; 1984;325-70.

143. Hunt AM, McEwen J, McKenna SP, et al. The Nottingham Health Profile: subjective health status and medical consultations. *Soc Sci Med.* 1981; **15A**:-221-9.

144. Davies AR, Ware JE Jr. *Measuring Health Perceptions in the Health Insurance Experiment.* Santa Monica, California: The RAND Corporation (R-2711-HHS); 1981.

145. Ware JE Jr. Scales for measuring general health perceptions. *Health Serv Res.* 1976;**11**:396-415.

146. Daut RL, Cleeland CS, Flanery, RC. Development of the Wisconsin Brief Pain Questionnaire to assess pain in cancer and other diseases. *Pain.* 1983;**17**:197-210.

147. Tarlov AR, Ware JE Jr, Greenfield S, et al. The Medical Outcomes Study: a new paradigm for evaluating medical care. *JAMA.* 1989; In print.

148. Lurie N, Ward NB, Shapiro MF, Brook RH. Termination from Medi-Cal — does it affect health? *New Engl J Med.* 1984; **311**:480-4.

149. Ware JE Jr. Standards for validating health measures: definition and content. *J Chronic Dis.* 1987;**40**:473-80.

150. Sackett DL, Chambers LW, MacPherson AS, Goldsmith CH, Mcauley RG. The development and application of indices of health: general methods and a summary of results. *Am J Public Health.* 1977;**67**:423-8.

151. Jette AM. Health status indicators: their utility in chronic-disease evaluation research. *J Chronic Dis.* 1980;**33**:567-79.

152. Fowler FJ, Wennberg JE, Timothy RP, et al. Symptom status and quality of life following prostatectomy. *JAMA.* 1988;**259**:3018-22.

153. Jette AM, Davies AR, Cleary PD, et al. The functional status questionnaire: reliability and validity when used in primary care. *J Gen Intern Med.* 1986;**1**:143-9.

154. Spitzer WO, Dobson AJ, Hall J, et al. Measuring the quality of life of cancer patients: a concise QL-index for use by physicians. *J Chronic Dis.* 1981;**34**:587-97.

155. Zola IK. Studying the decision to see a doctor: review, critique corrective. *Adv Psychosom Med.* 1972;**8**:216-36.

156. Mayou R. Chest pain, angina pectoris and disability. *J Psychosom Res.* 1973; **17**:287-91.

157. Mechanic D. The experiences and reporting of common physical complaints. *J Health Soc Behav.* 1980;**21**:146-55.

158. Pennebaker JW, Skelton JA. Psychological parameters of physical symptoms. *Person Soc Psychol Bull.* 1978;**4**:524-30.

159. Torrance GW. Social preferences for health states: an empirical evaluation of three measurement techniques. *Socio-Econ Plan Sci.* 1976;**10**:129-36.

160. Patrick DL, Sittampalam Y, Somerville SM, Carter WB, Bergner M. A cross-cultural comparison of health status values. *Am J Public Health.* 1985;**75**:1402-7.

161. Rubenstein LB, Calkins DR, Fink A, et al. How to help your patients function better. *West J Med.* 1985;**143**:114-7.

162. Bargmann E, Grove C. *Surgery in Maryland Hospitals 1979 and 1980: Charges and Deaths.* Washington, DC: Public Citizen Health Research Group; 1982.

163. U.S. Department of Health and Human Services, Health Care Financing Administration, HHS News, press release and untitled questions and answers accompanying *Medicare Hospital Mortality Information 1986.* Washington, DC: U.S. Government Printing Office; December 17, 1987.

164. Pennsylvania plans to release doctor and hospital outcome data. *Med World News.* 1987;**28**(23):8-9.

165. Bennett D, Campbell K. Most consumers show little concern in selecting health-services providers. *Marketing News.* August 15, 1986; 14.

166. Greenfield S, Aronow HU, Elashoff RM, Watanabe D. Flaws in mortality data: the hazards of ignoring comorbid disease. *JAMA.* 1988;**260**:2253-5.

167. Andrews LB. Informed consent statutes and the decision-making process. *J Legal Med.* 1984;**5**:163-217.

168. Kaufmann CL. Informed consent and patient decision making: two decades of research. *Soc Sci Med.* 1983;**17**:1657-64.

169. The President's Commission for the Study of Ethical Problems in Medicine and Biomedical and Behavioral Research. *Making Health Care Decisions. The Ethical and Legal Implications of Informed Consent in the Patient-Practitioner Relationship.* Volumes I-

III. Washington DC: U.S. Government Printing Office; 1982.

170. Thompson. Psychological issues in informed consent. *President's Commission for the Study of Ethical Problems in Medicine and Biomedical and Behavioral Research Making Health Care Decisions: The Ethical and Legal Implications of Informed Consent in the Patient-Practitioner Relationship.* Volume 3. U.S. Government Printing Office; 1982; 113.

171. Janis IL, Mann LI. *Decision-Making: A Psychological Analysis of Conflict, Choice and Commitment.* New York: Free Press; 1977.

172. Hogarth RM. *Judgement and Choice: The Psychology of Decision.* Chichester: Wiley; 1980.

173. Taylor SE. Hospital patient behavior: reactance, helplessness or control. *J Soc Issues.* 1979;**35**:156-84.

174. Barofsky I Compliance, adherence, and the therapeutic alliance: steps in the development of self-care. *Soc Sci Med.* 1978;**12**:369-76.

175. Tagliacozzo DL, Mauksch HO. The patient's view of the patient's role. In: Jaco EG, ed. *Patients, Physicians and Illness.* 2nd ed. New York: Free Press; 1972.

176. Lewis CE, Lewis MA, Lorimer AA, Palmer BB. Child-initiated Care: the use of school nursing services by children in an "adult-free" system. *Pediatrics* 1977;**60**:499-507.

177. Lewis CE, Lewis MA, Ifekwunigue M. Informed consent by children and participation in an influenza vaccine trial. *Am J Public Health.* 1978;**68**:1079-82.

178. Lewis CE, Lewis MA. Children's Health-related Decision-making. *Health Ed Quarterly.* 1982;**9**:225-37.

179. Lewis CE, Rachelefsky G, Lewis MA, de la Sota A, Kaplan M. A randomized trial of A.C.T. (asthma care training) for kids. *Pediatrics.* 1984;**74**:478-86.

180. Lewis C, Pantell RH, Kieckhefer GM. Assessment of childrens' health status: field test of new approaches. *Med Care.* 1989; In press.

181. Lewis CE, Lewis MA. A twelve-year follow-up of participants in a child-initiated care system. *Pediatrics.* 1989; In Press.

182. Wu WC, Pearlman RA. Consent in medical decision making: the role of communication. *J Gen Intern Med.* 1988;**3**:9-14.

183. Howard JM, DeMets D. How informed is informed consent? The BHAT experience. *Controlled Clin Trials.* 1981;**2**:287-303.

184. Louis Harris and Associates. Views of informed consent and decision-making: parallel, surveys of physicians and the public. In: *The President's Commission for the Study of Ethical Problems in Medicine.* Washington, DC: U.S. Government Printing Office; 1982: 113.

185. Cassileth BR, Zupkis RV, Sutton-Smith K, March V. Informed consent — why are its goals imperfectly realized? *N Engl J Med.* 1980;**302**:896-900.

186. Roter D. Patient participation in patient-provider interactions: the effects of patient question-asking on the quality of interactions, satisfaction and compliance. *Health Ed Monographs.* 1977;**5**:281-314.

187. Wright P. The harassed decision-maker: time pressures, distractions and the use of evidence. *J Applied Psych* 1974; **59**:555-61.

188. Fischoff B. Knowing what you want: measuring labile values. In: Wallsten TS, ed. *Cognitive Processes in Choice and Decision Behavior.* Hillsdale, New Jersey: Erlbaum; 1980.

189. Barbour GL, Blumenkrantz MJ. Videotape aids informed consent decision. *JAMA.* 1978;**240**:2741-2.

190. Tversky A. Kahneman D. Judgement under uncertainty: heuristics and biases. *Science.* 1974;**185**:1124-31.

191. Tversky A, Kahneman D. Causal schemas in judgments under uncertainty. In: Fishbeir M, ed. *Progression in Social Psychology, I.* Hillsdale, New Jersey: Erlbaum; 1980:49-72.

192. Nisbett RE, Ross R. *Human Inference: Strategies and Shortcomings of Social Judgment.* Englewood Cliffs, New Jersey: Prentice-Hall; 1980.

193. Morrow G, Gootnick J, Schmale A. A simple technique for increasing cancer patients' knowledge of informed consent of treatment. *Cancer.* 1978;**42**:793-9.

194. Johnson JE, Leventhal H. Effects of accurate expectations and behavioral instructions on reactions during a noxious medical examination. *J Pers Soc Psych.* 1974;**29**:710-8.

195. Egbert LD, Battit GE, Welch CE, et al. Reduction of post-operative pain by encouragement and instruction of patients. *New Engl J. Med.* 1964;**270**:825-7.

196. Wernick RL, Jaremko ME, Taylor PW. Pain management in severely burned adults: a test of stress innoculation. *J Behav Med.* 1981;**4**:103-9.

197. Mills RT, Kantz DS. Information, choice, and reactions to stress: a field experiment in a blood bank with laboratory analogue. *J Pers Soc Psychol.* 1979;**37**:608-20.

198. Andrew JM. Recovery from surgery, with and without preparatory instruction, for three coping styles. *J Pers Soc Psychol.* 1970;**15**:223-6.

199. Vernon DT, Bigelow, DA. Effect of information about a potentially stressful situation on responses to stress impact. *J Pers Soc Psychol.* 1974;**29**:50-9.

200. Wilson JF. Behavioral preparation for surgery: benefit or harm. *J Behav Med.* 1981;**4**:79-102.

201. Langer EJ, Rodin J. The effects of choice and enhanced personal responsibilities for the aged: a field experiment in an institutional setting. *J Pers Soc Psychol.* 1976;**34**:191-8.

202. Rodin J, Langer EJ. Long-term effect of a control-relevant intervention with the institutionalized aged. *J Pers Soc Psychol.* 1977;**35**:897-902.

203. Pauker SG, McNeil BJ. Impact of patient preferences on the selection of therapy. *J Chronic Dis.* 1981;**34**:77-86.

204. McNeil BJ, Pauker SG, Fox HC Jr, Tversky A. On the elicitation of preferences for alternative therapies. *N Engl J Med.* 1982;**306**:1259-62.

205. McNeil BJ, Pauker SG. The patients' role in assessing the value of diagnostic tests. *Radiology.* 1979;**132**:605-10.

206. Tversky A, Kahneman D. The framing of decisions and the psychology of choice. *Science.* 1981;**211**:453-8.

207. Kahneman D, Tversky A. Prospect theory: an analysis of decision under risk. *Econometrica.* 1981;**47**:263-91.

208. Kaplan SH, Greenfield S, Ware JE Jr. Impact of the doctor-patient relationship on the outcomes of chronic disease. In: Stewart M. Boter D, eds. *Communicating with Patients in Medical Practice.* Beverly Hills, California: Sage Publications; In press.

209. Schwartz CG, Kahne MJ. Medical help as negotiated achievement. *Psychiatry.* 1983;**46**:333-50.

COMMENTARY

Kaplan and Ware challenge one of the basic tenets of modern medicine — care is too technical and scientifically based to be evaluated by patients. They show, rather convincingly, that the evidence favors patients' abilities to judge not only the interpersonal skills of physicians (what used to be called bedside manner) but their technical prowess as well. Consumers of health care services have become more discerning shoppers; patients are demanding a more active decision-making role in their care. Clinicians ought to pay attention to these demands and to the skills patients demonstrate by evaluating what physicians do.

Not surprisingly, Kaplan and Ware point out that groups such as the American Board of Internal Medicine (ABIM) are studying the feasibility of using patients' evaluations of the interpersonal skills of residents as a potential element of the certification process. At the Harvard Community Health Plan in Boston, an academically oriented non-profit HMO, enrollees are being asked about their criteria for judging the quality of one hospital compared with another within the plan's referral network.

Some readers may register discomfort at the thought of patients evaluating the process of health care delivery. Yet, as the authors point out, only the patients can accurately report the impact of disease on their daily lives. Interestingly, the information on patients' functional status, their ability to perform usual daily activities, is not routinely gathered in traditional sites such as the medical record or insurance claims forms.

Kaplan and Ware argue that the functional status assessment, done largely by patients themselves, will become an important component of burgeoning quality assurance systems. That is, if patients can accurately assess how they are doing, this information can be codified and compared to some standardized data set. Once codified and standardized, the functional assessment ratings will be used to compare individual physicians and render a performance score based on the levels of reported functional status among their patients.

Related questions include, "When should physicians first be taught how to improve their interpersonal skills and consequently patient evaluations?" Groups such as the Society for General Internal Medicine (SGIM) have several major educational efforts and task forces aimed at improving physician-patient communications. Some observers (1) have called for a new contractual approach to the traditional physician-patient relationship. Others (2) have warned of a compensatory alliance forming with non-ill family members when there is a dysfunctional physician-patient relationship. It remains to be seen how these concepts will alter Kaplan' and Ware's analysis. Can dysfunctional physician-patient relationships still produce fair and accurate assessments of a physician's skill?

Kaplan and Ware mention the National Study of Medical Outcomes several times. As of this writing, only preliminary (and nonpublished) results are available. Perhaps with a national data set and simplified, validated, reporting methods, one can envision future office practice records to routinely include a post-visit evaluation form alongside the problem list and history. (The Editors)

References

1. Quill TE. Partnerships in patient care: a contractual approach. *Ann Intern Med.* 1983;**98**: 228-34.
2. Hahn SR, Feiner JS, Bellin EH. The doctor-patient-family relationship: a compensatory alliance. *Ann Inter Med.* 1988;**10**:884-9.

Chapter 3

Measuring the Severity of Illness and Case Mix

LISA I. IEZZONI, MD

INTRODUCTION

A resurgence of competition in many economic spheres, including the health care sector, has occurred in the 1980s. Many recent changes intended to contain the escalating costs of health care are based on increasing competition. However, information, which is crucial to competition, is not readily available in the health care industry. Unlike industries that clearly specify the characteristics and quality of their products, the health care industry generally supplies few clues about the relative merits of providers. To improve health care efficiency through competition, this situation must change (1).

What types of information about quality will fuel competition in the health care sector? Answers are coming from the most unlikely sources. In several states and regions, business communities, frustrated by tremendous growth in employee health benefit costs, are asking for more information concerning patients and their outcomes than that available through computerized billing records (2,3). One common refrain demands information concerning "severity of illness," to be used in computing the so-called "algebra of effectiveness" — the concept that patient outcome is a complex function not only of the services provided and other factors such as random events, but also of the patient's clinical attributes, including severity of illness (Figure 1).

Spurred by these requests, an entire industry has arisen to define and measure the severity of illness of hospitalized patients (Table 1). The common denominator is the transformation of from several to several hundred bits of clinical information into a summary score indicating "severity." But this industry also is competitive — information is needed to choose among vendors. However, its newness prompts more fundamental questions. What is meant by "severity of illness?" How is this information used to assess the quality of hospital care? Is this an appropriate way to judge the competence of health care providers?

Severity measurement systems hold important implications for physicians. At a minimum, they could standardize the content, structure, and terminology of the inpatient medical record. This record could become the main source of information for judging provider capabilities. At the outside, they could affect the choice and timing of diagnostic and therapeutic interventions. This chapter reviews aspects of severity measurement that are particularly relevant to physicians. The first section offers a historical perspective, in the belief that it is both comforting and instructive to know that some of the battles that today seem so pressing have been fought before. The second section

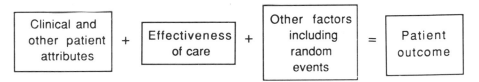

Figure 1. The "algebra of effectiveness," a schematic representation of the factors affecting patient outcome. Actual relationships are probably very complex, and may differ by type of outcome, diagnosis, or condition. Severity of illness information can appear on both sides of the equation as follows: Severity is part of the clinical and other patient attributes that contribute to patient outcome; and severity can define patient outcome, for example severity of illness on discharge from the hospital.

describes the policy context that has fostered the emergence of the severity measurement industry. The third section outlines the issues involved in defining severity; the fourth section outlines the role of severity information in quality assessment; and the fifth section introduces five of the leading severity measurement systems. The chapter concludes by suggesting the implications for physicians and medical practice.

HISTORICAL PERSPECTIVE

Perhaps the earliest severity of illness information was noted by Hippocrates, born around 460 B.C. Hippocrates believed in the prompt recording of clinical observations to avoid the inaccuracies inherent in memory (4). He did not list diagnoses, but focused on symptoms and syndromes from which he derived prognoses. The prognostic "epigrams" of Hippocrates describe the features of severely ill patients. For example, "It is a bad sign in all cases, when during high fever, the thirst subsides without obvious reason"; and "If the patients get startled when you touch them, they are in serious condition" (5).

Between the time of Hippocrates and the modern era, clinical information on individual patients was recorded fitfully, if at all. In the early 19th century, American hospitals began keeping records in bound volumes, organized chronologically by admissions (not by patients). Notations emphasized symptoms as described by the patient, with little information on physical findings, treatment, or diagnostic speculation (6). For example, a complete

TABLE 1. Characteristics of Five "Severity" Measurement Systems

Severity Measure	Basis of Severity Construct	Uses Diagnostic Framework	Data Requirements	Unit of Classification	Classification System
Acute Physiology and Chronic Health Evaluation (APACHE II)	Imminent risk of death	No	Medical record	Patient	Score from 0 to 71
Computerized Severity Index	Treatment difficulty	Yes	Medical record	Disease and patient	Score from 0 to 4
Disease Staging: Clinical Criteria Version	Risk of death or impairment	Yes	Medical record	Disease	Stage from 1 to 4 with substages
Disease Staging: Q-Scale	Resource use	No; variants consider patient DRG	Discharge abstract	Patient	Percentage compared with an average of 100
MedisGroups	Imminent risk of organ failure	No	Medical record	Patient	Score from 0 to 4
Patient Management Categories	Resource use	Yes; also considers major surgery	Discharge abstract	Disease and patient	Cost-based relative weight compared with an average of 1.0

note on a patient from the August 18, 1824, Massachusetts General Hospital records stated, "Skin nearly natural, tongue rather dry, with moist red edges. Countenance good. Took hasty pudding at 10 a.m." (7). Even in the late 19th century, the Mayo brothers in Rochester, Minnesota, generally failed to record results of physical examinations, diagnoses, or treatments; in most cases, their note contained only the date, the patient's age, residence, and phrases such as "gas on the stomach and poor sleep" and "night terrors — wetting bed" (8). The unit medical record, which accumulates all information on a patient in a single place, was not fully implemented until 1916, at the Presbyterian Hospital in New York (4).

In 1917 The American College of Surgeons Conference on Hospital Standardization expounded, "If good records are kept, it is almost certain that good work will be done" (9). The Conference called the medical record "valueless" at 75% of hospitals, intimating that the lack of diagnostic information was an intentional "cover up" of the surgeon's inability to make a diagnosis. Ernest Amory Codman, one of the founders of the College, suggested a new and heretical use for the medical record: "Our record system should enable us to fix responsibility... for the success or failure of each case treated" (10). Today, much of the use of severity data and other medical record information for quality assessment is based on Codman's ideas.

Codman and the "End Result Idea"

A self-described "eccentric" practicing surgery at the Massachusetts General Hospital in the early 1900s, Codman developed the "end result idea... which was merely the common-sense notion that every hospital should follow *every* patient it treats, long enough to determine whether or not the treatment has been successful, and then to inquire 'if not, why not' with a view to preventing similar failures in the future" (11). He believed that to improve, hospitals "must compare their results with those of other hospitals" and "must welcome publicity not only for their successes, but for their errors," and he noted that "such opinions will not be eccentric a few years hence" (12). In assessing these end results, Codman acknowledged the importance of adjusting for patient risk of bad outcomes. He observed (13):

> For the man who practices surgery, there are two kinds of mortality — chance and intentional.
> Chance mortality is the kind which occurs unexpectedly, and which no amount of foresight can prevent. It is caused by unanticipated Calamities or Catastrophes. Death from pulmonary embolism is a good example.... Is it not possible to determine what this percentage of danger is, just as easily as it is to compute fire risk?...
> Intentional mortality is incurred by the chief surgeon when he attempts cases in which the condition is acknowledged to be grave. It is speculative — like gambling against known chances in a game in which skill, judgment, and luck all count.

Protesting the seniority system of promotion, Codman resigned from the Massachusetts General Hospital in 1914 to start his own small, surgical hospital. He periodically published an introspective series of its end results, grouping the failures under such headings as "errors due to lack of technical knowledge or skill," "errors possibly due to lack of judgment," "errors due to incorrect diagnosis," and "cases in which the nature and extent of the disease was the main cause of failure" (12). Codman was particularly concerned about the handling of this last class of failure, and he asked (12):

> Shall I say in the future?:
> 1. You are too bad a risk; go to a first-class surgeon.
> 2. You are a bad risk; I must double my usual fee.
> 3. You are a bad risk; you need not pay unless you live.
> All are logical. I like the last best.

Codman Hospital was not a financial success.

Statistics and Standardization

In the late 1800s hospitals began to publish statistics, such as number and types of cases treated and number of deaths. An original intent of these statistics was to prove that charitable contributions were not misappropriated (13). But the diverse content, structure, and terminology of case records hampered production of these statistics. Campaigns for standardization of the medical record were mobilized on two fronts, one for terminology and another for structure.

The desire for standardized nomenclature for causes of death was first voiced at the First Statistical Congress in Brussels in 1853 (14), and the first international classification was adopted in Paris in 1855. Americans did not embrace this early version of what has become the *International Classification of Diseases*. Bellevue Hospital and the American Medical Association had each developed diagnostic lexicons, and the Massachusetts General Hospital had its own classification system (15). In 1911 the American Medical Association recommended adoption of the *International List of Causes of Death*. The accompanying American manual indicated "undesirable" terms that should be avoided, for example, the term ". . . 'heart failure' is a recognized synonym, even among the laity, for ignorance of the cause of death on the part of the physician" (14).

The movement for standardization of medical records was spearheaded by the American College of Surgeons and individuals such as Raymond Pearl, the statistician to The Johns Hopkins Hospital. Pearl suggested standardized, printed history forms, with information in a format that could be readily punched onto cards for quick analysis (13). The College recommended that all records be preceded by a summary, indicating chief complaint, initial diagnosis, operation, final diagnosis, and complications, and in 1918 they stated, "Consistent and fearless review of case records by the hospital staff... is a just and effective means to deal with incompetent medical and surgical work in a hospital. Facts are not debatable..." (16). Opponents of the standardization movement argued that it would hinder the individual physician's expression (6).

Thus, debates in the early 20th century foreshadowed some of the controversies of today. Three such controversies are using the medical record to assess quality of care, standardizing the information in that record, and suggesting that hospitals compare their performance to that of their peers. Perhaps the most prescient idea was voiced by Codman — that hospitals judge their efficiency by their therapeutic successes, *appropriately adjusted for patient risk*. More than 70 years ago, the American College of Surgeons warned, "... all hospitals are accountable to the public for their degree of success... If the initiative is not taken by the medical profession, it will be taken by the lay public" (16). Today this admonition sounds curiously familiar.

POLICY CONTEXT

Reimbursement and Case Mix

Interest in severity of illness and cross-hospital comparisons arose after changes in hospital reimbursement. These changes were first seen with adoption of prospective payment, first for all payers in New Jersey and then nationally by Medicare in 1983. This reimbursement method redefined the hospital product from a series of services compensated separately, to the case as designated by the patient's Diagnosis Related Group (DRG). This tactic focused on the mix of services required for effective care of the hospital's new "product" or case type, and thus improved not only the efficiency of hospital care but also its quality (17).

Although DRGs originated over a decade earlier through efforts at Yale University to develop length-of-stay norms for utilization review, they received renewed attention with the change in payment policy. Developers of DRGs pursued several goals, including creating patient classes "interpretable medically" and based on variables commonly available on hospital abstracts (18). This latter goal led to the exclusive use of discharge abstract data to define more than 470 medical and surgical case types, relying on *International Classification of Diseases, Ninth Revision, Clinical Modification (ICD-9-CM)* diagnostic and surgical codes, age, and discharge status (in a limited number of classes). Diagnostic codes are viewed sequentially with the first code considered the "principal diagnosis" (reason for admission) and dictating medical DRG assignment in most cases. Additional codes are scanned for qualifying complications or comorbidities that define the more complex DRGs Although DRG categories were initially derived clinically, further empirical refinements used a database of over 1.5 million discharges and statistical techniques to group cases with similar lengths of stay.

The DRGs classification was immediately controversial, with critics claiming that DRGs are not sensitive to severity of illness. In his 1982 report (19) proposing the Medicare prospective payment system, Secretary of Health and Human Services Richard S. Schweiker acknowledged this dispute, but argued:

> The DRGs cover a wide range, from very expensive cases (e.g., heart transplant, kidney transplant, coronary bypass, and severe burn) to very inexpensive kinds of cases. Thus, the DRGs account for the major variations in severity of illness across patients.... Severity within DRGs is primarily a concern if certain hospitals tend to have more severe cases within DRGs compared to other hospitals, and if severity is positively associated with costs...
>
> No widely applicable method currently exists to make valid severity distinctions... DRGs have the distinct advantage of being based on available data. Nevertheless, severity is one dimension that may warrant further study.

As a partial response to the severity question, special reimbursement provisions were adopted, such as outlier payments for cases with very long stays or extraordinarily high costs, and the indirect teaching hospital adjustment, which provides extra payment to hospitals using a formula based on the number of resident physicians and hospital size.

The severity of illness controversy involved two issues. The first involved defining the data required to draw severity distinctions. Clinicians involved in DRG development, among others, argued that *ICD-9-CM* is unable to delineate severity differences (20-23). Others countered that much of the difficulty stemmed from the way *ICD-9-CM* had been used in DRG classification (24-26). Even those who contended that *ICD-9-CM* was inadequate to the task of severity adjustment urged caution in requiring additional data elements (such as clinical information from the medical record) for payment classification (22,23).

The second issue involved the question of whether severely ill patients are more expensive to treat appropriately. An empirical answer to this question has not been found. Various studies using severity measures have had conflicting results (27,28). A report to Congress issued by the Health Care Financing Administration in the spring of 1988 concluded, "The Department does not believe that any system to measure clinical severity of illness is currently an administratively feasible major improvement to or substitute for DRGs" (29). However, Congress took the severity controversy seriously. In P.L. 99-509 Congress mandated that by October 1988 the Secretary of Health and Human Services develop a proposal "to account for variations in severity of illness and case complexity which are not adequately accounted for by the current classification and payment system." The Secretary of Health and Human Services is likely to be drawing from ongoing, government-sponsored research using computerized discharge abstract data, such as a Yale University project, to refine the DRG complication and comorbidity classification. Thus, severity of illness remains a focal point of hospital reimbursement policy debates.

Focus on Quality

The prospective payment system aimed to promote efficient, good-quality care and contain escalating costs. When the system was first used in New Jersey, its proponents saw it as a program mainly to enhance the quality of hospital care. Others, given the monetary incentives of the system, were concerned that hospitals would have to cut services to profit under case-based payment. Those concerned about compromised quality questioned the location of the boundary between excessive services (which could be cut without fear) and necessary services.

These and other efforts at cost control heightened interest in assessing the quality of hospital care. Groups from the American Association of Retired Persons to the business community began showing interest in new directions. As Vladeck (30) observed:

> In keeping with contemporary mores, recent concerns with the quality of health services have focused largely on questions of measurement, comparison, public disclosure, and incentives and disincentives. An era that glorifies markets, deregulation, and the mythology of consumer sovereignty inclines the debate in that direction.

A new emphasis on competition was found in health care — quality and efficiency would reap their own pecuniary reward. A chief architect of this strategy, Walter McClure, touted the "buy right" principle: "Purchasers must reward efficient, high-quality providers with patients" (31). Under his program, quality is equated with patient satisfaction, effectiveness, and innovation. Medicare officials suggested that the third decade of their program adopt "value" as its by-word, stating that the government aims to "buy right" not "buy cheap" (32). However, the question of how to identify high-quality, efficient health care providers remains.

As with Codman's "end result idea," this era accepts patient outcome as a meaningful way to judge provider quality or the effectiveness of care. This perspective brought severity of illness to the forefront of the issue: One cannot adequately evaluate outcomes without first adjusting for patient risk; this requires knowledge of patient severity. The pitfalls in producing outcome data without adequate severity adjustment were exemplified by the first release of hospital mortality statistics by the federal government in March 1986. A front-page article in the *New York Times* proclaimed that the hospital that had the most egregious mortality experience according to the governmental model was a hospice in Las Vegas caring for terminally ill patients (33)!

Several regional and statewide programs have focused on collecting severity of illness information. McClure's "buy right" experiment relies on severity data generated through a commercial system, MedisGroups, which abstracts clinical variables from the medical record. According to McClure, "... there is no other way than to go in and abstract the clinical findings from the chart. Let's stop fooling ourselves that we can compare patient severity by claims" (that is, by discharge abstract data) (31).

Spurred by its business community, Pennsylvania adopted Act 89 in 1986. This law encourages the provision of "quality, cost-effective" health care services by providing information to consumers on the quality and cost of different providers. The law empowered a Health Care Cost Containment Council to collect and disseminate comparative "quality" data such as risk-adjusted outcomes. Section 3 of Act 89 defined severity as, "in any patient, the measurable degree of the potential for failure of one or more vital organs." Hence, Pennsylvania now requires all hospitals to collect information using the MedisGroups severity assessment system. It is not yet clear exactly how the data derived through MedisGroups severity reviews will be analyzed and published by the Health Care Cost Containment Council.

As a consequence of Regulation 87-3 adopted in January 1988, Colorado is developing its own "Uniform Clinical Data Set," which will be used to assess patient condition on admission ("severity") and at discharge ("outcome"). This project was scheduled to begin in 1989. Initial data collection will probably focus on a subset of conditions, requiring a broad range of clinical data, including procedural findings, laboratory results, and in-hospital drug use. Other states, including Iowa, Massachusetts, Ohio, and Washington, are considering following suit with Pennsylvania and Colorado, although none has specified an approach toward collection of severity of illness data.

In Rochester, New York, one experiment underway redistributes hospital payments to reward providers rendering higher quality care. Quality is assessed using MedisGroups severity measurements on admission and later in the hospital stay, to suggest the trajectory of the in-hospital course. The state's DRG payment will also be refined to reflect admission severity distinctions.

Thus, a series of initiatives has converged in an interest in severity measurement, both for hospital payment and for quality assessment. Despite the fervor of this interest, demanding questions remain unanswered. What is meant by "severity of illness?" How is severity information used to judge quality of hospital care? Is any particular severity measure better than another? These questions are explored below.

DEFINITION OF SEVERITY

Despite the growing interest in severity measurement, no accepted definition of severity of illness exists. As Gertman and Lowenstein (23) observed, " 'Severity' is what sociologists term a 'folk wisdom' word like 'satisfaction' or 'happiness,' operationally indefinable in a way that is perfectly acceptable to all parties." However, the potential applications and utility of a severity of illness measure arise from its definition of severity (34).

Not only do physicians have different definitions of severity, but other health care professionals do as well. Smits and colleagues (22) noted that physicians generally focus on the impact of a particular disease on the physiologic integrity of the patient, asking such questions as is a patient more likely to die, become disabled, or experience long-run sequelae than other patients. However, physicians disagree about whether it is important to place severity distinctions in a diagnostic structure, and whether severity should be distinguished by the use of various procedures, such as surgery or intensive care unit (ICU) monitoring. Psychiatrists concentrate more on cognitive dysfunctions, which may or may not include physiologic disturbances. Nurses may consider the physiologic perspective of physicians, while adding psychological and dependency attributes of the patient. Physical and occupational therapists target the functional capabilities of patients and their ability to perform the daily activities of living independently. Health care managers emphasize resource needs, implicitly correlating higher severity with higher "intensity" or costs.

Stein and associates (35) offered an inclusive framework for grading severity, consisting of three categories. The first, physiologic or morphologic severity, relates to the extent of biologic derangements or abnormalities that can be quantified by laboratory tests, pathologic reports, or other scientific means. Environmental influences, such as treatment, can affect this type of severity. The second, functional severity, involves the ability of the individual to conduct daily activities. This approach is independent of specific diagnoses and views the patient as a whole. The third category, burden of illness, concerns the impact of the condition on the family or on society. "Severe" illness generates large expenses, interferes with family function, or disrupts society.

Physiologic severity and financial burden are not always directly related: Higher severity does not always create greater costs. Very ill patients may be treated inexpensively for several reasons (22). Patients with severe physiologic or biochemical disorders often present significant surgical or procedural risks, and are therefore treated with less expensive, conservative approaches. Severely affected patients may be easier to diagnose, requiring fewer expensive tests. Terminally ill patients may choose not to be resuscitated or treated in expensive ICUs, thus lowering potential costs of treatment.

Regardless of one's perspective, a timeframe is required — an "episode of illness" over which severity is assessed. For example, if death is the endpoint, when should it occur? Physicians commonly adopt a long time horizon in judging severity. For instance, many staging systems used by oncologists to indicate the extent or severity of malignancy focus on distant prognosis, such as 5-year survival or recurrence risk. Physicians view higher blood pressures as more severe than lower pressures, because of the risk for catastrophic vascular or cardiac events in the near or distant future. In the ICU or trauma center, the timeframe may be immediate, involving the chance of surviving to the next day or week. The definition of episode of illness is especially important in the reimbursement context. Physiologically compromising, chronic diseases that require periodic admissions, such as congestive heart failure or sickle cell anemia, may be costly in the long run, whereas individual hospitalizations are relatively inexpensive.

Finally, in establishing a definition of severity, it is impossible to escape the practical bonds of data requirements. Information is necessary to draw severity distinctions; the type and nature of information used bounds the scope of such distinctions. But information is expensive, and trade-offs are inevitable. For example, will the measure rely exclusively on required discharge abstract data, such as age, sex, *ICD-9-CM* diagnostic and procedural codes, and discharge status, or will additional information be taken from the medical record? Obviously, the latter approach could permit more precise severity distinctions, but at a much higher cost. Such precision may not be as important for some applications as for others. Obtaining information from the inpatient medical record ties the severity assessment to a single admission, or to a series of admissions at a given hospital. Information drawn from various sources is necessary to extend the timeframe of the severity assessment.

In summary, examining patient severity is an important part of clinical research, and it guides many therapeutic decisions. However, in the policy arena, "severity of illness" has various meanings. Part of the difficulty in health policy discussions is that those debating the issue may be approaching it from different perspectives. Those supporting the use of severity of illness assessments for hospital payment may have a different conceptual framework than those advocating its use for quality assessment. For the former, severity is implicitly correlated with cost, and the episode of illness is the unit of payment (for example, the acute care admission for DRG-based reimbursement, a year of care for the health maintenance organization).

Advocates of severity measures as adjuncts to quality assessment generally adopt a physician's perspective on acute illness — acute, physiologic disorders that portend imminent risk of a poor clinical outcome such as in-hospital death or organ failure — not chronic conditions or functional or psychosocial impairments. The episode of illness is very short — the hospitalization or the 30 days after admission. Thus, several attributes that characterize a global assessment of the patient and could foreshadow poor outcome are absent. In discussing use of a severity measure for any purpose, the definition of severity must be clearly stated to understand both its scope and limitations, and its appropriateness for the intended goal.

SEVERITY OF ILLNESS MEASURES AND QUALITY ASSESSMENT

Severity of illness data have two major uses in hospital quality assessment. The first is to adjust for the risk of poor outcomes; the second is to generate outcome information. Both focus on judging the outcome of care and are intended for application as a screening tool across large numbers of cases.

Risk Adjustment

A conceptually appealing use for severity measurement is to adjust for the risk for undesirable outcomes. Poor outcomes in a given population (such as a hospital's or physician's caseload), or those not predicted after statistical adjustment for severity, could indicate poor quality of care (36,37). One such outcome is death; adjustments should be made based on the truism that more severely ill patients are more likely to die than those less affected. This use of severity adjustment parallels Codman's concept of "intentional mortality" — that certain grave illnesses present known and potentially quantifiable risks for death during surgery. The use of severity-adjusted mortality information to judge hospital quality is discussed further in Chapter 4. Risk adjustment can also apply to other adverse outcomes, such as surgical, procedural, or other therapeutic complications, unexpected admissions after outpatient surgery, nosocomial infections, readmission to the hospital shortly after discharge, and increased disability at discharge.

This use of severity information for risk adjustment generally relies exclusively on patient condition on admission to the hospital or during the initial contact with the provider. The purpose is to establish risk before therapeutic intervention, so as not to confound the risk assessment with iatrogenic mishaps that may arise from poor quality care. "Admission" severity therefore represents the clinical status of the patient before care; thus, eventual outcomes presumably stem from the combined influences of physiologic status (as shown by admission severity), other patient and random factors that may not be covered by the severity measure, and therapeutic efficacy. Putting aside patient and random factors, controlling for admission severity should help in the assessment of therapeutic efficacy when untoward outcomes occur.

By definition this approach must delineate the time of "admission" to distinguish admission severity findings from those occurring later, possibly due to poor quality care. One possibility is to record the first measurements on admission, a tactic that runs the risk of being influenced by possibly random differences in patient behavior (for example, a temperature may be artificially lower because the patient took aspirin before coming to the hospital). Another difficulty is that a full evaluation or complement of tests may not be done immediately on admission. Some measures have dealt with this by designating the first two days as the admission period and collecting the worst values from this timeframe. But this strategy may not work for conditions such as acute myocardial infarction or pulmonary edema in which outcome may be closely linked to immediate treatment.

A variant of the risk adjustment approach uses admission severity to examine the appropriateness of acute care hospitalization and the timeliness of admission. This approach presumes that patients at low severity are also at low risk, and may not need hospitalization. A corollary assumes that some cases of high severity at admission suggest substandard outpatient care or delays in diagnosis and appropriate treatment. Examples include ruptured appendix, perforated peptic ulcer, diabetic ketoacidosis, and status asthmaticus. These admission severity findings could flag quality shortfalls before admission.

Severity as an Outcome Measure

The second role for severity information in quality assessment is as a measure of outcome itself, again across large numbers of cases. Two such uses have generated the greatest interest. The first involves examining severity at discharge from the hospital. Proponents of this approach suggest that severity at discharge may be a sensitive measure of therapeutic efficacy. They suggest that this tactic identifies not only cases in which therapy was not effective, but also instances of premature discharge from the hospital. A major question about this strategy is whether the acute, physiologic model on which most severity measures are based adequately measures the chronic impairments, functional limitations, and dependencies pertinent to the period immediately before and after most acute care discharges.

The second method transforms severity of illness information into outcome data using the "clinical trajectory." This strategy involves examining severity at two points in time — for example, on admission and later during hospitalization — and looking at the trajectory of change in severity. Did the patient worsen, improve, or stay the same?

In 1975 Gonnella and Goran (38) advised comparing severity on admission and at discharge, saying this tactic "allows analysis of the contribution physician services make to any change in the stage of the clinical problem." More recent supporters of this approach suggest comparing severity on admission with a "maximum" or "peak" severity, the nadir of clinical status observed during hospitalization. In many cases "maximum" severity is synonymous with the admission rating, but proponents believe that this strategy is more useful than the focus on discharge because of the generally low severity at most discharges. Data from the Graduate Medical Education Study (39) launched in 1980 support the potential utility of this approach.

"Clinical trajectory" data could be aggregated across cases to permit cross-provider comparisons. For example, holding admission severity constant, the percent of patients worsening after admission could be contrasted across physicians or hospitals. Providers with a higher number of worsening trajectories presumably are more likely to have rendered substandard care. Statistical norms for different conditions could indicate standards for fractions of cases after the improvement trajectory.

Use as Screening Tools

Both approaches use severity-based data across large numbers of cases to highlight potential problems. The severity findings serve only as screening tools, flagging case types or patterns possibly resulting from faulty care. Neither approach is powerful or refined enough to judge specific cases. Part of the imprecision stems from the neglected "other patient factors" alluded to above — no severity measure accounts for all clinical characteristics associated with or indicating patient outcome. Codman's "chance" or random occurrences over which the provider has no control also intervene. A final factor involves the continuing perplexities of human biology and the limitations of medical therapeutics. Patients do not always respond predictably to even the highest quality of clinical intervention.

Given these limitations, the utility of severity-based information should be judged by the standards applied to other screening tools. What are the sensitivity, specificity, and predictive values of these strategies for identifying substandard care? These questions cannot yet be answered. Although the conceptual bases of these uses of severity-based measures for quality assessment seem reasonable, they need to be tested. One hurdle is the specification of the "gold standard" for evaluating quality of care in individual cases. Once the screening tool has identified potential instances of faulty care, a gold standard is required to pass final judgment on specific cases. Decades of study have not yet produced widely accepted standards for the practice of medicine in the United States.

Although several programs are ready to produce severity of illness information, it is not yet clear how valuable that information will be in assessing hospital quality of care. Because they seem to distinguish severity differences among patients, these data will receive clinical credibility never accorded the DRGs. Danger exists that these untested but clinically attractive data will be accorded greater weight than they deserve. Thoughtful and responsible interpretation of these data requires physician participation to suggest the strengths and limitations of the severity measurement approach.

SEVERITY MEASUREMENT SYSTEMS

Although the DRGs are used for hospital payment, various other systems have been developed as measures of illness severity. Five of the best-known systems are reviewed below, focusing on features of greatest interest to physicians. Several reviews of specific systems and relevant issues can be found in the clinical and research literature (27-29,34,40-42).

Overview

The five methods described in this chapter have various definitions of severity, classification approaches, and required data elements (Table 1). The measures are adapted for divergent goals and settings; no single system best meets all needs. The first step in choosing among systems involves specifying the goal of the severity information and the practical boundaries of cost and burden of data collection (license fees for these systems can range up to $45,000 per hospital per year). Judging which system is best suited to meet the delineated goals requires consideration of several dimensions.

From the physician's perspective perhaps the most important dimension is validity — the clinical credibility of the system, and the relationship between the classification scheme and the real severity of a patient's illness. Credibility must be judged in the clinical context. A valid system for a neonatal ICU may differ from one for a geriatric service or a psychiatric ward. All five systems were derived mainly for adult, medical and surgical cases, although one applies primarily to the ICU. All concentrate almost exclusively on acute medical conditions, as distinguished from functional disability or psychosocial impairment, and all focus on imminent risks (of death or organ failure) or immediate concerns (about treatment difficulty or cost). Thus, none of the measures deals comprehensively with patient status, either short or long term. A major difference among the methods involves the role of diagnosis. Two systems classify severity regardless of diagnosis; the remaining three systems require a diagnostic infrastructure in the belief that severity is a diagnosis-specific concept. One system uses procedure performance to define patient categories.

Clinical credibility is directly linked to the data used to define severity levels. The chief distinction is between systems that rely exclusively on discharge abstract information (*ICD-9-CM* diagnostic and procedural codes, age, sex, discharge status) and those requiring primary data collection from the medical record. Systems that depend solely on discharge abstract data are less expensive to implement, with a potential compromise of clinical scope and credibility.

Three factors suggest the nature of this compromise. The first involves intrinsic limitations of *ICD-9-CM*, which was never intended to characterize severity of illness (43). *ICD-9-CM* contains various codes, including "'problems' that are not diagnoses, many more symptoms, and 'other' reasons for seeking health care" (44). Some *ICD-9-CM* codes indicate severe illness, such as respiratory arrest, ruptured abdominal aortic aneurysm, hepatic encephalopathy, paraplegia, and thyrotoxicosis with thyroid storm. However, *ICD-9-CM* does not list the clinical criteria that define these conditions or offer a complete spectrum of severity information. For example, although *ICD-9-CM* offers 37 different four- and five-digit codes describing types of anemia, it does not specify absolute levels of hematocrit or rates of blood loss (43).

The second factor concerns the accuracy of *ICD-9-CM* coding. Several Institute of Medicine studies found high rates of inaccurate coding in the late 1970s (45,46); with the implementation of DRG-based payment in the early 1980s, hospitals became more likely to assign more complex principal diagnoses than warranted or juggle the sequence of codes to maximize payment (47). More recent studies have found persistent high rates of coding inaccuracies (48,49). Certain coding rules must also be considered. For example, the coding guidelines stipulate that diagnoses qualified as "probable," "question," or "rule out" must be coded as if they exist (50). Despite requirements for physician verification of the correctness of diagnostic codes before Medicare hospital payment, errors in *ICD-9-CM* coding remain a potential problem for systems based on these data.

Finally, discharge abstracts report on diagnoses pertinent to the entire hospital stay; conditions present on admission or early in the stay are not differentiated from those occurring later in the hospital course. For example, a secondary diagnosis of pneumonia in a surgical patient could represent a condition present on admission or a complication that occurred postoperatively. These two scenarios lead to different conclusions about the quality of hospital care; they could possibly be distinguished by looking at the dates of surgery (if surgery occurred on day 1 or 2, the pneumonia is more likely to be a complication). The concern about timing of a complication may be less pressing for certain conditions, such as distant cancer metastases, which are unlikely to develop during hospitalization. However, systems founded on discharge abstract data are structurally less suited for either use of severity data in quality assessment (risk adjustment by admission severity or measuring change in patient condition over time).

These limitations must be balanced against the lower cost of these data. In addition, reservations about the clinical credibility and accuracy of methods based on *ICD-9-CM* codes do not automatically ensure superior validity or utility in systems requiring primary data collection from the medical record. These approaches have their own complexities and greater implications for physicians and the practice of medicine. It is also important to remember that even the results of systems based on chart review are generally presented within a diagnostic structure (such as DRGs), often one dependent on *ICD-9-CM* codes.

From the physician's perspective, the availability of comprehensible documentation about the content and the logic of the methodology are important when choosing a system. Evaluating the clinical credibility of a measure and thus its potential utility requires understanding its inner workings. Available and intelligible documentation is a prerequisite to this task. The five systems reviewed here vary widely on this score.

APACHE

Knaus and colleagues (51) at the George Washington University Medical Center developed the acute physiology and chronic health evaluation (APACHE) system in 1978. They intended to develop a tool to facilitate evaluations of quality of care and efficacy of treatments rendered to critically ill patients in the ICU (51,52). The original goal was to describe the severity of illness of individual patients, independent of physician judgment or variations in practice style. All critically ill medical and surgical patients were considered, except those with acute myocardial infarctions and burns (for whom classification systems already existed).

Development. The initial APACHE system focused on 34 acute physiologic measurements grouped into seven systems (neurologic, cardiovascular, respiratory, gastrointestinal, renal, metabolic, and hematologic) and a chronic health assessment. Values of each of the 34 measurements were assigned a weight from 0 through 4, reflecting "how sick" a patient was (51). The 34 acute measurements were chosen after a review of the clinical literature, searching for variables that indicated illness severity and that were readily available in the ICU. The weights were derived through a nominal consensus process involving seven critical care specialists. Initial testing of the system on more than 500 George Washington ICU patients revealed a strong positive correlation between the acute physiology component of the APACHE score and the risk for in-hospital death (51,53).

APACHE II, a simplified version developed in 1982, uses 12 commonly measured, physiologic measurements, chosen for breadth of organ system coverage, objectivity, and validity (52). The weights assigned to various values of these 12 measurements were slightly modified from those derived through clinical consensus and used in the original version. Subsequent tests on 5,815 ICU patients in 13 hospitals showed a strong positive correlation between APACHE II scores and risk for in-hospital death (52,54,55).

Definition of Severity. APACHE aims to predict risk for in-hospital death among critically ill patients. Score computation and data elements are independent of the patient's diagnosis. This independence is founded on the concept of "homeostasis" expounded by Walter B. Cannon in 1929 — that "the body's major physiologic systems interact to maintain internal balance and rapidly correct disturbances" (55). Despite this framework, APACHE's developers suggest that additional indicators of severity may be necessary to evaluate more completely the severity of patients with certain diagnoses (54). However, a study of the ability of APACHE II to predict in-hospital death in 18 nonsurgical conditions found a fairly consistent relationship between scores and risk for death across 17 of the conditions (the exception was diabetic ketoacidosis) (55).

Classification Approach. APACHE II assigns a score from 0 to 71 to each case. The highest score yet recorded is 55; in a study of 5,815 ICU admissions, 36% of cases had scores less than 10 and 62% had scores less than 15 (54). APACHE II scores combine three components: the acute physiology score, generating up to 60 points; patient age, grouped into five categories, with age over 74 years receiving the maximum 6 points; and chronic health status, with 5 points assigned if a patient has one or more of five chronic conditions (severe liver, cardiovascular, respiratory, renal disease, or immunocompromised state). The acute physiology score is computed by adding the weights assigned to each of the 12 acute physiologic measurements from the patient. Eleven of twelve physiologic measurements generate from 0 points (for normal values) to 4 points (for very deranged values). The twelfth, the Glasgow Coma Score, yields from 0 to 12 points. The points assigned to serum creatinine are doubled if acute renal failure is present. Information sufficient to produce APACHE scores is readily available from numerous publications in the clinical literature.

Data Elements.   APACHE II requires information on age, chronic health status, and 12 physiologic measurements: temperature, mean arterial pressure, heart rate, respiratory rate, arterial oxygenation, arterial pH, serum sodium, serum potassium, serum creatinine, hematocrit, leukocyte count, and Glasgow Coma Score. Because these data do not appear on the discharge abstract, they must be collected from medical records or other primary sources. In the study of 5,815 ICU admissions, values for all 12 physiologic measurements were available in 87% of cases, with serum creatinine and arterial blood gas findings missing most commonly (54). In the original APACHE, in which 34 values were measured, missing values were assumed to be normal and were assigned a weight of 0. APACHE II developers describe measurement of all 12 physiologic findings as "mandatory" except "when clinical judgment strongly suggests the results would be within normal limits" (54).

Timing of Reviews.   APACHE II focuses on the most deranged values for each of the 12 physiologic measurements within the first 24 hours of a patient's ICU stay. Although APACHE's developers recommend use of the most abnormal value in the first day of ICU treatment, studies of cases at their own institution showed that in 88% of the physiologic measurements, the worst value was the value *on admission* to the unit (54).

Potential Applications.   APACHE is used to assist in assessing the efficacy of specific clinical interventions in gravely ill patients (56,57). Its developers suggest additional uses for their system, such as determining the appropriateness of ICU admissions (58) and assisting in identifying the source of quality shortfalls in ICUs (59,60). They also propose that hospital-level mortality data be adjusted for admission physiologic status before public release (61). APACHE II forms the core of Medicare's Mortality Predictor System for stroke, pneumonia, acute myocardial infarction, and congestive heart failure cases (62). However, use of APACHE across a range of hospitalized patients could prove problematic. Important characteristics of patients not in the ICU may not be adequately captured by APACHE (63).

One application that sparks debate is using APACHE to make therapeutic decisions on individual patients. Although the system was not originally intended to aid decision making in individual situations, some believe that the measure is sufficiently powerful to guide clinicians in making treatment choices for critically ill patients, such as deciding which patients to admit to a unit in facilities with limited intensive care resources (56,64). Several institutions across the country already use APACHE II for this purpose.

Computerized Severity Index

With its introduction in 1987, the Computerized Severity Index (CSI) became the newest tool for widespread measurement of severity of illness. The CSI was developed by Horn and colleagues (65-67) at the Johns Hopkins

Medical Institutions during the period of controversy in which DRGs were introduced as the classification system for hospital payment. The goals ascribed to the CSI reflect this heritage. It aims specifically to meet policy needs, such as improving fairness of hospital payment and severity-adjusting outcome data for quality assessment, and for helping hospitals manage in the era of cost containment (65-67).

Development.   The CSI is a descendant of the "manual severity of illness index," a system also developed by Horn and colleagues in 1980. Its original purpose was to help a particular hospital respond to state regulatory agency questions about the hospital's length of stay and patient charges (68). The manual severity of illness index scored patients on a four-point scale, independent of diagnosis. It required review of the medical record to rate the patient along seven dimensions: stage of principal diagnosis at admission; complications of principal diagnosis; interactions with comorbidities; patient dependency on intensive services; nonoperating room procedures (life support services received the highest rating); rate of response to therapy; and residual symptoms at discharge. Ratings on these seven dimensions were considered in producing the overall score. The manual severity of illness index was the methodologic cornerstone of a series of studies demonstrating differences in patient mix across hospitals and physicians and linking these differences to resource needs (68-71).

Critics of the manual severity of illness index were concerned about subjectivity of the chart review process and the inability of the severity rating to identify consequences of poor quality care (72). In 1984 Horn initiated development of the CSI, aiming to remove controversial dimensions by using "explicit" clinical criteria. The intention was to produce a system also independent of diagnosis. However, as work progressed, the researchers became convinced that they could not achieve their desired degree of validity and accuracy without a diagnostic structure. They reoriented to develop severity indicators for over 700 conditions.

To identify the condition-specific severity indicators, nurse researchers scanned textbooks and clinical literature. Indicators were reviewed by more than 100 physicians to confirm that the criteria were medically meaningful and reflected current medical practices. Using physician judgment, each indicator was placed along a four-point scale (mild, moderate, severe, life-threatening). Relevant clinical indicators were combined to form a severity matrix for each disease. Tests of the draft CSI were first done on 1,200 cases representing 60 common conditions, drawn from a tertiary teaching hospital, and subsequently on 1,000 cases from six hospitals across the country. Empiric validation of the weighting scheme was performed on these data using regression techniques. The CSI is continually updated, based on user comments. Because the system is new, no empiric work using the CSI has appeared in the literature. CSI documentation and software are developed and marketed by Health Systems International (the purveyors of DRGs) in New Haven, Connecticut.

Definition of Severity.   The CSI defines severity of illness as the treatment difficulty presented to physicians due to the extent and interactions of a patient's disease. A basic assumption of the system is that knowledge of diagnosis is crucial to severity measurement. The system aims to capture the "total burden of illness," viewed as twofold: first, the severity of the "clinical problem" or principal diagnosis that brought the patient to the hospital, and second, the severity of the "clinical context/environment" or the complications and comorbidities that the patient experiences while hospitalized (66).

Classification Approach. The computerized CSI algorithm assigns a score from 0 through 4 reflecting increasing severity to each of the patient's diagnoses. In addition, an overall score (also from 0 to 4) is computed, which considers the interaction of the principal diagnosis with each of the secondary diagnoses. This overall score accords different weights to different secondary diagnoses (for example, a secondary diagnosis of "broken finger" is not weighted as heavily as one of "chronic obstructive pulmonary disease"). The pattern of clinical variables identified for each diagnosis dictates its score. For a diagnosis to be assigned to a severity level, at least two clinical findings from that level must be present (for example, at least two level 3 clinical indicators must be present to assign the diagnosis a score of 3).

The CSI uses the *ICD-9-CM* as its diagnostic framework. More than 10,200 *ICD-9-CM* diagnostic codes were collapsed into approximately 700 conditions. Its developers recommend that the CSI be used simultaneously with *ICD-9-CM* coding in the medical record department to avoid duplicating reviews. The CSI principal and secondary diagnoses thus reflect hospital *ICD-9-CM* coding practices. The system demands *complete* diagnostic coding. For example, the severity matrix for lung cancer does not indicate whether metastases are present — a secondary diagnosis of metastatic malignancy must provide that information. The severity score assigned to each condition becomes the sixth digit added to the standard five-digit *ICD-9-CM* code. A severity score of 0 for a given diagnosis indicates that no clinical criteria were met, and questions the accuracy of the *ICD-9-CM* code. In this way, the CSI aims to improve chart documentation and *ICD-9-CM* coding practices.

Data Elements. The CSI encompasses more than 600 clinical characteristics across all conditions. These clinical indicators require abstraction from the medical record. They include patient history (for example, degree of weight loss, number of stools per day); symptoms (for example, nausea, chest pain, confusion, vertigo); physical examination findings (for example, rales, papilledema, ascites, jugular venous distention, nodular abdominal tumor); vital signs; laboratory tests (serum chemistries, enzymes, hematology findings, urinalysis, air blood gases, cerebrospinal fluid analysis); and basic radiology studies (for example, chest, abdominal, and bone roentgenograms). The diagnosis-specific data collection approach recognizes that not all clinical findings are relevant for all conditions. *ICD-9-CM* codes assigned to the patient are entered into the computer first. Then the software algorithm prompts the reviewer to collect information on the specific clinical indicators relevant for that condition. For example, with an *ICD-9-CM* diagnosis of bacterial meningitis, information on intracranial pressure is collected, whereas with an *ICD-9-CM* diagnosis of abdominal aneurysm, information on the degree of widening of the aorta is collected. According to the developers of the CSI, the software asks 32 questions on the average patient. A "help" file of alternative definitions facilitates reliable and correct data collection across different settings.

Timing of Reviews.   The CSI can be applied at several points over the hospital stay. Measurements on admission (first 48 hours) and at discharge (last 48 hours) are particularly common. The most abnormal values during these periods are gathered. In addition, the CSI computes a "maximum" severity over the entire hospital stay. Maximum severity computation requires collection of the most deranged values obtained over the entire hospital stay, regardless of timing (for example, the most abnormal hematocrit could apply to day 1 and the most abnormal pulse rate to day 3).

Potential Applications.   The CSI arose in an era of cost containment and its attendant concerns. The purposes for the system consequently span from health policy to hospital management issues. Adjusting DRGs for severity of illness to improve the fairness of hospital payment is one goal that began being tested in New Jersey in the summer of 1988. This test involves collection of *maximum* CSI scores on 80,000 cases in 24 volunteer hospitals throughout the state. These data will be used to generate severity-adjusted DRG payment weights.

The developers of the CSI see their system as being particularly helpful in facilitating quality assessment. Risk-adjusted hospital mortality data based on admission CSI severity is one use. In addition, they suggest examining change in severity of illness over time, for example, comparing an admission and a maximum score. Deterioration from admission status could indicate a *possible* shortfall in quality of care, but such analyses should be performed over groups of cases. The system does not aim to identify substandard quality in individual instances, but rather to flag cases that should be reviewed in greater depth.

Disease Staging

Gonnella and colleagues (73) at the Jefferson Medical College in Philadelphia began work on Disease Staging in 1974 as part of a project to evaluate quality of ambulatory care in California's Medicaid program. Their goals included the desire to assess physician diagnostic efficiency, facilitate prognostication, evaluate therapeutic effectiveness, and design clinical trials at the typical, short-term general hospital in the United States (74).

Development.   Twenty-three physician consultants participated in initial specification of Disease Staging. Two specialists worked independently on each disease. Four generic levels of severity ("stages") served as guidelines for modeling a disease. Using clinical judgment, they specified clinical criteria to define each stage, and designated additional substages to describe each disease's progression. The consultants provided common descriptions for each stage and substage, noting synonymous terms, and the "supporting evidence" (clinical variables required to prove its presence. Each physician listed references from the clinical literature that supported the classification system. The original specifications were reviewed by other physicians engaged in Disease Staging development, and through a consensus process, final clinical staging criteria were established. To make the system computer-accessible, a team of medical records professionals translated the clinical stage and substage definitions into *ICD-9-CM* codes, and a Disease Staging software program was produced.

Since its initial form, the Disease Staging clinical criteria and *ICD-9-CM* translations have been reviewed and revised by many physician consultants and coding specialists. In addition, empiric research has led to further refinements and the development of new, computerized Disease Staging algorithms (75-77). The most recent study (78) examined resource use for nearly 7 million patients discharged from hospitals across the United States, to develop a patient-level "severity" measure, "Q-Scale," which is independent of diagnostic code sequencing and is predictive of resource consumption. Documentation of the Disease Staging clinical criteria and the associated software products are owned and marketed by SysteMetrics, a division of McGraw-Hill based in Santa Barbara, California.

Definition of Severity.   Disease Staging considers severity within the context of specific diseases. The conceptual foundation of the system starts with the definition of disease (74):

> A disease is a well-defined model of a process of disruption in the normal homeostasis of psychological-physiological systems... Each disease should be defined in terms of some specific organ or organ system involved... Every disease must specify some characteristic pathophysiological change... An etiologic factor or set of factors causing the pathophysiological changes must be given.

Within this framework, severity is the final factor considered necessary to establish a "diagnosis." Clinical Disease Staging views severity as the risk for death or temporary or permanent impairment. The software-based Q-Scale "severity" measure was designed to allow patient-level classification, to predict resource use, and to refine the DRGs for hospital payment.

Classification Approach.   Disease Staging focuses on aproximately 400 diseases that are common in short-term, U.S. acute care hospitals. Most of these diseases are separated into four main stages using a rubric borrowed from the staging concept of oncology. The stages reflect increasing disease severity, as follows: stage 1 — conditions with no complications or problems of minimal severity; stage 2 — problems limited to an organ or organ system, significantly increased risk for complications; stage 3 — multiple site involvement, generalized systemic involvement, poor prognosis; stage 4 — death.

Substages within these major stages indicate more subtle clinical distinctions. For example, stage 2 appendicitis contains four substages: 2.1, appendicitis with perforation causing localized peritonitis or peritoneal abscess; 2.2, appendicitis with perforation causing generalized peritonitis; 2.3, intestinal obstruction; and 2.4 pylephlebitis with or without liver abscess. Within diseases, increasing numerical stages represent increasing severity, but these numerical values cannot be compared across conditions. For analyses focusing on risk for death, cases are assigned to the highest stage attained without consideration of discharge status.

Higher stages of diseases are defined by complications of increasing severity. Unrelated secondary diseases or diagnoses (that is, those that are *not* complications as designated by the Disease Staging criteria) represent comorbidities. For example, in a patient with a principal diagnosis of essential hypertension, a secondary diagnosis of hypertensive heart disease would represent a complication, whereas a secondary diagnosis of alcoholic cirrhosis would represent a comorbidity. The Disease Staging Q-Stage software assigns a stage to each of the listed diagnoses and indicates whether secondary diagnoses are related to the principal diagnosis (disease complications) or not (comorbidities). This process permits a single patient to have several staged conditions.

The Q-Scale software assigns a single value to a patient, regardless of the number of diagnoses. This scale is used to predict resource need, and it is independent of the order of diagnoses. This scale expresses "severity" as a percentage centered around a referent group's average of 100. For example, a within-DRG Q-Scale value of 150 indicates that the particular case is 50% higher in "severity" or resource need, than the national average within that DRG. The software can also compute this figure independent of DRG.

Data Elements.   Because of the economy of its application, the most popular version of Disease Staging is the computerized product that relies exclusively on standard discharge abstract information. The software runs on mainframe computers or in batch or interactive mode on microcomputers.

The clinical criteria version of Disease Staging requires abstraction from the medical record of the designated "supporting evidence or clues" for each disease (77). These clinical variables are specific to each condition, and represent symptomatic, physical examination, laboratory, and other findings available in the medical record. For example, the supporting evidence or clues required to assign stage 2.2 appendicitis include generalized abdominal pain; fever (greater than 38.5 °C); diffuse tenderness and rigid abdomen, paralytic ileus; leukocytosis (greater than $15 \times 10^9/L$) with increased neutrophil count; and findings of intestinal obstruction confirmed by surgical or pathologic examination.

Timing of Reviews.   The computerized version of Disease Staging is a retrospective system, applied to standard discharge abstract data after hospital admission. However, the clinical criteria version can be applied at several points during the hospital stay. Its developers recommend comparing admission, peak, and discharge severity to facilitate quality assurance activities.

Potential Applications.   Disease Staging is a diverse system. Applying it directly to medical records and its several software products offers many uses. A recent focus of its developers has been severity refinement for DRG-based hospital payment. However, with its roots in efforts by Gonnella and colleagues to evaluate medical practice, the system is also used to assess quality, especially to determine the timeliness of admission. The comments of Gonnella and Goran from 1975 remain very pertinent: Disease Staging could be used as a tool to direct the scarce resources available for quality assurance "into areas where intervention will be most productive" (38).

MedisGroups

The MedisGroups severity system evolved out of concerns of physicians at Saint Vincent Hospital, a 578-bed facility in Worcester, Massachusetts, that mortality statistics alone did not represent the entire patient experience at their institution. The severity measure has since been linked with various software and data collection packages, such as procedure appropriateness and nosocomial infection monitoring, to provide a comprehensive quality assurance tool for hospitals (79,80). Recent efforts at widespread implementation of MedisGroups, such as the Pennsylvania mandate, require only the severity component, the focus of the ensuing discussion.

Development. Two Saint Vincent physicians, Karlin and Brewster, responded to the concerns of their colleagues by identifying clinical variables that reflected patient severity. They focused on the "key clinical finding." Over 9 months in 1979, Karlin and Brewster observed the morning report of medical residents, noting which clinical variables were the basis of severity assessments by residents (80,81). These observations led to an initial list of key clinical findings. Karlin and Brewster linked each key clinical finding to a severity level, based on its perceived association with actual or potential organ failure. Chiefs of service and attending physicians at the hospital reviewed this list and the severity assignments. During the next 2 years, this list was expanded to include surgery, obstetrics, and pediatrics, starting with an examination of patient records to identify pivotal clinical variables. The resulting system, which links several key clinical findings to produce a single severity score, became MedisGroups, a registered trade name owned by MediQual Systems, Inc., in Westborough, Massachusetts. The system is proprietary, and thus, information about its inner workings is not published.

Although initial system development was based on clinical judgment, subsequent refinements have relied largely on a database of hundreds of thousands of cases in hospitals licensed to use MedisGroups. Using these data, MediQual clinical staff annually examine each key clinical finding, looking at its relationship to risk for in-hospital death. Additional refinements are suggested by outside clinical specialists and by physicians at MedisGroups-member hospitals. When possible, these additional changes are also evaluated empirically.

Definition of Severity. MedisGroups produces severity scores independent of patient diagnoses based on risk for imminent "organ failure," with the most severe cases actually experiencing "organ failure." Because of the independence from diagnosis, failures in different organ systems are equated (81-83). For example, the following key clinical findings are weighted equally by MedisGroups, indicating a similar level of risk within each respective organ system: skin infection, joint effusion, gastrointestinal hemorrhage identified through endoscopy, and cardiac valve area less than 1.0 cm^2 determined by cardiac catheterization. However, MedisGroups is structured so that patients with several, severe key clinical findings receive higher scores. Thus, for example, patients with cardiac disease or gastrointestinal hemorrhage are more likely to have several key clinical findings than patients with skin infections or joint effusions. Although the system scores patients independent of diagnosis, its developers recommend that MedisGroups data be analyzed within broad diagnostic categories, such as DRGs.

Classification Approach and Timing of Reviews. The MedisGroups system has two major types of reviews. The "admission" review records not only acute derangements, but also more chronic conditions that may affect clinical status. Admission scores range from 0 to 4, indicating increasing risk for imminent organ failure. For medical cases, the admission period encompasses the first two calendar days of the hospital stay; for surgical cases, the timing of the admission review depends on the scheduling of surgery. The surgical admission review encompasses all aspects of the surgery, including the pathologic findings, as part of the admission period. Special provisions are made for patients who have surgery late in their hospital stays.

A "mid-stay" review is done only on patients who stay in the hospital the required length of time. This review identifies "morbidity" that arises acutely during the hospital stay — chronic derangements are not considered in mid stay reviews (scoring for this review focuses on relatively severe or acute subsets of key clinical findings). The mid-stay review produces three tiers of scores: "no morbidity," "morbidity," and "major morbidity." For medical cases, the mid-stay review encompasses days 3 through 7 of the hospital stay. For surgical cases, this review generally covers the 5 days after surgery. Although most key clinical findings can be drawn from any time during this period, information on vital signs and 10 specified laboratory key clinical findings must be taken from the last 48 hours of the mid-stay review. Although MediQual uses the term "morbidity" for this mid-stay review, it merely represents an additional severity score. Other information is required to attribute this "morbidity" to a problem with quality of care.

Data Elements. The 1987 version of MedisGroups contained 260 possible key clinical findings representing clinical abnormalities drawn from patient history, physical examination, laboratory, pathology, radiology, and other procedural findings from the medical record. Because the system is independent of diagnosis, the chart abstractor must look for any key clinical finding. From 5 to 10 key clinical findings are identified in the average admission review.

Some key clinical findings represent continuous variables, such as hematocrit, serum sodium, total bilirubin, and systolic blood pressure. The reviewer records the "worst" value for these variables observed during the review period; "normal" values, as designated by MedisGroups, are not recorded. Other key clinical findings are dichotomous: They are either present or absent according to standards set by the MedisGroups Glossary (a lexicon designed to facilitate consistent interpretation of terms found in the medical records by the chart abstractors). Many dichotomous key clinical findings relate to specific diseases rather than general physiologic function; some require performance of certain procedures. Examples of dichotomous key clinical findings include coma or stupor on neurologic examination, congestive heart failure on chest radiograph, colonic polyp on colonoscopy, urinary retention found through intravenous pyelogram, spinal cord compression identified through computed tomography, and aortic dissection identified through arteriography.

Each key clinical finding is assigned to a "severity group" from 0 to 3, based on its association with actual or imminent organ failure. The MedisGroups software designates ranges of continuous key clinical findings that prompt severity group assignments. The admission score considers all key clinical findings. Scores are assigned by an algorithm based on the number of key clinical findings and their severity group assignments. For example, two or more group 3 key clinical findings lead to an admission score of 4; one group 3 or two or more group 2 findings result in an admission score of 3 (83). Only certain group 2 or 3 key clinical findings result in mid-stay "morbidity."

Potential Applications.   MedisGroups was developed in a hospital, and has subsequently been used in individual facilities. In conjunction with the other software and data collection products marketed by MediQual, the MedisGroups severity system aims to facilitate in-house quality assurance activities by identifying physicians whose experience deviates from the norm, and inappropriate use of particular procedures. Using data submitted by participating hospitals, MediQual produces normative data for its clients by which the performance of their institution can be judged.

However, the adoption of MedisGroups by the "buy right" and Pennsylvania programs elevated the system out of the sphere of intrainstitutional quality assurance into the realm of cross-hospital comparisons and widespread quality assessment. Its envisioned role in this application is twofold: first, to use the admission score to adjust for risk for poor outcomes such as in-hospital death; and second, to focus on "morbidity" as an outcome of hospital stay. The experiment in Rochester, New York, will indicate whether this approach toward quality assessment can be combined successfully with hospital reimbursement (84).

Patient Management Categories

Patient Management Categories (PMCs) are the only patient classification system to focus on the implications of clinical presentation on specific service and resource needs of groups of patients. As such, PMCs were not intended primarily as a measure of severity of illness. Instead, their goal was " ... to identify and incorporate clinical and severity distinctions among patient types where those distinctions reflect expected differences in patient management and, consequently, hospital resource requirements" (85). The PMCs draw from diagnostic, severity, and procedural information to structure their classification system, and they are viewed as an alternative, not an adjunct, to the DRGs.

Development.   Young and colleagues at Blue Cross of Western Pennsylvania developed the PMCs in 1978. The Health Care Financing Administration supported initial development of the system, and the research objective was to capture the cost of a hospital's case mix in a fashion consistent with the process of care (86). The researchers viewed their task as twofold:

first, identification of "clinically homogeneous patient categories," and second, derivation of "relative cost weights" reflecting the costliness of these patient types (87). Another goal was to produce an efficient system that would not require additional data collection.

To accomplish these goals, Young worked with approximately 50 disease-specific panels, each made up of four to six physicians (generalists and specialists) experienced in the treatment of a particular condition. Using clinical judgment, the physician panels specified case types, then delineated the diagnostic and therapeutic services required to care for the "typical" patient within each type (85). The panels formulated flow diagrams, or patient management paths, moving from reason for admission (for example, signs and symptoms), to diagnostic components of care (for example, specified laboratory tests), to diagnosis, to components of treatment required.

To avoid the need for additional data, discharge abstract information was used to produce the PMC software. The clinical data thus includes diagnostic and procedural codes, discharge status (alive compared with dead), patient age, and sex. The latter three variables were used sparingly in PMC classification, and the former support most of the algorithms. *ICD-9-CM* diagnostic codes were linked to approximate the case types specified by the physician panels; when major surgery was done, appropriate procedural codes were added to define the PMC.

Finally, relative cost weights were specified for each PMC using cost data for relevant services derived through a detailed accounting procedure at six western Pennsylvania hospitals. Unit costs for the components of care specified by the physician panels for each patient type were totaled, then compared with the average cost category. A method was also developed to assign one relative cost weight to each patient, based on the comorbidities associated with that particular case.

The original set of PMCs has been updated, and the most recent version includes nine new PMCs specifically for acquired immunodeficiency syndrome cases. PMC software and documentation are available through the Pittsburgh Research Institute, a nonprofit affiliate of Blue Cross of Western Pennsylvania.

Definition of Severity.   PMCs consider severity of illness a disease-specific concept. According to the developers of PMCs, it is common "to assume that there is a direct relationship between severity and costs — that the more severe cases should cost more. This relationship can be tested..." (86). As mentioned above, the PMCs aimed to capture severity distinctions, insofar as such distinctions contributed to different resource needs. Although developers of PMCs state that "sicker" cases are not always more expensive, in general, PMCs with higher cost-based relative weights indicate greater illness severity than those with lower weights. This generalization relies on the process of care specified through each patient management path.

Classification Approach.   The PMC computer algorithm uses standard discharge abstract data to assign each patient to one or more PMCs. The software differs from the DRGs in that it considers the clinical inter-relations of diagnostic codes, disregarding their order. Therefore, it uses the diversity available through *ICD-9-CM* to define case types. For example, if three *ICD-9-CM* codes are present, indicating gastrointestinal hemorrhage, diverticular disease, and hypertension, the software recognizes the hemorrhage to be a complication of the diverticular disease, whereas it considers the hypertension a separate process (or comorbidity). Two PMCs would be assigned — one PMC for diverticular disease with bleeding, and a second PMC for hypertension. The PMC assigned with the first code is the principal PMC; other categories indicate comorbidities.

The most recent release contains 848 PMCs, but 280 PMCs account for about 90% of cases. Each PMC has its associated relative cost weight. For cases with several comorbidities, an algorithm assigns a single relative cost weight that considers the impact of the coexisting conditions on resource needs. For example, the cost-based relative weight for stable angina is 0.481, whereas for chronic obstructive pulmonary disease, the figure is 0.619; a weight of 1.0 represents the average cost of a patient in the population base. A patient assigned to both PMCs has a "comorbid combination weight" of 0.813. There is no upper bound on the value of comorbid combinations; the highest such weight recorded in a statewide, Maryland database was 23.0.

Another algorithm adjusts cost-based relative weights for cases based on the different use of resources of patients discharged alive compared with patients who died. The developers of PMCs found that the cost implications of discharge status varies by condition. For some conditions, patients who die have higher costs than those discharged alive; for other case types the reverse is true. The cost-based relative weights adjusted by discharge status reflect these differences (88).

Data Elements. The PMCs rely on standard discharge abstract information. The software can accommodate up to 20 *ICD-9-CM* diagnosis and procedure codes, and it can be executed on various computers, including mainframes, minicomputers, and microcomputers.

Timing of Reviews. The PMCs were designed as a retrospective system. To achieve their goal of economy, they would be applied after discharge to the data routinely collected in processing the patient bill. Therefore, the assigned PMCs would reflect the entire hospital stay, not particular points during the stay.

To facilitate the use of PMCs in quality assurance, however, their developers suggest that the necessary *ICD-9-CM* diagnostic and procedural data could be abstracted at several points over the hospitalization. The precise timing (for example, on admission, midway through the stay) would depend on the intended application. This process would depart from the usual coding for billing purposes and would add to the cost of the system.

Potential Applications. The PMCs are an alternative to the DRGs, and as such, they can fulfill the roles currently played by the DRGs in hospital payment, case mix indexing, and other functions. Their developers suggest examining PMC-specific death rates and looking at other outcomes that could potentially indicate quality of hospital care. For example, PMCs have been designed for wound dehiscence, wound infection, and postoperative hematoma.

Frequent assignment to such PMCs could reflect substandard care. If PMCs are assigned at several points over the hospital stay through extra *ICD-9-CM* coding activities, events such as infections later in the hospitalization could suggest shortfalls in quality of care.

One important feature of the PMCs is the associated patient management pathways, the strategy specified by the physician panels for effective care of the typical patient. Developers of PMCs state that these pathways "do not represent standards of care, but they can be used as a basis for utilization review and quality assessment" (86). This focus on the process of care is unique to the PMCs.

HANDLING OF CLINICAL CASES

The conceptual foundations of these severity measures involved careful thought. However, rating severity requires balancing various patient presentations with data limitations. How do these systems really rate severity? A preliminary answer is offered through the summary of cases involving diabetic ketoacidosis, acute myocardial infarction, and intertrochanteric fracture of the femur. These cases, abstracted from actual medical records, represent several dimensions important in comparing the severity measures (medical compared with surgical, in-hospital death compared with discharged alive, acute illness with and without concomitant chronic disability).

The first case is a 17-year-old girl with diabetes mellitus who was admitted with somnolence, an arterial pH of 6.96, and "large" urine ketones, but who responded quickly to therapy and was discharged after an uncomplicated 5-day stay. This patient is generally rated as moderately to severely ill on admission by systems that depend on clinical items abstracted from the medical record. These clinically detailed systems focus on the low arterial pH on admission and other physiologic derangements. These systems vary in their use of more descriptive findings; for example, the CSI notes "Kussmaul breathing," whereas MedisGroups describes the patient as "lethargic." Although the clinically detailed systems view the patient as moderately to very sick, the two approaches based exclusively on *ICD-9-CM* codes and whose purpose is to suggest resource needs — the Disease Staging Q-Scale and the PMCs — rate the patient as lower than a national average, both suggesting that this patient type is approximately 20% less resource-intensive than the average patient. Given that both approaches equate severity and cost, their view of patient severity is very different from that of the clinically detailed measures. None of the systems suggest a quality of care review — the patient is discharged alive with a relatively brief length of stay.

The second case is a 66-year-old man admitted with an anterior acute myocardial infarction, whose course was complicated by rapid atrial fibrillation, congestive heart failure, pneumonia, and oliguria; the patient died on the eleventh hospital day. The clinically detailed systems rate this patient as moderately ill on admission. They focus on various clinical attributes although most note electrocardiogram and chest radiograph results and creatine kinase values. Again, the Disease Staging Q-Scale and PMCs yield similar results. The maximum Q-Scale finds this patient type 290% more expensive than a national average; the PMCs find this patient type 285% more expensive. The systems differ in their decision about whether to conduct a quality of care review. The CSI automatically flags the case for quality review, because the maximum severity is higher than the admission value. Disease Staging considers a quality review because of steady worsening over a fairly prolonged stay; if death had occurred early in the stay, a quality review may not be indicated. APACHE II, MedisGroups, and the PMCs depend more on normative data to guide their judgments. For example, if within an institution or across a reference database, acute myocardial infarction cases with admission MedisGroups scores of 2 often died, a quality review may not be instituted.

The third case is an 81-year-old man with a history of dementia, chronic obstructive pulmonary disease, and recurrent aspiration pneumonias, who fractured his hip in a fall; his course was complicated by a pneumonia, but he was discharged and improved on the tenth hospital day. The clinically detailed systems view this patient as moderately ill on admission, although the diagnosis-dependent systems consider the hip fracture to be of low severity. For example, the CSI assigns a score of 1 to the hip fracture *ICD-9-CM* code and the clinical criteria version of Disease Staging assigns the fracture to stage 1.0. The clinical indicators focus only on the presence of the fracture in judging the fracture severity. The CSI alone broaches functional status, but this effort involves only a gross assessment ("requires assistance" or "completely dependent"). In contrast, the two measures founded on resource needs rate this patient as much more costly than average — 230% more costly for the Disease Staging Q-Scale, and 165% more costly for the PMCs. These values are less than the ratings for the acute myocardial infarction case, but only 60% less for the Q-Scale. None of the systems suggests a quality of care review.

These cases show that, despite some similarities, the systems offer various approaches for judging patient severity. Many of the details of their assessment strategies vary, as do the data elements on which ratings are based. Before choosing among these systems, it is important to understand the implications of these differences for the intended purpose. The most obvious choice is between systems founded on resource need and those derived from a more clinically based severity model; very different perceptions may emerge with these two tactics. Another major decision is between systems offering ratings of specific conditions and those providing only an overall assessment. Finally, an important difference involves the variables available through the measure to assess quality of care directly. For example, PMCs are the only system to suggest components of care for given patient management paths. These components could serve as possible guideposts for the next task — actually judging quality of care for cases flagged by the severity screen. The complexities of severity measurement may seem minor compared with the complexities of judging quality.

IMPLICATIONS FOR PHYSICIANS

Regardless of the approach adopted, once severity-based information is produced, there will be an irresistible urge to use it — appropriately or not. The severity data yielded by any of the tools described will be helpful but unlikely to solve the quality assessment problem completely. The data must be used responsibly and intelligently; the benefits and limitations must be recognized, and physicians are uniquely suited for this task. In addition, widespread use of a severity of illness measure will affect medical practice in other ways.

Documentation of the Medical Record

Adoption of a severity measure that requires primary data collection may lead to standardization of the medical record similar to that seen 70 years ago. The medical record will serve not only as a medicolegal document and a chronicle of clinical observations and decisions, but also as the main source of information for judging the skill and proficiency of the physician and hospital. If a medical record-based severity system is implemented, the structure, content, and nomenclature of this record may evolve to facilitate the severity review and perhaps influence severity findings. Three major issues arise.

The first issue concerns the accuracy and reliability of information in the medical record. A growing number of studies have focused on the "reliability" of severity measures, examining the extent to which different abstractors reviewing the same medical record produce like results (41,89,90). Systems that require subjective interpretation of record information are presumably less reliable than those that require abstraction of straightforward "objective" clinical data, such as laboratory values, electrocardiographic findings, or specified terms from radiology or pathology reports.

None of these studies has assessed the reliability of the "objective" clinical values, such as the evaluation of jugular venous distention requested by the CSI and the congestive heart failure on chest radiograph noted by MedisGroups. Yet the clinical literature is full of examples of interphysician variations in such "scientific" pursuits as reading electrocardiograms and evaluating pathology specimens (91,96). This body of literature suggests that much of the medical art remains subjective, open to interpretation, and inherently unreliable.

In clinical practice, this subjectivity and uncertainty are constant companions to the diagnostic and therapeutic process, and many issues are clarified or become evident in retrospect. The adoption of a severity measure would spotlight these supposedly "objective" clinical findings. This leads to the second concern about medical record documentation — the potential for manipulation.

Manipulation could take two forms — that of commission or omission. This manipulation does not necessarily represent blatant inaccuracies. Given the uncertainty inherent in so many clinical encounters, the presence or absence of a finding is often arguable; thus, its recording is similarly open to debate. One example involves the recording of the diastolic blood pressure. In a manual reading, pinpointing the termination of the Korotkoff sounds is difficult. If this termination occurs around 104 to 106 mm Hg, and the provider knows subconsciously or consciously that 105 mm Hg is the cutoff for a change in severity score, this knowledge could affect his or her choice of diastolic blood pressure. In certain circumstances (such as admission severity), it may be desirable to have a higher reading; in other situations (such as "maximum" severity), a lower reading would be preferred. Explicit or subliminal manipulation could compromise the integrity of medical record documentation and defeat the purpose of severity measurement. The pressure for manipulation will relate to the uses of the severity data. If the data are considered carefully and fairly, with appropriate guidelines concerning their limitations, such pressure will be minimized.

The final issue concerns who is documenting the medical record, raising the question of impact of hospital type on severity assessment. For example, at tertiary teaching hospitals many physicians comment in the chart, whereas at small community hospitals, such notations are comparatively sparse. This might affect relative severity assessments across hospitals for systems such as MedisGroups, which require most information to be drawn from physician notations. Another concern involves the inevitable differences in opinion among physicians evident in many medical records.

Impact on Procedure Use

Severity measurement systems vary in the extent to which procedures and test results are used to produce patient scores. APACHE II is at one extreme, relying on testing routinely performed on ICU patients, although such tests as air blood gases are not routine outside the unit; at the other extreme are MedisGroups, which specifies certain types of technologies to define its key clinical findings (including such sophisticated procedures as angiography and computed tomography), and the PMCs, which define many patient classes by surgery types. Will adoption of such severity measures affect procedure use?

An answer to this question probably depends on the type of severity. At admission, a high severity may be preferable for certain analyses, thus causing tests to be performed in which abnormal results are anticipated during admission. The severity measure could even dictate the type and timing of testing. This possibility also raises questions about the timeframe of the "admission" period, given the goal of capturing severity before medical intervention. Conversely, higher severity later in the admission or at discharge would be less desirable; hence, less testing may be pursued late in the hospital stay.

Of greatest concern is the potential for indiscriminant testing, to identify unexpected abnormalities. This possibility could generate costs beyond the price of the testing itself, including the expense of evaluating false-positive findings, iatrogenic threats to patients from unnecessary diagnostic procedures, and the discomfort and anxiety produced by the process. Although excessive testing is conceivable, countervailing forces could come from programs that monitor procedure use (which could prove costly) and from concerns about the costs of hospitalizations under case-based payment. Nonetheless, widespread adoption of a severity measure could alter the scope, nature, timing, and extent of diagnostic testing.

Access to Care

The severity measures that have gained prominence in policy debates are largely related to acute, medical, or surgical illnesses, with little or no consideration of functional impairments, chronic disabilities, and psychosocial dysfunctions. This could create difficulties for physicians whose caseloads include a large number of chronically ill or handicapped patients, or patients from nursing homes or chronic disease hospitals. Although these conditions may not always produce acute physiologic derangements, they could foreshadow poor outcomes (such as complications from the inability to ambulate postoperatively). This risk is not captured adequately by these severity measures, possibly jeopardizing physicians with large numbers of such patients. For these physicians, adverse outcomes beyond their control may not be predicted by the severity measure.

Will this cause physicians or hospitals to avoid chronically ill or disabled patients? The response to this question depends on the fairness and sensitivity with which the severity information is considered. The limitations of the severity data yielded by these systems must be acknowledged, with a special emphasis on the lack of information on chronic ailments and disabilities. Otherwise access to care for this vulnerable population could be compromised.

CONCLUSIONS

Will severity-based information answer the need for intelligence to foster increasing competition and improve quality among health care providers? A complete answer is not yet known. But an educated guess hazards that severity information, as defined in the current policy context, will assist in but not single-handedly fulfill this *need*. The severity-based data generated by the measures described offer substantial improvements in clinical credibility over prior approaches to large-scale analyses of hospital quality. However, the benefits of these data must be weighed against their costs. For example, gathering and analyzing severity information from the medical record could be expensive, adding another administrative cost not related to direct patient care to an already overburdened system (97). Hidden costs involve increasing diagnostic testing and the consequences of using these data to make unwarranted judgments about provider quality.

Given these warnings, this area should be pursued actively but cautiously. However, in several regions, the political winds have already whipped up a major maelstrom, sometimes pitting those desiring information against those about whom information is to be provided. The touchstone that must guide this area is the common goal of improving health care quality. Codman's hope that providers would willingly compare and publicize both their successes and failures has yet to be realized. But willingly or unwillingly, providers are being pushed to this end. The 1918 exhortation of the American College of Surgeons that physicians participate in this process is particularly pertinent. Only through physician insight can these severity-based data provide their maximal benefit. Physicians can help answer the topical and persistent question, is severity of illness-based information the most efficient and meaningful way to screen for shortfalls in quality of inpatient care?

Acknowledgments: The author thanks Douglas P. Wagner, PhD, George Washington University Medical Center, Washington, DC; Susan D. Horn, PhD, The Johns Hopkins University, Baltimore, Maryland; Jonathan E. Conklin and Cathleen A. Barnes, SysteMetrics/McGraw-Hill, Santa Barbara, California; Daniel Z. Louis, MS, Jefferson Medical College, Philadelphia, Pennsylvania; Elizabeth Estabrook, RN, MediQual Systems, Inc., Westborough, Massachusetts; Wanda W. Young, ScD, and Dorothy Z. Joyce, Pittsburgh Research Institute, Pittsburgh, Pennsylvania; and Jennifer Daley, MD, Beth Israel Hospital, Boston, Massachusetts.

References

1. Ginsburg PB, Hammons GT. Competition and the quality of care: the importance of information. *Inquiry*. 1988;**25**:108-15.

2. Kaple JG. Using severity indices to assess quality of care. *Bus Health*. 1987;**4**(10):23-8.

3. Aquilina D, McLaughlin B, Levy S. Using severity data to measure quality. *Bus Health*. 1988;**5**(8):40-2.

4. Kurtz DL. *Unit Medical Records in Hospital and Clinic*. New York: Columbia University Press; 1943:2-10.

5. Siegel RE. Clinical observations in Hippocrates: an essay on the evolution of the diagnostic art. *J Mt Sinai Hosp*. 1964;**31**:285-303.

6. Reiser SJ. *Medicine and the Reign of Technology*. Cambridge: Cambridge University Press; 1978:205-10.

7. Massachusetts General Hospital. Medical case records. August 18, 1824.

8. Clapesattle H. *The Doctors Mayo*. Minneapolis: The University of Minnesota Press; 1941:385.

9. Hornsby JA. The hospital problem of today — what is it? *Bull Am Coll Surg*. 1917;**3**:4-11.

10. Codman EA. Case-records and their value. *Bull Am Coll Surg*. 1917;**3**:24-7.

11. Codman EA. *The Shoulder. Rupture of the Supraspinatus Tendon and Other Lesions in or about the Subacromial Bursa*. Boston: Thomas Todd Company, Printers; 1934:v-xi.

12. Codman EA. *A Study in Hospital Efficiency as Demonstrated by the Case Report of the First Five Years of a Private Hospital*. Boston: Thomas Todd Company, Printers; 1917.

13. Pearl R. Modern methods in handling hospital statistics. *Bull Johns Hopkins Hosp*. 1921;**32**:184-94.

14. Bureau of the Census, Department of Commerce and Labor. *Manual of the International List of Causes of Death*. Washington, DC: Government Printing Office;1911:14-6,40.

15. Hollings B. Record keeping at the Massachusetts General Hospital. *Mod Hosp*. 1914;**2**:94-8.

16. American College of Surgeons. Standard of efficiency for the first hospital survey of the College. *Bull Am Coll Surg*. 1918;**3**:1-4.

17. Vladeck BC. Medicare hospital payment by diagnosis-related groups. *Ann Intern Med*. 1984;**100**:576-91.

18. Fetter RB, Shin Y, Freeman JL, Averill R, Thompson JD. Case mix definition by diagnosis-related groups. *Med Care.* 1980;**18**(2 suppl):1-53.

19. Schweiker RS. Report to Congress. *Hospital Prospective Payment for Medicare.* Washington, DC: U.S. Department of Health and Human Services;1982:74-5.

20. Mullin RL. Diagnosis-related groups and severity: ICD-9-CM, the real problem. *JAMA.* 1985;**254**:1208-10.

21. McMahon LF Jr, Smits HL. Can Medicare prospective payment survive the ICD-9-CM disease classification system? *Ann Intern Med.* 1986;**104**:562-6.

22. Smits HL, Fetter RB, McMahon LF Jr. Variation in resource use within diagnosis-related groups: the severity issue. *Health Care Financ Rev.* 1984; Suppl:71-8.

23. Gertman PM, Lowenstein S. A research paradigm for severity of illness: issues for the diagnosis-related group system. *Health Care Financ Rev.* 1984;Suppl: 79-80.

24. Iezzoni LI, Moskowitz MA. Clinical overlap among medical diagnosis-related groups. *JAMA.* 1986;**255**:927-9.

25. Gonnella JS. Case mix classification: the need to reduce inappropriate homogeneity [Editorial]. *JAMA.* 1986;**255**:941-2.

26. Young WW. Substitution permissible [Editorial]. *JAMA.* 1986;**255**:942-3.

27. Jencks SF, Dobson A. Refining case-mix adjustment: the research evidence. *N Engl J Med.* 1987;**317**:679-86.

28. Cretin S, Worthman LG. *Alternative Systems for Case Mix Classification in Health Care Financing.* Santa Monica, California: The Rand Corporation (R-3457-HCFA);1986.

29. Health Care Financing Administration, Office of Research and Demonstrations. *Report to Congress: DRG Refinement: Outliers, Severity of Illness, and Intensity of Care.* Baltimore:U.S. Department of Health and Human Service (HCFA pub. no. 03254);1987:15.

30. Vladeck BC. Quality assurance through external controls. *Inquiry.* 1988;**25**:100-7.

31. McClure W. Competition and the pursuit of quality: a conversation with Walter McClure [interview by John K. Iglehart]. *Health Aff (Millwood).* 1988;**7**:79-90.

32. Roper WL, Hackbarth GM. HCFA's agenda for promoting high-quality care. *Health Aff (Millwood).* 1988;**7**:91-8.

33. Brinkley J. U.S. releasing lists of hospitals with abnormal mortality. *New York Times.* March 12, 1986:1.

34. Hornbrook MC. Hospital case mix: its definition, measurement and use: Part I. The conceptual framework. *Med Care Rev.* 1982;**39**:1-43.

35. Stein RE, Gortmaker SL, Perrin EC, et al. Severity of illness: concepts and measurements. *Lancet.* 1987;**2**:1506-9.

36. Blumberg MS. Risk adjusting health care outcomes: a methodologic review. *Med Care Rev.* 1986;**43**:351-93.

37. U.S. General Accounting Office. Medicare. *Improved Patient Outcome Analyses Could Enhance Quality Assessment.* Washington, DC (GAO/PEMD-88-23);1988.

38. Gonnella JS, Goran MJ. Quality of patient care — a measurement of change: the staging concept. *Med Care.* 1975;**13**:467-73.

39. Richards T, Lurie N, Rogers WH, Brook RH, Monsivais GI, Meredith L. *Measuring Case Mix and Quality of Care: Validity Studies for the Graduate Medical Education Study.* Santa Monica, California: Rand Corporation (R-3509 HHS);1987:65-78.

40. Hornbrook MC. Hospital case mix: its definition, measurement and use: Part II. Review of alternative measures. *Med Care Rev.* 1982;**39**:75-123.

41. Thomas JW, Ashcraft MLF, Zimmerman J. *An Evaluation of Alternative Severity of Illness Measures for Use by University Hospitals.* Ann Arbor, Michigan. Department of Health Services Management and Policy, School of Public Health, University of Michigan;1986.

42. McMahon LF Jr, Billi JE. Measurement of severity of illness and the Medicare prospective payment system: state of the art and future directions. *J Gen Intern Med.* 1988;**3**:482-90.

43. U.S. Public Health Service, Health Care Financing Administration. *The International Classification of Diseases, 9th Revision, Clinical Modification.* Washington, DC: U.S. Department of Health and Human Services (PHS 80-1260);1980.

44. Slee VN. The *International Classification of Diseases: ninth revision (ICD-9)* [Editorial]. *Ann Intern Med.* 1978; **88**:424-6.

45. Institute of Medicine. *Reliability of Hospital Discharge Abstracts.* Washington, DC: National Academy of Sciences; 1977.

46. Institute of Medicine. *Reliability of Medicare Hospital Discharge Records.* Washington, DC: National Academy of Sciences; 1977.

47. Simborg DW. DRG creep: a new hospital-acquired disease. *N Engl J Med.* 1981;**304**:1602-4.

48. Hsia DS, Krushat WM, Fagan AB, Tebutt JA, Kusserow RP. Accuracy of diagnostic coding for Medicare patients under the prospective-payment system. *N Engl J Med.* 1988;**318**:352-5.
49. Lloyd SS, Rissing JP. Physician and coding errors in patient records. *JAMA.* 1985;**254**:1330-6.
50. American Hospital Association. *ICD-9-CM Coding Handbook for Entry-Level Coders, With Answers.* Chicago: American Hospital Publishing, Inc.;1979.
51. Knaus WA, Zimmerman JE, Wagner DP, Draper EA, Lawrence DE. APACHE — acute physiology and chronic health evaluation: a physiologically based classification system. *Crit Care Med.* 1981;**9**:591-7.
52. Wagner DP, Draper EA. Acute physiology and chronic health evaluation (APACHE II) and Medicare reimbursement. *Health Care Financ Rev.* 1984; Suppl:91-105.
53. Wagner DP, Knaus WA, Draper EA. Statistical validation of a severity of illness measure. *Am J Public Health.* 1983;**73**:878-84.
54. Knaus WA, Draper EA, Wagner DP, Zimmerman JE. APACHE II: a severity of disease classification system. *Crit Care Med.* 1985;**13**:818-29.
55. Wagner DP, Knaus WA, Draper EA. Physiologic abnormalities and outcome from acute disease: evidence for a predictable relationship. *Arch Intern Med.* 1986;**146**:1389-96.
56. Knaus WA, Zimmerman JE. Prediction of outcome from intensive care. *Clinics Anaesthes.* 1985;**3**:811-29.
57. Wagner DP, Draper EA, Abizanda Campos R, et al. Initial international use of APACHE: an acute severity of disease measure. *Med Decis Making.* 1984;**4**:297-313.
58. Knaus WA, Draper EA, Wagner DP. Toward quality review in intensive care: the APACHE system. *QRB.* 1983;**9**:196-204.
59. Knaus WA, Draper EA, Wagner DP, Zimmerman JE. An evaluation of outcome from intensive care in major medical centers. *Ann Intern Med.* 1986;**104**:410-8.
60. Wagner DP, Knaus WA, Draper EA. Identification of low-risk monitor admissions to medical-surgical ICUs. *Chest.* 1987;**92**:423-8.
61. Wagner DP, Knaus WA, Draper EA. The case for adjusting hospital death rates for severity of illness. *Health Aff (Millwood).* 1986;**5**:148-53.
62. Daley J, Jencks S, Draper D, Lenhart G, Thomas N, Walker J. Predicting hospital-associated mortality for Medicare patients: a method for patients with stroke, pneumonia, acute myocardial infarction, and congestive heart failure. *JAMA.* 1988;**260**:3617-24.
63. Coulton CJ, McClish D, Doremus H, Powell S, Smookler S, Jackson DL. Implications of DRG payments for medical intensive care. *Med Care.* 1985;**23**:977-85.
64. Zimmerman JE, Knaus WA, Judson JA, et al. Patient selection for intensive care: a comparison of New Zealand and United States hospitals. *Crit Care Med.* 1988;**16**:318-26.
65. Horn SD. Physician profiling: how it can be misleading and what to do. *Consultant.* 1987;**27**:86-94.
66. Horn SD, Backofen JE. Ethical issues in the use of a prospective payment system: the issue of a severity of illness adjustment. *J Med Philos.* 1987;**12**:145-53.
67. Horn SD, Horn RA. The Computerized Severity Index: a new tool for case-mix management. *J Med Syst.* 1986;**10**:73-8.
68. Horn SD. Validity, reliability and implications of an index of inpatient severity of illness. *Med Care.* 1981;**19**:354-62.
69. Horn SD, Horn RA, Sharkey PD, Chambers AF. Severity of illness within DRGs: homogeneity study. *Med Care.* 1986;**24**:225-35.
70. Horn SD, Bulkley G, Sharkey PD, Chambers AF, Horn RA, Schramm CJ. Interhospital differences in severity of illness: problems for prospective payment based on diagnosis-related groups (DRGs). *N Engl J Med.* 1985;**313**:20-4.
71. Horn SD, Sharkey PD, Chambers AF, Horn RA. Severity of illness within DRGs: impact on prospective payment. *Am J Public Health.* 1985;**75**:1195-9.
72. Schumacher DN, Parker B, Kofie V, Munns JM. Severity of Illness Index and the Adverse Patient Occurrence Index: a reliability study and policy implications. *Med Care.* 1987;**25**:695-704.
73. Gonnella JS, Louis DZ, McCord JJ. The staging concept — an approach to the assessment of outcome of ambulatory care. *Med Care.* 1976;**14**:13-21.
74. Gonnella JS, Hornbrook MC, Louis DZ. Staging of disease: a case-mix measurement. *JAMA.* 1984;**251**:637-44.
75. Conklin JE, Lieberman JV, Barnes CA, Louis DZ. Disease staging; implications for hospital reimbursement and management. *Health Care Financ Rev.* 1984;Suppl:13-22.

76. Gonnella JS, ed. *Disease Staging Clinical Criteria.* Third edition. Santa Barbara, California: SysteMetrics/McGraw-Hill;1987.

77. Conklin JE, Houchens RL. *DRG refinement Using Measures of Disease Severity.* Santa Barbara, California: SysteMetrics/McGraw-Hill;1987.

78. SysteMetrics. *Disease Staging Q-Scale.* Santa Barbara, California: SysteMetrics/McGraw-Hill;1988.

79. Brewster AC, Jacobs CM, Bradbury RC. Classifying severity of illness using clinical findings. *Health Care Financ Rev.* 1984;Suppl:107-8.

80. Brewster AC, Karlin BG, Hyde LA, Jacobs CM, Bradbury RC, Chae YM. MEDISGRPS: a clinically based approach to classifying hospital patients at admission. *Inquiry.* 1985;**22**:377-87.

81. Iezzoni LI, Ash AS, Moskowitz MA. MedisGroups: a clinical and analytic assessment. Report prepared for the Health Care Financing Administration, Cooperative Agreement No. 18-C-98526/1-03. Boston: Health Care Research Unit, Boston University Medical Center; 1987.

82. Iezzoni LI, Moskowitz MA, Ash AS. The ability of MedisGroups and its clinical variables to predict cost and in-hospital death. Report prepared for the Health Care Financing Administration, Cooperative Agreement No. 18-C-98526/1-04. Boston: Health Care Research Unit, Boston University Medical Center; 1988.

83. Iezzoni LI, Moskowitz MA. A clinical assessment of MedisGroups. *JAMA.* 1988;**360**:3159-63.

84. Iezzoni LI, Ash AS, Cobb JL, Moskowitz MA. Admission MedisGroups score and the cost of hospitalizations. *Med Care.* 1988;**26**:1068-80.

85. Young WW. Incorporating severity of illness and comorbidity in case-mix measurement. *Health Care Financ Rev.* 1984;Suppl:23-31.

86. Pittsburgh Research Institute. *Information on Patient Management Categories.* Pittsburgh, Pennsylvania: Pittsburgh Research Institute; undated.

87. Young WW, Swinkola RB, Zorn DM. The measurement of hospital case mix. *Med Care.* 1982;**20**:501-12.

88. Young WW. *Measuring the Cost of Care Using Patient Management Categories. Final Report to the Health Care Financing Administration* (Grant No. 18-P-97063/3). Pittsburgh, Pennsylvania: Blue Cross of Western Pennsylvania, May 1985.

89. Richards T, Lurie N, Rogers WH, et al. *Measuring Case Mix and Quality of Care. Rater Training and Reliability in the Graduate Medical Education Study.* Santa Monica, California: Rand Corporation (R-3446-HHS);1987.

90. Charbonneau D, Ostrowski C, Poehner ET, et al. Validity and reliability issues in alternative patient classification systems. *Med Care.* 1988;**26**:800-13.

91. Eddy DM. Variations in physician practice: the role of uncertainty. *Health Aff (Millwood).* 1984;**3**:74-89.

92. Smyllie HC, Blendis LM, Armitage P. Observer disagreement in physical signs of the respiratory system. *Lancet.* 1965;**2**:412-3.

93. Raftery EB, Holland WW. Examination of the heart: an investigation into variation. *Am J Epidemiol.* 1967;**85**:438-44.

94. Wiener S, Nathanson M. Physical examination: frequently observed errors. *JAMA.* 1976;**236**:852-5.

95. Gjørup T, Bugge PM, Jensen AM. Interobserver variation in assessment of respiratory signs: physicians' guesses as to interobserver variation. *Acta Med Scand.* 1984;**216**:61-6.

96. Johnson JE, Carpenter JL. Medical house staff performance in physical examination. *Arch Intern Med.* 1986;**146**:937-41.

97. Himmelstein DU, Woolhandler S. Cost without benefit: administrative waste in U.S. health care. *N Engl J Med.* 1986;**314**:441-5.

COMMENTARY

The amiable community hospital internist and her chief of medicine are locked in a rancorous argument about practice patterns. The internist claims her patients are "sicker" than those of her colleagues, necessitating above-average expenditures and excessive (by two standard deviations from national data) lengths of stay. The wily chief pulls a report from his desk drawer detailing the internist's cases, which have now been codified using a new severity of illness case mix index. The internist is shocked to learn that more than 70% of her "sick patients" fall into a category normally reserved for patients considered to be only slightly ill. She retreats from the chief's office ashen-faced.

Perhaps a bit too melodramatic, yet this exchange of information is happening with increasing frequency across the country. Dr. Iezzoni continues on our theme of "the flow of information" as she expertly reviews five current measures of clinical severity and their use in quality assurance activities. As she says, "Because they seem to distinguish severity measures among patients, these data will receive clinical credibility never accorded the DRGs. Danger exists that these untested but clinically attractive data will be accorded greater weight than they deserve."

We believe that Dr. Iezzoni has been able to offer the reader, for the first time anywhere, a crisp discussion of these five systems often viewed with a mixture of skepticism and dread by clinicians. The inner machinery of the systems is explained for the nonexpert — not in an exposé-like format but in a clear and comprehensive fashion.

In a truly path-breaking section, Dr. Iezzoni outlines at least three major areas where these measures will have a great impact on clinical practice: the possibility of further standardization of the medical record; the extent to which the sequence and type of procedures could be used to influence patient severity scores; and the potential difficulties encountered by clinicians whose practices include a preponderance of patients with chronic disease — inadequately captured by the severity of illness scoring systems. Dr. Iezzoni correctly points out that these systems are potentially helpful but not complete screens for shortfalls in hospital quality.

In the conclusion, Dr. Iezzoni calls for physician insight and vigilance as to the limitations of these systems. In a recent editorial (1), one of the editors has suggested a battle plan to cope with these changes for clinicians, including: learning as much as possible about these systems; becoming involved in their hospitals' selection and implementation of a system; participating in coalitions whose primary focus is the evaluation of these systems in medical care purchasing; volunteering to participate in pilot projects for further refinements; and subjecting their own clinical performance to evaluation as soon as possible to provide adequate time for improvement.

Clearly, these severity of illness indices will be powerful tools for comparing clinical practice. They carry with them the potential for abuse (2). In the final analysis, physicians knowledgeable in their use will have an advantage with their practice directors and hospital presidents that their uninformed colleagues will lack. (The Editors)

References

1. Couch JB, Nash DB. Severity of illness measures: Opportunities for clinicians [editorial]. *Ann Intern Med.* 1988;**109**;771.
2. Horn SD, Horn RA, Moses HG. Profiles of physician practice and severity of illness. *Am J Public Health.* 1986;**76**:532-5.

Chapter 4

Hospital Mortality as an Indicator of Quality

ROBERT W. DUBOIS, MD, PhD

INTRODUCTION

On March 12, 1986, the *New York Times* published a landmark article titled: "U.S. Releasing Lists of Hospitals With Abnormal Mortality Rates" (1). Never before had a newspaper printed the names of hospitals with detailed descriptions of their death rates. These hospitals had death rates that were either higher or lower than expected. This article and related ones that followed implied that hospitals with higher-than-expected death rates might provide worse care than other hospitals.

Before this *New York Times*' story, discussions about the utility of modeling death rates appeared primarily in journals dealing with health services research. After publication of this article, death rates began to attract increasing attention among policymakers and consumers. It has become fairly common to peruse a local newspaper and find the death rates of hospitals in the area.

Do hospital death rates deserve this attention? Do studies support the assertion that hospitals with higher-than-expected death rates provide worse care? If the literature cannot firmly support or refute this assertion, how should practicing clinicians, hospital directors, and public policymakers deal with these increasingly common lists of death rates?

This chapter will address these and other issues pertaining to hospital mortality.

HISTORY OF DEATH RATES AND RATIONALE FOR THEIR USE

As mentioned above, death rates became a focus of attention after the *New York Times*' article. However, this was not the first time that mortality data received such notoriety. Over a century ago, Florence Nightingale drew attention to death rates to influence public policy decisions.

In 1854 Florence Nightingale joined the British forces in Crimea to help their sick and wounded. During her first winter, she documented a startling statistic: 46% of the soldiers who entered the army infirmaries died there. By publicizing this fact, she was able to mobilize support for her cause: to improve the infirmaries' hygiene, obtain more nurses, and provide better supervision and training (2).

In 1856 Nightingale returned to England. Her attention now focused on the British health care system, specifically the death rates of hospitals in London. She again discovered and publicized disturbing data; general hospitals had death rates of 7.9%, whereas death rates in workhouses and special hospitals were 9.4% and 11.5%, respectively (3). Prompted by these statistics, she asked questions that remain unanswered over a century later: Did the hospitals with high death rates care for sicker patients or did they provide a different standard of care?

More than 100 years ago, Florence Nightingale realized that a hospital's death rate may be influenced by the type of patients it admitted. She also hypothesized that hospital care might influence mortality. Today, researchers, policymakers, and consumers still wonder whether a hospital's death rate reflects the quality of care it provides. Although few studies have shown a definite relationship between unexpectedly high death rates and poor quality, other studies suggest that this relationship could exist.

Conceptually, if a hospital's quality affects its death rate, then some deaths must be preventable. Crudely stated, certain patients die in hospitals with higher-than-expected death rates who would not die in hospitals with lower-than-expected death rates. Four studies suggest that some deaths occur unnecessarily.

Rutstein and colleagues (4) developed a list of "sentinel health events," or medical conditions that should never occur if patients receive high-quality care. When they do occur, it implies that the patient had received inadequate care. For example, because proper immunizations protect patients against tetanus, this condition should never arise.

Rutstein and colleagues (4) also identified avoidable outcomes. They listed several surgical conditions that should never result in death, including elective tonsillectomies and elective hernia repairs. They suggested that if even a single patient dies after one of these procedures, one should ask why. In most instances, the response would probably be that the patient's death was unnecessary and untimely (4). These researchers presented a conceptual framework suggesting that some deaths occur unnecessarily, but they did not provide empiric data.

In contrast, Landefeld and associates (5) showed that some deaths could have been avoided. They reviewed 233 autopsies done by two Massachusetts hospitals. Eleven percent (26 of 233) of these autopsies were felt to have "major unexpected findings that would probably have led to a change in therapy and improved survival, had they been diagnosed before death" (5).

Landefeld and associates (5) provide empiric evidence that hospitals may have control over *some* of the deaths that occur within them. This study does not, however, provide data to determine how often preventable deaths occur. Landefeld's study hospitals did autopsies on a minority of patients who died (University Hospital, 37%; Community Hospital, 26%); these deaths may not be representative of all deaths. In general, physicians do autopsies on patients whose clinical course had peculiarities or where the diagnosis may have been uncertain. Therefore, the 11% rate of major unexpected findings cannot be used to suggest how often typical hospital deaths could be avoided.

Two studies (6,7) provide data about how often certain deaths may be prevented. The first study (6) examined deaths from asthma. The investigators reviewed the hospital care received by 35 patients who died from this condition and compared it with the care received by a sample of patients who survived. They found that 46% of the deaths from asthma were potentially avoidable and reflected inadequate monitoring (including failure to monitor arterial blood gas values) and inadequate use of nebulized beta agonists.

The final set of studies (7) examined deaths during childbirth. In the 1930s, the New York City Department of Health reviewed all pregnancy-related deaths. A committee of obstetricians examined women's hospital charts and where applicable interviewed the providers of care. They found that the physician or midwife could have prevented 47% of the deaths (7). In a related study (7), the New York Academy of Medicine examined maternal mortality in 67 hospitals. Excluding hospitals with less than 1,000 deliveries during this period, the rate of preventable maternal deaths varied almost sixfold: One hospital had a 14% rate of preventable deaths, another had an 82% rate of preventable deaths (7).

As a group, these studies provide some important evidence. First, some hospital deaths can probably be prevented. Second, certain hospitals have more preventable deaths than others. These studies do not show that hospitals with unexpectedly high death rates provide worse care. Rather, they provide the rationale to suggest that these hospitals *might* provide worse care.

USES OF MORTALITY DATA

In 1958 a new anesthetic agent, halothane, was introduced into clinical anesthesia. Soon thereafter, scattered reports of massive postoperative hepatic necrosis began to appear in the literature. By 1963 the manufacturer had issued a drug warning. In that same year, the National Academy of Sciences began investigating (8) the potential relationship between halothane anesthesia and massive hepatic necrosis. This investigation examined the surgical experience in 34 hospitals by reviewing 1 million operations that resulted in 17,000 deaths. The investigators concluded that halothane had an excellent record for safety, but in rare circumstances may have contributed to liver damage.

As a byproduct of this study, the investigators noticed a 24-fold difference in mortality rates among these hospitals. After adjusting the death rates for various factors (age, gender, prior operation, duration and severity of surgery, and physical status), a 3-fold variation in death rates persisted (8). What accounted for these differences? Was it inadequate adjustment for differences in the types of patients cared for by these hospitals or did certain of these hospitals provide different quality of care?

The observation that postoperative mortality rates varied significantly among hospitals in the National Halothane Study triggered a follow-up investigation (9,10). These investigators used a large database (Professional Activity Study of the Commission on Professional and Hospital Activities) to examine the surgical death rates in 1,224 hospitals. They built a model that used 15 variables to adjust for differences in surgical patients among hospitals. This model determined an expected death rate for each hospital that was compared with the hospital's actual death rate. They found that significant variability in surgical death rates persisted despite the detailed adjustment factors used in the modeling (9,10).

The National Halothane Study (8) and the Stanford Institutional Differences Study (10) examined surgical death rates. In a related endeavor, Williams (11) developed a model to investigate hospital deaths that occurred in the neonatal period. Using data from 504 California hospitals, he built a model that used newborn birth weight, gender, race, and plurality to determine an expected death rate for each hospital. His model explained most of the variability in perinatal mortality.

Unfortunately, the studies discussed thus far had a significant limitation: They could only provide information about surgical or neonatal deaths. These patients account for a very small portion of all in-hospital deaths. Most deaths occur in adults admitted with medical conditions.

In contrast, other studies (12-17) modeled death rates using data from nonsurgical and surgical patients. The models also used a wide array of variables to account for case mix, including age, gender, diagnosis, length of hospital stay, admission from a nursing home, and admission from an emergency department. Like the surgical and neonatal studies, these investigators determined a predicted death rate for each hospital and compared it with the actual death rate. Some hospitals had higher-than-expected death rates; others had lower-than-expected death rates.

The most widely discussed models have been developed by the Health Care Financing Administration (HCFA) (18). These models used the Medicare claims database, which has information from approximately 5,500 U.S. hospitals. The 1986 model used data aggregated to the hospital level and included the following variables: age, gender, race, average length of stay, and the proportion of admissions within certain frequent Diagnosis Related Groups (DRGs). The model explained 59% of the variance in mortality and determined an expected death rate for each hospital.

The model also identified several outlier hospitals where the actual death rate significantly differed from the expected death rate. As described above, the *New York Times* published this list of outlier hospitals. Unfortunately, the list was not carefully examined before publication. One hospital with an actual death rate that greatly exceeded its expected rate was a hospice, an oversight frequently sighted by HCFA's critics. Outlier hospitals with high death rates used this example to argue that their death rates merely reflected a sicker population.

It is interesting to note that the outlier hospitals with low death rates had less criticism about this model and its data. They felt that lower-than-expected death rates reflected high quality, and not merely healthy patients. At least one hospital even advertised these data. The Eisenhower Medical Center in California ran an advertisement in the *Los Angeles Times* that said: "If you are considering heart surgery, read this . . . the Eisenhower Medical Center had the lowest death rate in the country" (19).

From a methodologic view, the 1986 HCFA model had various flaws: aggregated data, inadequate adjustment for case mix, and no mechanism to identify deaths that occurred soon after discharge. In spite of these problems, the 1986 HCFA death rate release probably advanced the field more rapidly than any other previous study. Immediately after its publication, researchers, policymakers, and consumers began to ask that more data be analyzed more extensively. The HCFA responded by consulting with researchers, meeting with policy groups, and beginning the modeling anew.

By the fall of 1987, HCFA had developed a new, more statistically sophisticated model that examined not only in-hospital deaths, but also any death that occurred within 30 days of admission. Hospitals could not show lower death rates by transferring patients to a nursing home or another acute care hospital. The model also included various measures of patient complexity (hospital admission during the previous year and comorbid conditions). Before publishing these data, HCFA allowed each hospital to respond in writing and explain why their death rates were either higher or lower than expected. These responses were published with the data (20).

In spite of the methodologic improvements, various hospitals (usually the high outliers), researchers, and policymakers still argue that the data should be disregarded. The HCFA acknowledged the lack of severity of illness adjustment in its model, but felt that the publication provided important information to providers and consumers.

The 1988 HCFA mortality data model did not incorporate a severity of illness measure. However, HCFA has developed a medical records review instrument that will allow hospitals to determine more precise expected death rates for several key conditions (myocardial infarction, cerebrovascular accident, pneumonia). Using this instrument, hospitals would randomly select medical records of patients admitted with one of these conditions. Medical records personnel, nurses, or physicians would review the hospital course and collect the necessary historical information, physiologic measurements, findings on physical examination, and laboratory test results. They would insert these data into condition-specific equations that would determine the expected death rate for the hospital based on the illness severity of its patients.

The HCFA has begun pilot tests with these instruments and hopes to have them calibrated and validated in time for the next report. Outlier hospitals will then have the opportunity to respond scientifically to the mortality data by showing that they have sicker patients. If the high outlier hospital cannot document a sicker patient population, they will have to look very carefully at the care they provide.

The HCFA models identified hospitals where the actual death rate differed significantly from the expected rate. These studies posed the following question: Are there specific hospitals that potentially provide very high- or very low-quality care that should undergo closer examination? Here, death rates function as a screening tool.

Death rates have also been used to explore several other questions. First, do hospitals that perform high volumes of a given procedure have lower mortality rates for that procedure than hospitals performing lower volumes? Or as Flood (21,22) titled an article, "Does Practice Make Perfect?" This question has important policy ramifications. If practice does make perfect, then all hospitals should not perform all procedures. Rather certain procedures should be regionalized to selected sites (23).

Most studies that have addressed this issue used a similar methodologic approach. The investigators chose a surgical condition to study and a database from which to obtain relevant information. They built a death rate model with the typical adjustment variables (age, gender, race, and comorbid conditions). These models also incorporated a measure of volume, typically the yearly number of similar procedures performed by a hospital (24,25). Most studies found an inverse relationship between volume and death rate; hospitals that performed high volumes of a procedure had lower mortality. Coronary artery bypass surgery and intestinal operations showed strong relationships; stomach operations and repair of femur fractures did not (27,28).

Figure 1 shows many of these volume-outcome studies (18). Procedures that appear above the line have more studies showing the expected relationship than studies showing inconsistent findings. At a glance, only two procedures appear below the line. How should these studies be interpreted? Viewed in their entirety, the literature appears to support the hypothesized relationship. However, the interpretation of this phenomenon may not be straightforward.

Does practice make perfect? Do hospitals where higher volumes of a procedure are performed actually provide a better service, or do these hospitals merely attract healthier patients? Like all of the studies discussed, they did not use precise measures of illness severity. However, most of the study procedures are performed on an elective basis, and therefore the patients usually are clinically stable at the time of surgery. This would suggest that illness severity may not explain all of the discrepancies in surgical death rates.

If hospitals where high volumes of procedures are performed provide better care, who or what is the critical factor? Is it the surgeon for whom practice significantly improves skill (the data have been inconclusive in this regard)? Of is it the operating room staff, the intensive care unit (ICU) staff providing postoperative care, or another set of personnel? Perhaps, these hospitals can afford certain costly equipment that improves patient outcome? Similarly, does a threshold volume exist? Perhaps hospitals must perform a minimum number of procedures per year to achieve salutary effects. Beyond that threshold, additional procedures may provide no further improvement in outcome. The answers to these questions await further study.

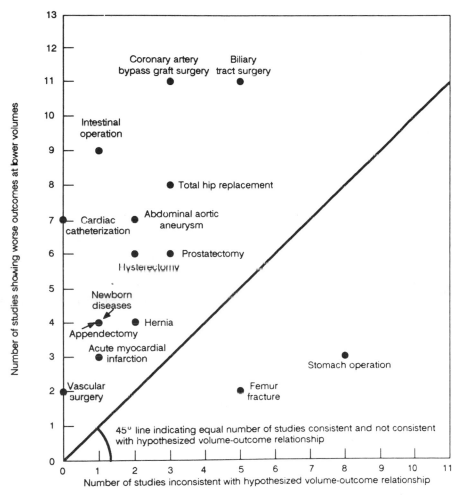

Figure 1. Number of studies showing either worse outcomes at low hospital volume or no effect. From U.S. Congress, Office of Technology Assessment. *The Quality of Medical Care: Information for Consumers*. Washington, DC: U.S. Government Printing Office, June 1988 (OTA-H-386).

Mortality data have been used to explore whether teaching hospitals achieve better outcomes than nonteaching hospitals. In a British study, Lipworth and coworkers (28) examined the death rates in a large series of hospitals. After adjusting for differences in age and gender, the death rates in the nonteaching hospitals exceeded those in the teaching hospitals for various conditions (ischemic heart disease, prostatic hypertrophy, and peptic ulcer disease). Whether this finding reflects better care or a different mix of patients is not known.

The last study (29) in this sampling of mortality models investigated whether cost-containment pressures influenced hospital performance. Shortell and Hughes (29) developed a death rate model based on 1983 to 1984 data from 981 hospitals. In addition to adjusting for case mix (similar to the models described above), they added variables dealing with state regulations. They found that hospitals in states with stringent certificate of need legislation and stringent programs to review hospital rates had higher death rates. These two regulatory activities were associated with a 5% increase in death rates (29). The study also examined whether a competitive environment had an adverse influence on hospital death rates. Using enrollment in health maintenance organizations (HMOs) as a proxy for local area competition (higher HMO enrollment suggests a more competitive environment), they found a significant relationship.

In summary, hospital death rates have been used to screen a group of hospitals and identify facilities that appear to provide very high- or very low-quality care; and to examine whether certain characteristics of hospitals or their environment are associated with improved health care outcomes.

BUILDING A DEATH RATE MODEL

The results derived from hospital death rate models can have far-reaching consequences. Hospitals with higher-than-expected death rates in HCFA's model became the focus of increased scrutiny. The HCFA formally asked them for explanations, and newspapers publicly questioned their performance. Potentially, these hospitals could lose market share or have lawsuits brought against them. Do death rate models have sufficient accuracy to allow these consequences? Similarly, death rate models suggest that hospitals that perform large volumes of coronary artery bypass surgery achieve better outcomes. Do death rate models have sufficient accuracy to allow policymakers to forbid hospitals from performing bypass surgery if they perform low volumes of that procedure?

With the potential impact of these models, it is critical that physicians, hospital administrators, insurance company executives, employers, and politicians understand their inherent strengths and limitations. This section will examine how death rate models are built, how outlier hospitals are identified, and how to differentiate appropriate use of mortality data from abuse.

The Database

All death rate studies begin with a database. The ideal database should include the elements shown in Table 1. However, no database has all of these capabilities. To understand why they lack certain key items, it is important to recall why these databases arose.

The typical database containing hospital information was developed by insurers, fiscal intermediaries, or the government to process and pay claims. Hospital personnel reviewed medical records and collected only that information that the payer required (patient name, social security number,

TABLE 1. Characteristics of an Ideal Database

1. Large number of hospitals
2. Large number of patients from each hospital
3. Many years of data
4. Accurate data
5. Patient age
6. Patient gender
7. Patient race
8. Patient socioeconomic status
9. Key historical data (admission comorbidities)
10. Diagnoses
11. Procedures performed during the hospitalization
12. Detailed clinical data (physical examination, laboratory studies)
13. Outcome (disability, death)
14. Hospital characteristics (nurse: bed, board certification %)
15. Be computerized

length of hospitalization, procedures performed). Until the advent of Medicare's Prospective Payment System, the diagnosis had little impact on payment; thus, it was not recorded. The reader should remember that hospitals collected and submitted data to facilitate reimbursement, not to provide information for mortality studies. For that reason, these databases contain little clinical information. Table 2 lists the elements in the Uniform Hospital Discharge Dataset, which represents the capability of most currently available databases.

Unfortunately, these databases have an additional limitation: The information contained within them may be inaccurate. These inaccuracies were carefully studied by The Institute of Medicine (IOM) during the 1970s. In these studies, a registered records administration reabstracted medical records from a series of hospitals. The investigators compared the reabstracted data with the data from the original discharge face sheet. On the positive side, they found excellent reliability for certain items: age (96% agreement), gender (99.5% agreement), and disposition (93% agreement). Unfortunately, in certain areas they found significant rates of disagreement. The procedure listed on the face sheet had 25% disagreement with the reabstracted procedure (30,31). The diagnosis showed even greater disparity. At the time of the IOM studies, hospitals used a four-digit diagnostic coding system. In this system, the fourth digit describes the diagnosis in greater detail than the third digit. The IOM study found 73% agreement at the third digit but only 63% agreement at the fourth digit (30,31).

TABLE 2. Elements in a Typical Computerized Database

1. Admission date
2. Discharge date
3. Date of birth (or age)
4. Gender
5. Race
6. Marital status
7. Principal expected source of payment
8. Additional expected source of payment
9. Patient disposition
10. Principal diagnosis (and secondary diagnoses)
11. Principal procedure (and secondary procedures)

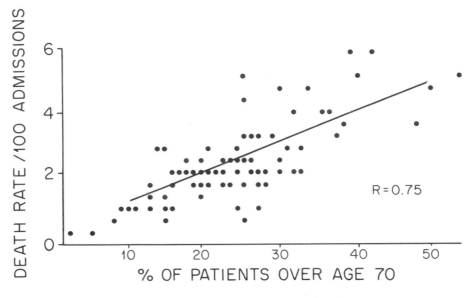

Figure 2. Hospital death rate as a function of the percent of patients who were over age 70 at admission. Reprinted with permission. Dubois RW, Brook RH, Rogers WH. Adjusted hospital death rates: a potential screen for quality of medical care. *Am J Public Health.* 1987;**77**:1162-6.

It could be argued that hospitals had little incentive to code diagnoses accurately during the 1970s because reimbursement did not depend on it. This changed in 1983 when the HCFA began the Prospective Payment System (PPS). Under PPS, HCFA paid hospitals on the basis of the patient's admission diagnosis (DRG). Thus, since 1983 hospitals had a financial incentive to more accurately list the diagnoses.

A recent study by the Inspector General (32) examined whether hospital discharge abstracts have become more accurate. They reabstracted 7,050 medical records from 239 hospitals. Once again, significance discrepancies were documented. The reabstracted DRG differed from the hospital DRG 20.8% of the time.

The studies by the IOM and the Inspector General showed frequent database errors in both procedure and diagnosis. The California Peer Review Organization (33) found that databases also contained inaccurate discharge status. Twenty-three percent of the patients in their sample who supposedly died in the hospital had been discharged alive.

These investigators have repeatedly shown that hospital records contain certain data that are accurate and other data that are not. This fact should persuade the reader to maintain a healthy skepticism when examining mortality information. Because both the diagnosis and the outcome (dead or alive) may be inaccurate, the diagnosis-specific death rate may be inaccurate as well.

A DEATH RATE MODEL CASE STUDY

This section will examine the mechanics of modeling death rates. A hospital death rate model developed by myself and my colleagues will be used as a case study. In brief, we obtained a computerized database, built a death rate model, and identified a group of outlier hospitals (16,17). The database for this study came from an investor-owned chain of 93 hospitals in the Western, Southwestern, and Southeastern United States. It contained all of the usual Uniform Hospital Discharge Data Set elements (Table 2) and a few additional items (admissions from a nursing home and admissions from an emergency department). The study used 205,000 admissions from a 6-month period in 1985. The data were aggregated to the hospital level.

Initial examination showed that the 93 hospitals differed in many ways: They ranged in size from 40 to 586 beds; had markedly differing proportions of nursing home patients (0% to 15%); had different patterns of admissions (admissions through the emergency department ranged from 0% to 58%); and had death rates that varied widely. Although the death rate for these hospitals averaged 2.3%, it varied almost 20-fold (0.3% to 5.8%).

We next explored whether hospitals with very high death rates differed in straightforward ways from hospitals with very low death rates. Several variables correlated with a hospital's death rate. Age had the strongest relationship ($r = 0.75$). As Figure 2 shows, hospitals with a higher percentage of elderly patients almost uniformly had higher death rates. This has strong clinical appeal because the elderly have less resilience to sickness and thus have a greater likelihood of dying in the hospital.

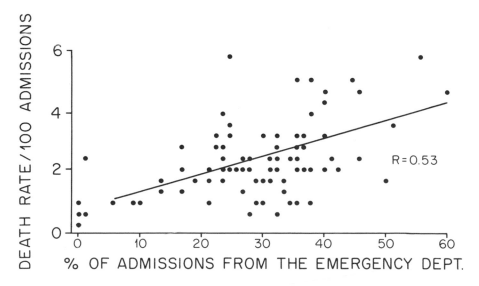

Figure 3. Hospital death rate as a function of the percent of patients admitted from the emergency department. Reprinted with permission. Dubois RW, Brook RH, Rogers WH. Adjusted hospital death rates: a potential screen for quality of medical care. *Am J Public Health.* 1987;77:1162-6.

Figure 3 shows a similar relationship between admissions from the emergency department and death rate ($r = 0.53$). This also has a clinical explanation: Patients admitted from an emergency department usually have a more guarded immediate prognosis than an electively scheduled patient. Thus, they also have a greater likelihood of an in-hospital death. We found two other variables that significantly correlated with the death rate: nursing home patients, $r = 0.29$; and hospital case mix index, $r = 0.55$). Once again, the statistical relationship reflected clinical expectations. Nursing home patients frequently have several, often chronic, medical problems, and higher case mix indices reflect greater need for resources and often more severely ill patients.

It is interesting to note where relationships did not occur. In this database, hospitals that cared for larger proportions of Medicaid patients did not have higher death rates. The univariate analysis showed four variables that *individually* were strongly associated with death rates. During the next analytic step, we combined these four variables using multivariate statistics (multiple regression) to develop our hospital death rate model (adjusted r-squared = 0.64). Using the coefficients from this model, we could predict the death rate for each of the 93 hospitals in the study.

Figure 4 compares each hospital's actual death rate with the model's predicted death rate. Most hospitals fell very close to the prediction line. However, death rates significantly exceeded their predicted value at 11 hospitals (high outliers) including one that exceeded its expected value by four standard deviations and another by five standard deviations. Nine hospital death rates

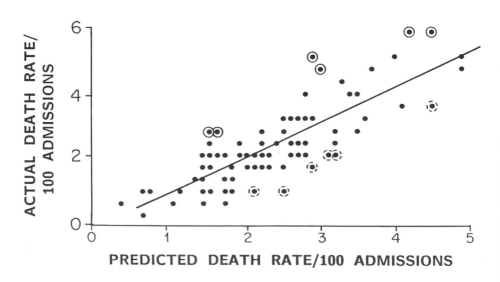

Figure 4. Predicted hospital death rate compared with actual hospital death rate. Reprinted with permission. Dubois RW, Brook RH, Rogers WH. Adjusted hospital death rates: a potential screen for quality of medical care. *Am J Public Health*. 1987;77:1162-6.

TABLE 3. Comparison of Death Rates within Specific Diagnostic Groups for High and Low Outlier Hospitals

Diagnosis	Death Rate			95% CI
	Low Outliers	High Outliers	High Outliers- Low Outliers	
Cerebrovascular accident	28/276	60/225		
DRG 14	0.10	0.27	0.17	0.10–0.24
Complicated respiratory infection*	10/59	30/90		
DRG 79	0.17	0.33	016	0.02–0.3
Pulmonary edema/respiratory failure	16/124	28/143		
DRG 87	0.13	0.19	0.06	−0.02–0.14
Simple pneumonia*	17/229	42/308		
DRG 89	0.07	0.17	0.10	0.04–0.16
Acute myocardial infarction	42/348	76/362		
DRG 121, 122, 123	0.12	0.21	0.09	0.03–0.15
Heart failure/shock	25/395	34/419		
DRG 127	0.06	0.08	0.02	0–0.04
Cardiac arrhythmias	6/267	10/151		
DRG 138, 139	0.02	0.07	0.05	0.01–0.09
Nutritional/metabolic	6/243	25/212		
DRG 296, 297, 298	0.02	0.12	0.10	0.06 0.14
Urinary tract infection	4/216	10/189		
DRG 320, 321, 322	0.02	0.05	0.03	−0.01–0.07
Septicemia: age > 17	14/74	32/93		
DRG 416	0.19	0.34	0.15	0.01–0.29

*Age greater than 70 years and/or complications and/or comorbidities.
Reprinted with permission. Dubois RW, Brook RH, Rogers WH. Adjusted hospital death rates: a potential for quality of medical care. *Am J Public Health*. 1987;77:1162-6.

fell significantly below the value predicted from the regression model (low outliers). Overall, there were 20 hospitals where actual death rates differed from predicted death rates by more than two standard deviations. Only 5 should be observed by chance alone.

Closer examination of the outlier hospitals showed that 49% of all deaths occurred within 10 diagnostic categories. In each of these categories, the death rate in the high outlier hospitals exceeded the death rate in the low outlier hospitals (Table 3). Why did these outlier hospitals arise? Over a century ago, Florence Nightingale suggested two possible explanations: They cared for a sicker group of patients or they provided worse quality care. Can outlier hospitals arise for other reasons?

CAUSES OF HOSPITAL DEATH RATE OUTLIERS

After HCFA's release of mortality data, high outlier hospitals claimed that they cared for sicker patients than other hospitals. Various policymakers questioned whether these hospitals might instead provide a lower standard of care. Too often, discussions about outlier hospitals focus only on these two explanations. Yet, at least four other explanations should be considered. This section will examine the most widely discussed and the most widely overlooked causes of death rates in outlier hospitals (Table 4).

TABLE 4. Causes of Death Rates in Outlier Hospitals

1. Statistical selection effects
2. Time frame (in-hospital compared with 30-day mortality)
3. Diagnostic coding errors
4. Severity of illness
5. Ethical decisions
6. Quality of care

First, outlier hospitals can arise due to statistical selection effects. In essence, death rates have a random component and a hospital could become an outlier due to these random events. A common clinical observation clarifies this concept. Clinicians frequently care for hospitalized patients who appear to have similar illnesses on admission and who also appear to receive similar therapy. Yet, sometimes these patients survive the hospitalization and at other times, for no obvious reason, they do not.

This observation suggests that an *individual* patient's chance of living or dying during hospitalization has a random or unpredictable component. If true, then a hospital's *overall* death rate must also have a random component. During some periods, patients who usually live will by random chance die in the hospital. Because mortality models choose hospitals where the death rate exceeds its predicted value, it seems logical that some outlier hospitals will arise merely due to bad luck. On an ongoing basis, they provide adequate care to moderately ill patients and will usually have an actual death rate that closely matches its expected death rate. Occasionally, however, the actual death rate will significantly exceed the expected death rate *by chance alone*.

To illustrate, a coin falls on heads, on average, 50% of the time. Periodically, a coin will fall on heads 10 times in a row. If every time a coin landed on heads 10 times in a row it was assumed to be "loaded," then a significant number of coins would be considered "loaded" coins when in fact they were not. Using this rationale, how many of the HCFA outliers arose due to chance?

Two methods can address these statistical selection effects. The first method examines the stability of an outlier hospital over time. If an outlier hospital arose due to bad luck alone, the death rate of that hospital should fall within the expected range during subsequent observation periods. The second method identifies the outlier hospital in 1 year (such as 1986) and examines the care provided in that facility during another year (1985 or 1987).

Second, outlier hospitals can arise due to the time frame selected for observation. Some models use in-hospital deaths (in-hospital mortality), whereas others use all deaths that occur within 30 days of hospital admission, regardless of where that death actually occurs (30-day mortality). If the model uses in-hospital deaths, then discharge practices could greatly affect the results. Does the hospital transfer its most ill patients to a referral center? If so, many of these patients will die in another hospital. The transferring hospital will maintain a low death rate despite its ill patients.

The availability of nursing homes and family wishes may also determine where the patient dies. If a hospital routinely discharges its terminally ill patients to a local nursing home, its in-hospital death rate will remain low. Another hospital that either has no nearby nursing home or where the patients choose to spend their final days in the hospital may have an extremely high death rate.

Thirty-day mortality rates have been used as an alternative to in-hospital death rates. This statistic means that deaths that occur within 30 days of admission in any other setting, are attributed to the admitting hospital. Unfortunately, 30-day mortality rates have limitations. Deaths that occur after the patient leaves the hospital may not reflect the quality of care rendered by that hospital. Certainly, discharging a patient prematurely from the hospital can lead to an undesirable outcome. But, other factors determine the patient's health 2 weeks after discharge, including the follow-up care rendered by the physician, patient compliance with prescribed treatment plans, and whether the patient returns for care if new symptoms arise. The hospital may have little control over these events. No study has determined how often deaths after discharge reflect poor antecedent care and how often they reflect nonhospital factors.

In summary, hospital death rate models have routinely used either in-hospital or 30-day death rates. Problems can arise with either outcome variable. As a solution, HCFA or another agency should examine the stability of the hospital rankings before publishing the information. Does a hospital's performance vary significantly between a model that uses in-hospital death rates from one that uses 30-day death rates? It would be unwise to implicate quality as the primary factor if the hospital appears as an outlier using one model but within the expected range using the other model.

Third, outlier hospitals can arise due to diagnostic coding errors. Inaccurate hospital discharge abstracts can arise from errors by physicians or medical records personnel. It is not known who has responsibility for most of them. As discussed above, various studies have documented that hospital discharge abstracts frequently contain errors. For example, a discharge abstract may indicate that a patient was hospitalized with pneumonia, when the patient actually had bronchitis, an illness with lower expected mortality. Similarly, physicians and hospitals may interchange the terms asthma and chronic obstructive pulmonary disease when these two conditions have different pathophysiologies and very different short- and long-term outcomes.

As a numeric example, two hospitals care for similar patients; 100 have a stroke and 100 have a transient ischemic attack. Twenty of the stroke patients die in each hospital, whereas none of the transient ischemic attack patients die. The physician and medical records department *should* differentiate the patients with a stroke from those with a transient ischemic attack. However, the first hospital separates these two groups and has a stroke death rate of 20%. The other hospital labels both conditions "stroke" and has a death rate of 10%. This hospital could appear inappropriately on the low end of a death rate list.

In the second phase of our hospital death rate study, we examined the medical records from six high outlier hospitals and six low outlier hospitals. We used the following diagnostic criteria for patients admitted with stroke:

TABLE 5. Clinical Findings in High and Low Outlier Hospitals

Clinical Findings	High Outliers	Low Outliers
Cerebrovascular accident		
APACHE II score*	14.9†	12.1
Glasgow coma score*	2.8‡	1.5
Heart rate	89	83
Age	78	75
Body-system score§	1.7	1.3
Mass effect on head CT scan (prevalence)*	0.09‡	0.02
Pneumonia		
APACHE II score*	16.2†	13.4
Heart rate	99†	87
Respiratory rate	28†	24
Age	76	75
Body-system score§	1.9	1.7
Myocardial infarction		
APACHE II score*	14.8†	11.4
Heart rate	85†	93
Respiratory rate	21	20
Age	72	71
Killip class*	1.35	1.34
Body-system score§	1.4	1.5

*A higher score indicates a greater severity of illness at the time of admission.
†Significant at $P<0.05$.
‡Significant at $P<0.10$.
§Number of body systems affected by the patient's comorbid conditions.
Reprinted with permission. Dubois RW, Rogers WH, Moxley JH, Draper D, Brook RH. Hospital inpatient mortality: is it a predictor of quality? *N Engl J Med.* 1987;**317**:1674-80.

acute onset of symptoms (over minutes to hours), a neurologic deficit that lasted at least 24 hours, and a presumed vascular cause. To be classified as a stroke, the case needed to meet all three diagnostic criteria. We found that approximately 20% of the cases listed as a "stroke" did not meet these criteria. However, in this study, the rate of misclassification did not differ significantly between the high and low outlier groups (17). Despite our finding similar rates of diagnostic misclassification, a hospital could potentially become an outlier because of inaccurate listing of diagnoses.

Fourth, outlier hospitals can arise due to unmeasured severity of illness. Theoretically, hospitals that care for sicker patients will have higher death rates. Furthermore, current death rate models do not adjust for severity of illness; they merely use proxies such as age, admission from a nursing home, or comorbidity. These latter measures cannot fully describe a patient's likelihood of death during a hospital stay. This task requires more detailed data.

Several studies have examined whether hospitals with high and low death rates care for different types of patients. In one study, Pollack and coworkers (34) found that unadjusted death rates varied almost sixfold (3% to 17.5%) among nine neonatal ICUs. However, patients in these neonatal ICUs differed greatly, with average age ranging from 15 to 36 months, medical admissions ranging from 39% to 81%, and the percentage of patients with serious underlying chronic disease ranging from 18% to 48%. They also collected severity of illness data from 2,394 patients and found marked differences among hospitals. Using a severity of illness measure (Physiologic Stability Index), the sixfold difference in death rates vanished; the actual death rate for each neonatal ICU closely matched the value predicted from the model (34).

Our mortality study addressed severity of illness in a similar manner (17). We reviewed patients' medical records from a set of outlier hospitals in which the actual death rate differed greatly from the rate predicted by our demographic and diagnostic model. We reviewed cases of stroke, pneumonia, and myocardial infarction because they accounted for a large fraction (36%) of deaths in outlier hospitals. For each of these conditions, the death rate in the high outlier hospitals was approximately twice the death rate in the low outlier hospitals. We reviewed medical records, tabulated the patients' comorbid conditions, and quantified the severity of their illnesses at hospital admission.

For example, we obtained the following information from medical records of patients admitted with stroke: admission comorbidity, evidence of mass effect on cranial computed tomography (CT) scan, and an APACHE II score. APACHE II is a severity-of-illness measure that incorporates the most abnormal value within the first 24 hours after admission for 12 objective physiologic variables (for example, heart rate, blood pressure, serum potassium level, and serum pH). APACHE II also uses age and the presence of severe chronic disease. For patients with pneumonia and myocardial infarction, we collected similar information. This clinical information showed impressive differences in patient populations between the high and low outlier hospitals (Table 5).

We used this information to build a more clinically accurate model. The predictions from this model closely matched the actual hospital death rates. Most of the twofold difference in death rates between the high and low outliers disappeared with better adjustment for severity of illness (Table 6).

TABLE 6. Hospital Death Rates in High and Low Outlier Hospitals Adjusted for Complexity and Severity of Illness

Condition	Outlier	Actual Death Rate	Predicted Death Rate*	Actual/Predicted Death Rate*
		%	% (CI)†	
Cerebrovascular accident	High	22	20.8 (17.3–24.3)	1.05 (0.73–1.37)
	Low	10	11.7 (5.9–17.5)	0.85 (0.51–1.19)
Pneumonia	High	18	17.5 (15.9–19.1)	1.03 (0.93–1.13)
	Low	9	10 (7.7–12.3)	0.90 (0.7–1.1)
Myocardial infarction	High	21	19 (16.9–21.1)	1.10 (0.96–1.24)
	Low	12	13.9 (11.9–15.9)	0.86 (0.74–0.98)

*The predicted death rate was derived from a logistic-regression model based on the comorbidity and severity of illness of the patients.
†CI denotes confidence interval (±1.96 SE).
Reprinted with permission. Dubois RW, Rogers WH, Moxley JH, Draper D, Brook RH. Hospital patient mortality: is it a predictor of quality? N Engl J Med. 1987;317:1674-80.

These results suggest that the hospitals in our study that had higher death rates than expected cared for sicker patients than the hospitals with death rates that were lower than expected. Although this clinical model explained most of the differences in death rates between the high and low outlier hospitals, it did not account for all the differences. For each condition, the actual death rate exceeded the rate predicted on the basis of the case complexity at the high outlier hospitals by 3% to 10% and fell short of the predicted rate at the low outlier hospitals by 10% to 15%. Thus, after we used substantial clinical information to control for severity of illness, an excess of mortality at the high outlier hospitals and a shortfall at the low outlier hospitals of about 10% remained unexplained ($P < 0.01$) (17). Although we used several separate measures of severity for each condition, the observed difference in death rates in this study may still reflect unmeasured severity of illness. In our judgment, however, after an adjustment for demographic characteristics and diagnoses at the hospital level, and a further adjustment for severity of illness at the patient level based on detailed clinical information, any differences in severity of illness that remain are probably small.

In our study, better adjustment for severity of illness explained most of the differences in death rates between the *group* of high and the *group* of low outlier hospitals. It is possible that an *individual* hospital could become an outlier due to its mix of patients. Our study examined the outliers as a group. Due to small sample sizes, we could not accurately predict condition-specific death rates for individual hospitals.

The fifth cause of outlier hospitals is more subtle. In some communities, families wish to bring their loved ones home to die. In other communities, families do not wish their loved ones to die at home or in a nursing home. Instead, they admit them to a hospital. These social or community differences may have an impact on a hospital's death rate.

Similarly, the "do not resuscitate" status of patients can influence a hospital's death rate. Patients with debilitating conditions or severe dementia frequently develop acute illnesses. Some families may want the hospital to provide aggressive care; others may not. A hospital would have a higher death rate if it allowed "do not resuscitate" patients to die. A hospital would have a lower death rate if it tried to resuscitate all patients, even those whose long-term functional status appeared grim. In our outlier study, we reviewed 182 deaths. Forty-nine percent of them had a "do not resuscitate" status. If the prevalence of "do not resuscitate" status varies significantly among hospitals, it may affect the outlier list (17).

Finally, a hospital could also become an outlier due to the care that it provides. Several studies have examined this relationship. Knaus and associates (35) reviewed the care and outcome in 13 ICUs. They used the APACHE II score to adjust for differences in severity of illness. One hospital had the lowest adjusted mortality rate (actual death rate/predicted death rate = 0.59). In that hospital, several indicators of very high-quality care were found. This hospital had a high therapeutic intervention score (more frequent dressing changes, chest physiotherapy, increased use of laboratory studies)

They also had a comprehensive nursing education program, 24-hour in-unit physician coverage, and a full-time ICU director.

In contrast, the hospital with the worst adjusted mortality rate (actual death rate/predicted death rate = 1.58) had neither 24-hour in-unit physician coverage nor a full-time unit director that participated in decisions regarding patient therapy. Knaus and associates (35) showed a relationship between death rates and quality.

In our study, we used two methods to compare the quality of care between high and low outlier hospitals (17). In the explicit (or structured) review, we developed a list of process of care criteria for the three conditions studied (myocardial infarction, pneumonia, and cerebrovascular accident). Each condition had approximately 125 separate quality of care criteria. Many of them used branching logic.

A physician collected information that allowed all the cases to be assessed according to the structured criteria. We compared the high and low outlier hospitals in terms of 31 process of care scales: 11 for pneumonia and 10 each for cerebrovascular accident and myocardial infarction. The results for high and low outlier hospitals did not significantly differ on 26 of 31 scales (Table 7). The results shown in Table 7 are not very different from what would have been expected with the hypothesis that there was no difference in the average process score between high and low outlier hospitals.

Our study also examined the quality of care in these hospitals using implicit or subjective review. One physician reviewed and dictated case summaries

TABLE 7. Relation of Hospital Outlier Status to the Quality of Care as Judged by Explicit Process Scales*

Process Scale	Cerebrovascular Accident	Pneumonia	Myocardial Infarction
Admission history	H	L†	H
Admission physical examination	H	L	H
Admission laboratory tests	L†	H	L
Initial therapy	L	L	H
Choice of antibiotic	NA	H	NA
Management of new symptoms	H	L	H
Management of abnormal laboratory values	H	L	L
Adverse-outcome scales‡			
Laboratory intensity	H†	H	L
Treatment intensity	H	H†	L
Follow-up of abnormal laboratory results	H†	H	L
Doctor-nurse interaction	H	H	L

*H indicates that high outlier hospitals had better process scores than low outlier hospitals, L indicates that low outlier hospitals had better process scores than high outlier hospitals, and NA denotes not applicable.
† Statistically significant at $P<0.05$.
‡ Adverse-outcome scales apply only to patients who died and reflect the process of care during the 24 hours before death.
Reprinted with permission. Dubois RW, Rogers WH, Moxley JH, Draper D, Brook RH. Hospital patient mortality: is it a predictor of quality? *N Engl J Med.* 1987;**317**:1674-80.

TABLE 8. Preventable Deaths in High and Low Outlier Hospitals

Outlier	Condition			All Three Conditions
	Cerebro-vascular Accident	Pneumonia	Myocardial Infarction	
High				
Rate of preventable death among patients who died	6/25 (24%)	14/44 (32%)*	11/37 (30%)	31/106 (29%)
Estimated rate of preventable death in total patient population†	5.8%*	5.5%*	5.7%	5.7*
Low				
Rate of preventable death among patients who died	3/25 (12%)	3/26 (12%)*	12/25 (48%)	18/76 (24%)
Estimated death of preventable death in total patient population†	1.2%*	1.0%*	6.7%	3.2%*

*The difference between the values in the high and low outlier hospitals was significant at $P<0.05$.
†This rate reflects the probability of a preventable death among all patients admitted with this condition (adjusted for severity of illness).
Reprinted with permission. Dubois RW, Rogers WH, Moxley JH, Draper D, Brook RH. Hospital inpatient mortality: is it a predictor of quality? *N Engl J Med.* 1987;**317**:1674-80.

of 182 patients who died during hospitalization. These case summaries were evaluated by one of three expert panels (on cerebrovascular accident, pneumonia, and myocardial infarction). At least three panel members reviewed each case summary. The reviewers evaluated the hospital stay and judged whether the death might have been prevented. The panel members were instructed to focus only on the care received by the patient after arrival at the outlier hospital or its emergency department. The expert panels determined that 9 of 50 (18%) deaths due to cerebrovascular accident, 17 of 70 (24%) deaths due to pneumonia, and 23 of 62 (37%) deaths due to myocardial infarction were possibly preventable (36).

For patients with myocardial infarction, the study showed no difference in the rate of preventable deaths between the high and low outlier hospitals. However, for patients with cerebrovascular accident, pneumonia, and all three conditions combined, the study showed a significantly higher rate of preventable deaths in the high outlier hospitals. Thus, of 100 patients admitted with pneumonia to a low outlier hospital, about 1 would be expected to have a preventable death. Alternatively, of the same 100 patients admitted to a high outlier hospital, about 5 would be expected to have a preventable death (Table 8 and statistical appendix).

In summary, we found differences in quality between the high and the low outlier hospitals using implicit assessments, but found no significant difference for any condition with explicit criteria. This discrepancy has several potential explanations.

First, the discrepancy between the structured and subjective reviews of quality may reflect differences in emphasis of these two techniques. Structure reviews stress compliance with specified criteria, whereas subjective reviews allow physicians to use their judgment in an unspecified manner. Other investigators have found similar discrepancies between structured and subjective process reviews of the same case.

Second, the structured approach may have lacked adequate sensitivity to detect a difference. One patient died soon after a feeding tube was inadvertently introduced into the right lung instead of the stomach. The structured review had 125 criteria, none of which dealt with this event. In other cases, preventable deaths may have occurred in patients who became hypoxic and did not receive a timely workup or treatment. In these instances, the patients had become lethargic or their complexions had become dusky. Our structured criteria defined the need for intervention based on more precise clinical features, such as a rapid respiratory rate, which may not have occurred or may not have been documented. Thus, by their very nature, structured and subjective reviews may differ in their ability to identify certain errors in performance.

This study provided the first evidence that high outlier hospitals might provide a lower standard of care than low outlier hospitals. At least for one group of hospitals, a death rate model differentiated hospitals that provided different types of care.

The above discussion identified six reasons why outlier hospitals might arise. It should be understood that not all outlier hospitals arise for the same reasons. One hospital with higher-than-expected death rates may have sicker patients; another might provide worse care; and a third may have somewhat sicker patients and provide somewhat worse care.

WHAT HAPPENS AFTER OUTLIER HOSPITALS ARE IDENTIFIED?

As shown in Table 4, there are at least six reasons to explain why a hospital's actual death rate differed from its expected death rate. To understand which reason (or reasons) applies to an individual hospital, the following activities should be done. First, examine intertemporal stability. Does the hospital remain an outlier when examined during two separate periods? If so, then the hospital's outlier status did not arise due to random events or what was termed statistical selection effects. Next, compare the hospital's ranking using in-hospital and 30-day mortality. Does the hospital have a similar ranking using both end-points? If not, then one of the explanations discussed previously may apply.

After performing these two analyses, medical records must be examined. Using criteria to exclude cases that do not have the relevant diagnosis, what is the "true" death rate for that condition? A hospital's death rate may no longer fall outside of the expected range.

The next step involves adjusting for severity of illness. As described above, ＾FA has developed a medical records abstraction instrument. If successful, ﾟitals could use this instrument to collect clinical values and could calculate an expected death rate for their patients. Comparison of the actual death rate with the expected death rate will allow the hospital to determine whether sick patients accounted for the initial discrepancy.

A hospital should also examine how many deaths occurred in patients with "do not resuscitate" orders at admission. Finally, the hospital or review group should assess the process of care provided to its patients. This could entail an implicit review of deaths or an explicit review of randomly sampled admissions.

HOSPITAL DEATH RATES: REFLECTIONS AND PREDICTIONS

In 1856 few individuals besides Florence Nightingale knew that death rates significantly differed among hospitals. Today, most health care policymakers, providers, and purchasers understand that these differences exist. Why these differences exist is less understood. In this environment, the following situations have become increasingly common: A hospital administrator needs to respond to government inquiries about a hospital's high death rate; a patient has elective surgery scheduled in a hospital that the local newspaper recently listed as a high outlier; and a physician is asked by the hospital administrator or by a patient to explain what these death rates mean.

As discussed earlier, outlier hospitals arise for many reasons, including hospital discharge practices, ethical choices by patients and their families, case mix, and quality of care. To respond appropriately to each of the situations listed above, an individual must systematically pursue each possibility. In essence, hospital death rate models merely raise a flag over certain facilities that need further investigation.

This chapter has identified various situations where a hospital with a higher-than-expected death rate might not provide inadequate care. In other words, the death rate screen has a false-positive rate. These same death rate screens also have false-negative determinations; that is, there are hospitals that provide poor care but whose death rates do not significantly differ from expected. A hospital might provide poor care but also have a relatively healthy patient population. These two factors could produce a death rate that falls very close to that predicted by the model. Users of mortality data must understand that current models can falsely incriminate and falsely exonerate hospitals.

Future models will inevitably have greater capabilities. As an example, death rate models currently lack measures of severity of illness. During the next several years, this may change as hospitals pressure the government to give them higher payments for sicker patients. Under the current Prospective Reimbursement System, hospitals receive similar payments for all patients with the same admission diagnosis. Yet, in most instances, sicker patients need more (and more costly) services. If hospitals begin to collect clinic data to substantiate higher reimbursements (that is, a severity-adjusted DRG), this same information could be used to build more sophisticated death rate models.

Future models will also have wider uses. Currently, HCFA releases mortality data by hospital. This same modeling process could also be applied to individual surgeons performing coronary artery bypass surgery or individual cardiologists providing care to patients with myocardial infarction. Once again, the models would determine a predicted death rate, only this time by physician. Outlier physicians would have death rates that significantly differed from expected.

Various limitations (small sample sizes and no measure of severity of illness) make physician-specific death rates currently inappropriate. However, in the not too distant future, local newspapers may well publish the actual and predicted death rates for physicians in key specialties.

Although widely publicized, mortality data probably have not influenced many health care decisions; however, this will change. Today, HMOs and preferred provider organizations (PPOs) use cost as the primary criterion in choosing hospitals, because no well-accepted measures of quality exist. However, as mortality models become more sophisticated, these organizations may use this information in their choice of providers. Hospitals and physicians with higher-than-expected death rates may be excluded from provider networks.

Despite their inherent limitations, death rate models will inevitably have wider exposure and greater influence in the coming years. Purchasers and users of health care services want a system to identify high-quality providers to pursue and low-quality providers to avoid. At the very least, death rate models may represent a partial step toward achieving this goal.

STATISTICAL APPENDIX

This appendix clarifies the statistics used in Table 8, which compares rates of preventable deaths between the high and low outlier hospitals. The discussion will focus on cerebrovascular accident to provide an example of the rationale and calculations.

Six of twenty-five deaths due to cerebrovascular accident were possibly preventable in the high outlier hospitals compared with 3 of 25 in the low outlier hospitals. This difference, although suggestive, does not reach statistical significance due to the small denominators. Yet, on the population level (the proportion of all patients admitted with this condition who ultimately experience a preventable death), the difference between 5.8% in the high outlier hospitals and 1.2% in the low outlier hospitals becomes statistically significant. The statistical significance of the latter comparison reflects the larger effective denominators that arise as follows:

In the low outlier hospitals, there were 276 cerebrovascular accident admissions during the sample frame with 28 deaths ($28/276 = 10\%$ death rate for cerebrovascular accident). Of the 28 total deaths, we reviewed the medical records of 25 of them (and an equal number of patients who did not die). Thus, we have detailed knowledge about 50 of 276 cases. However, even though we did not review the medical records of the remaining 226 patients, we know critical information about 223 of them from the claims data review. We know that they *did not die*. Because they did not die, they could not have experienced a "preventable death."

By design, we greatly oversampled the deaths to collect the information about the cases that truly mattered. In essence, we sampled almost all of the cases that could have experienced a preventable death, namely the 25 of 28 patients who died. We did not need to examine the medical records of the patients who were discharged alive to know that they did not experience a preventable death. For statistical comparison, the effective denominator should not be 25 (the patients who died in the sample) but rather 246. The reasoning goes as follows:

1. The death rate in the low outlier hospitals was 10%, based on an effective sample size of 276 (28/276).

2. To determine preventability, we sampled 90% (25/28) of the deaths.

3. The effective sample size for the population rate of preventable deaths becomes 90% of 276 or 246.

Using similar reasoning, the effective cerebrovascular accident denominator for the high outlier hospitals was 119. With these denominators, the difference between the preventable death rate of 5.8% in the high outliers and 1.2% in the low outliers is statistically significant.

References

1. Brinkley J. U.S. releasing lists of hospitals with abnormal mortality rates. *New York Times*. March 12, 1986:1.
2. Smith FB. *Florence Nightingale: Reputation and Power*. London: Croom Helm Ltd;1982.
3. Cope Z. *Florence Nightingale and the Doctors*. Philadelphia: J.B. Lippincott Co.;1958.
4. Rutstein DD, Berenberg W, Chalmers TC, Child CG 3d, Fishman AP, Perrin EB. Measuring the quality of medical care: a clinical method. *N Engl J Med*. 1976;294:582-8.
5. Landefeld CS, Chren MM, Myers A, Geller R, Robbins S, Goldman L. Diagnostic yield of the autopsy in a university hospital and a community hospital. *N Engl J Med*. 1988;318:1249-54.
6. Eason J, Markowe HL. Controlled investigation of deaths from asthma in a hospital in the North East Thames region. *Br Med J [Clin Res]*. 1987;294:1255-8.
7. Donabedian A. *Explorations in Quality Assessment and Monitoring. Volume III: The Methods and Findings of Quality Assessment and Monitoring*. Ann Arbor, Michigan: Health Administration Press;1985.

8. Summary of the National Halothane Study: possible association between halothane anesthesia and postoperative hepatic necrosis. *JAMA*. 1966;197:775-88.
9. Moses LE, Mosteller F. Institutional differences in postoperative death rates: commentary on some of the findings of the National Halothane Study. *JAMA*. 1968;203:492-4.
10. Stanford Center for Health Care Research. *Study of Institutional Differences in Postoperative Mortality*. Springfield, Virginia: U.S. Department of Commerce, National Technical Information Service, December 15, 1974 (publication No. PB-250-940).
11. Williams RL. Measuring the effectiveness of perinatal medical care. *Med Care*. 1979;17:95-110.
12. Roemer MI, Moustafa AT, Hopkins CE. A proposed hospital quality index: hospital death rates adjusted for case severity. *Health Serv Res*. 1968;3:96-118.
13. Goss ME, Reed JI. Evaluating the quality of hospital care through severity-adjusted death rates: some pitfalls. *Med Care*. 1974;12:202-13.
14. Duckett SJ, Kristofferson SM. An index of hospital performance. *Med Care*. 1978;16:400-7.

15. Hebel JR, Kessler II, Mabuchi K, McCarter RJ. Assessment of hospital performance by use of death rates: a recent case history. *JAMA.* 1982;**248**:3131-5.
16. Dubois RW, Brook RH, Rogers WH. Adjusted hospital death rates: a potential screen for quality of medical care. *Am J Public Health.* 1987;**77**:1162-6.
17. Dubois RW, Rogers WH, Moxley JH 3d, Draper D, Brook RH. Hospital inpatient mortality: is it a predictor of quality? *N Engl J Med.* 1987;**317**:1674-80.
18. U.S. Congress, Office of Technology Assessment. *The Quality of Medical Care: Information for Consumers.* Washington, DC: U.S. Government Printing Office, June 1988 (OTA-H-386).
19. Advertisement. *Los Angeles Times.* June 2, 1987.
20. U.S. Department of Health and Human Services, Health Care Financing Administration. *Medicare Hospital Mortality Information, 1986.* Washington, DC: U.S. Government Printing Office; December 17, 1987.
21. Flood AB, Scott WR, Ewy W. Does practice make perfect? Part I: the relation between hospital volume and outcomes for selected diagnostic categories. *Med Care.* 1984;**22**:98-114.
22. Flood AB, Scott WR, Ewy W. Does practice make perfect? Part II: the relation between volume and outcomes and other hospital characteristics. *Med Care.* 1984;**22**:115-25.
23. Luft HS, Bunker JP, Enthoven AC. Should operations be regionalized? The empirical relation between surgical volume and mortality. *N Engl J Med.* 1979;**301**:1364-9.
24. Luft HS, Hunt SS. Evaluating individual hospital quality through outcome statistics. *JAMA.* 1986;**255**:2780-4.
25. Luft HS, Hunt SS, Maerki SC. The volume-outcome relationship: practice-makes-perfect or selective-referral patterns? *Health Serv Res.* 1987;**22**:157-82.
26. Showstack JA, Rosenfeld KE, Garnick DW, Luft HS, Schaffarzick RW, Fowles J. Association of volume with outcome of coronary artery bypass graft surgery: scheduled vs nonscheduled operations. *JAMA.* 1987;**257**:785-9.
27. Riley G, Lubitz J. Outcomes of surgery among the Medicare aged: surgical volume and mortality. *Health Care Financ Rev.* 1985;**7**:37-47.
28. Lipworth L, Lee JA, Morris JN. Case-fatality in teaching and non-teaching hospitals 1956-59. *Med Care (London).* 1963;**1**:71-6.a.
29. Shortell SM, Hughes EF. The effects of regulation, competition, and ownership on mortality rates among hospital inpatients. *N Engl J Med.* 1988;**318**:1100-7.
30. Demlo LK, Campbell PM, Brown SS. Reliability of information abstracted from patients' medical records. *Med Care.* 1978;**16**:995-1005.
31. Demlo LK, Campbell PM. Improving hospital discharge data: lessons from the National Hospital Discharge Survey. *Med Care.* 1981;**19**:1030-40.
32. Hsia DC, Krushat WM, Fagan AB, Tebbutt JA, Kusserow RP. Accuracy of diagnostic coding for Medicare patients under the prospective-payment system. *N Engl J Med.* 1988;**318**:352-5.
33. California Medical Review Inc., San Francisco, California. Premature discharge study prepared for the Health Care Financing Administration, U.S. Department of Health and Human Services, undated.
34. Pollack MM, Ruttimann UE, Getson PR. Accurate prediction of the outcome of pediatric intensive care: a new quantitative method. *N Engl J Med.* 1987;**316**:134-9.
35. Knaus WA, Draper EA, Wagner DP, Zimmerman JE. An evaluation of outcome from intensive care in major medical centers. *Ann Intern Med.* 1986;**104**:410-8.
36. Dubois RW, Brook RH. Preventable deaths: who, how often, and why? *Ann Intern Med.* 1988,**109**:582-9.

COMMENTARY

No doubt, many readers will find Dr. Dubois' chapter very unsettling. We believe, however, that his contribution is critical. He deftly cuts through the layers of publicity that surrounded the publication of his initial work on hospital mortality (1) and provides us with a clear description of his methods, results, and goals for his research.

Dubois explains that Florence Nightingale first drew attention to differences in hospital mortality more than a century ago. Today, building on his computerized database, Dubois and his colleagues at RAND were able to construct a death rate model for the study hospitals. Using a consensus panel of expert clinicians, albeit a flawed but widely accepted research method, he was able to retrospectively review representative patient cases and, in turn, assign hospitals to an "outlier" status for an excessive number of so-called preventable deaths.

Apparently, there are at least six contributing factors that may result in assigning a hospital to a high-death-rate, outlier, status. These include statistical selection effects; the time frame involved; diagnostic coding errors; severity of illness; ethical decisions; and the quality of care.

This kind of research is coming at a time when our country is beginning to compare hospital performance through the public release of nationwide mortality rates. "Today, we predict the risk of an acutely ill patient surviving treatment; tomorrow, the length and quality of that survival" (2).

There are some important caveats here. It appears that Dubois may be mired in synecdoche — judging an entire hospital's staff by a series of unfortunate cases or judging one clinician by some series of untoward patient events.

More frightening to many is the possibility that evaluation might one day include an objective and reproducible estimate of the patient's predicted mortality risk as a guide to therapy and clinical decision making (2). This raises the specter of a defacto rationing tool and cost containment programs based on "predicted" poor outcomes.

Lastly, predicting preventable deaths and ranking hospitals by their mortality rates may cause us to take a closer look at a more fundamental issue — the appropriateness of care. While newspaper headlines blare the trumpet of alarm (3), the work of Dubois and colleagues will allow for a more thoughtful review and questioning of some of medicine's most tightly held shibboleths. (The Editors)

References

1. Dubois RW, Roger WH, Moxley JH, Draper D, Brooks RH. Hospital inpatient mortality: is it a predictor of quality? *N Engl J Med.* 1987;**317**:1674-80.
2. Knaus WA, Nash DB. Predicting and evaluating patient outcomes. *Ann Intern Med.* 1988;**109**:521-2.
3. Drake DC. Medicine's jagged edge: volumes of unnecessary care. *The Philadelphia Inquirer.* September 19, 1988:1-8.

Chapter 5

Industrial Models of Quality Improvement

PAUL B. BATALDEN, MD
E. DAVID BUCHANAN

INTRODUCTION

Three years ago the Hospital Corporation of America initiated a process to adapt the concepts of continuous quality improvement to the way we manage the delivery of health services to our patients. The quality improvement process is based on principles that an increasing number of successful companies worldwide are initiating as the most effective method for raising quality and productivity while reducing the total cost of use of either service or product. The following discussion sets out the principles that support the quality improvement process with an emphasis on how they relate to the practices of physicians.

HEALTH CARE AND HOSPITALS TODAY

A new style is emerging in the American health care system. One characteristic of this style is the increasing impact of organizations on the way the system functions. Not only have financing and governmental entities adopted distinctly different roles regarding their policies affecting payment and regulation of the system, but the care process itself is evolving into new structures. Typically patient care requires coordinated efforts of many health care professionals and workers. More and more the quality and effectiveness of an individual practitioner depends on developing frictionless interfaces with the other components of the system. In addition, patients today are more inclined to ask "why," search for alternative interventions, and participate actively in care decisions when choices are available.

These factors increase the amount of accountability expected of the medical care system: accountability to patients in terms of quality, choice, and value;

accountability to external audiences including payers, employers, and regulators; and accountability to peers and coworkers for communication and participation.

In this environment of accountability rather than authority, a professional leadership opportunity for improvement is clearly desired and can be professionally satisfying as less time is required to cope with deficiencies of the system, and more time is available to do the things that matter most to patients. For many physicians the realization that they have helped things improve will be the most satisfying reward.

Commitment

The concept of quality improvement being adopted by organizations throughout the United States involves a few basic characteristics: The quality of service or product is determined from a careful understanding of the needs and expectations of "customers"; the organization's leaders have a responsibility for quality that cannot be delegated to a quality department or quality committee; the improvement of the quality of the product or service is continuous and neverending; and everyone in the organization is involved in improving quality because everything can be improved (1-4).

As we apply quality improvement techniques to the delivery of medical services, we should remember that the commitment to improve precedes attempts to measure current performance. It is common to assume the reverse, that measurement can drive the intent to improve. In practice, however, this merely leads to defensive maneuvering and self-justifying behaviors. The commitment to improve must determine the nature and content of the measurement process, not the reverse.

Quality improvement is a continuous process to understand the needs and expectations of customers and to search for ways they can be better met. It is proactive not reactive; it tries to get ahead of problems by preventing them rather than waiting until a problem has gotten out of hand. Although problems need to be solved, quality improvement is not just an exercise in problem solving. One veteran of quality improvement implementation notes that "problem solving" only gets you back to where you should have been in the first place. Quality improvement is what you do from there, taking a system that runs reasonably well and making it superior.

Quality improvement is not something to be done when a customer complains or the outputs do not meet the specifications. Quality improvement is a way of life. Participation is regular and ongoing, crises are prevented before they arise, the quality of output is predictable, and systems anticipate problems rather than react to them. The quality of the output is continuously improving and the customer's needs and expectations are known, met, and then exceeded.

In a quality improvement organization, improving quality is everyone's job. It is not something assigned to one person or a small group. Everybody has a part of the action and everybody works to improve the way his or her part of the process contributes to a better whole (5). Some individuals readily accept the concepts; others take longer. Quality improvement involves a change in how one gets through the day, week, or month. At the beginning some groups within an organization will be moving forward while others are still learning the basics. Eventually, however, everyone in the organization will need to participate for the full potential to be realized.

According to the leaders of this approach to quality improvement, a "statistical way of thinking" is necessary, even though the techniques often require little beyond basic arithmetic skills (6). A statistical way of thinking includes an understanding that variation is a natural part of every process and that, to understand the variation and be able to take appropriate action, it should be measured over time. (7,8). For example, a mortality rate of 7.5% that is consistently declining over the years is different from a rate of 7.5% that has been increasing for several years, and both are different from a rate that is erratic — one year at 2%, one year at 20% and another year at 7.5%. The pattern of the variation provides significant information for those who wish to improve quality.

THE ORIGINS OF QUALITY IMPROVEMENT

Before the 1920s when most manufacturing was done in small shops, the quality of work was monitored by the people running the production process or by an inspector here and there. As the industrial revolution settled into the assembly lines of mass production, however, the cost of having inspectors grew, and the idea of measuring samples and of statistical process control emerged as an alternative to inspection of every piece. The theory was refined during the 1930s and the concepts were widely adopted during the expansion of United States industry in support of the war effort of the early 1940s.

For some time after that the technology did not advance significantly in the United States. Many companies used statistical process control on their production lines, but there was no effort to use the concepts in the decision-making processes of management. Quality was the responsibility of the quality department, not an element of the strategic development of most companies (9).

Some say American industry was lulled into a false sense of superiority. After the war when most other industrialized countries were rebuilding their economies, demand for American products was high. Because energy was inexpensive and raw materials were readily accessible, American firms could produce a particular level of quality at a lower cost than other countries. Americans had a clear competitive advantage and no incentive to develop more efficient ways of doing business. Besides, there were technologic improvements that contributed to improved quality and lower costs. Not until the mid 1970s did it become apparent that others had been moving at a different pace, particularly the Japanese.

After the war American forces occupying Japan were anxious to help the Japanese economy and to make their industrial firms competitive with foreign suppliers. The Japanese in turn saw the occupation forces as a major potential customer and were striving to produce equipment according to American specifications. As a result several experts from the United States were invited to Japan to teach statistical process control to Japanese engineers. Among the earliest advisors to the Japanese were W. Edwards Deming, Joseph M. Juran, and somewhat later, Armand V. Feigenbaum, all respected experts in the application of statistical techniques to production processes (10).

That the Japanese were able to install the statistical process control technology in their emerging production lines and become suppliers to the American occupation force is not the story. Rather, with the guidance of their American advisors, the Japanese were able to see that quality meant more than just meeting the specifications for the physical characteristics of a part or a product. They understood that with their geographic and geologic handicaps they would need to find other ways to produce equivalent or greater quality at a price that met international competition if their economy was to grow.

Statistical process control was only the beginning of what has become a comprehensive approach to quality making in Japanese industry. The techniques they have discovered range from listening carefully to their customers, designing products that reflect and anticipate the customers' needs, designing manufacturing processes that are simple to operate and maintain, obtaining total involvement of the entire work force in continuously improving the systems within which they work, and applying these concepts to every aspect of the business — the planning, management, administrative, and service functions as well as operations and manufacturing. The sum of it has come to be known as Total Quality Control or organization-wide quality control and improvement. It is what improved the Japanese competitive position in international trade to the point that they now dominate the world market for a wide variety of products and, more recently, services (11,12).

There is a story about a group of Japanese businessmen who visited the United States in the early 1950s and were astonished by the sophistication of the modern American factories. A similar group of Japanese businessmen visited the United States 25 years later and were astonished again — this time by the fact that almost nothing had changed during the intervening period. While the Japanese were building an economy based on quality and the long-term success of their companies, Americans had adopted a management style that emphasized short-term gains to the near exclusion of long-term considerations. The failure to continuously improve the physical plant was the most obvious of management's focus on short-term financial returns (13).

American industry is now changing. Several major American firms directly adopted the model of quality making from their Japanese subsidiaries, and many others credit the Japanese origins of their new Total Quality Control programs. The literature has been dominated by Japanese authors or Americans who guided them. In June 1980, NBC television aired a 90-minute program titled "If Japan Can Why Can't We?". That program is often used to mark the beginning of the American resurgence of interest in quality; the last 15 minutes of the program were devoted to Dr. W. Edwards Deming (14).

The development of quality improvement at Hospital Corporation of America has been guided largely by the work of Dr. Deming. He was born in 1900 and at this writing still consults widely and conducts a 4-day seminar monthly. He understood that statistical process control alone was not sufficient to produce consistent quality. He convinced Japanese managers that it was important to listen to the customer, understand what the customer needed, and then make the best possible product to suit that need. In doing so he brought them a new and much more complex concept of "customer" that included an "internal" customer as well as the usual "external" customers (15).

Simply meeting specifications is not enough if better is possible. The Japanese learned to reduce the amount of waste by minimizing the number of times specifications are not met; make the product or deliver the service with such consistency and predictability that inspection and its costs can be reduced substantially and often avoided entirely; reduce warranty costs by preventing early failure of the product; and please the customer in the process. Dr. Deming also points up the unknown costs of poor quality. The most important of these costs is the amount of business that is lost because of the number of people one dissatisfied customer may tell about an unhappy experience with your service or product (16).

DEMING'S 14 POINTS

Dr. Deming has gathered his beliefs about quality improvement techniques into a set of principles that he refers to as "the 14 points" (17). He has said that if he had to reduce his message to managers to just a few words, "I'd say it all had to do with reducing variation" (18). His 14 points reflect his insights about the causes of variation and how to reduce it. The validity of the points is reinforced by the fact that they also express a good deal of common sense about the attitudes that should exist within an organization and the nature of the relationships that are seen among people in successful organizations. Dr. Deming may not have had hospitals and medical care in mind when these concepts were formulated, but health care professionals run organizations in very much the same way as any other endeavor that employs people, operates processes, and produces a service or product for an ultimate customer, in our case the patient. In this organizational context the 14 points are applicable to anyone, including the administrators and professionals who work in all types of health care organizations, a 500-bed hospital with 2000 employees, or a solo practitioner's four-person office staff. The 14 points are as follows:

1. Create Constancy of Purpose

Every organization involves people working together. Whatever the organization is able to produce depends on the interactions of these people.

This also applies to physicians, who rely on others to perform various tasks that support the goals for a patient. For these individuals to perform up to their capacity, however, they must understand what the goals are, and be committed to quality of service and quality of patient care. If that sounds platitudinous, consider how often physicians or other professionals think about these issues when they join organizations, apply for medical staff privileges, or seek a place in a professional partnership or group practice?

When physicians direct their own employees, is there clarity and constancy about the purpose of the practice? What is meant by quality? Are employees ready to act correctly when questions of finance and patient care intermingle? Or, is there the possibility that employees might not be certain about the intentions of the physicians or the organizations in which they work? What would the effect be if there was any uncertainty?

There is evidence that given a basic level of professional skill, the environment within which patient care is provided is the single most important determinant of a successful outcome for the patient. An environment that places quality above all other considerations is the one patients and other customers will choose.

2. Adopt the New Philosophy

If a physician has a specialty and has been successful in helping patients with a particular condition — heart disease, Parkinson disease, arthritis — the physician reinvests in further knowledge and improvements in performance because he or she knows that is the way to secure the future. These same attitudes can be incorporated into the entire process of patient care. Better value and quality always attract people whenever there is a choice.

3. Cease Dependence on Inspection

Physicians have always known that they could not inspect quality into the services they provided — they had to design quality in. Given this perspective it is ironic that at the same time American and other competitive firms who adopt the quality improvement process are searching for ways to reduce the amount of inspection, the medical care system sees a continually growing amount of it. Peer review organizations (PROs), the Joint Commission for the Accreditation of Healthcare Organizations (JCAHO), state licensing agencies, state data commissions, and so forth seem to be a major growth industry. Furthermore, the purpose of inspection in health care seems increasingly directed toward adversarial proceedings rather than toward data gathering for improvement and redesign. We seem to want to inspect to establish sanctions. That occurs in PROs, in state governments, and in hospital quality assurance programs, and makes things difficult for even the best intentioned physicians.

Some inspection will always be necessary in quality assurance: We must know that the services we create and deliver are provided as intended. Failing that test we must encourage people to use the inspection information to redesign what they do. The form of inspection that emphasizes redesign must be directly linked to what is important and necessary for the customers. Currently how do we test the customer-relevance of the inspection processes we maintain? Do we inspect the health care system to measure whether the needs and expectations of patients have been met? Do we design our inspection efforts to understand the nature and causes of variation so it can be reduced? Or, have we fallen into the trap of measuring and inspecting what is conveniently available in the form of data gathered for essentially other purposes? We must rethink how we should inspect and how we should use inspection — we have never been able to depend on it as the means to quality health care.

4. Cease Awarding Business on the Basis of Price Alone

The organizational issue here relates to the tendency of bureaucracies to believe they can write specifications that will exactly define the quality of items or materials to be purchased from vendors. They then buy from the bidder who meets the specifications at the lowest price. But in this kind of relationship between the vendor and the user, the vendor does not have a chance to understand how the item may be used and whether there would be a way to improve the specifications so that the item could be more suitable, last longer, or be made less expensively.

In this sense, physicians understand that the impact of an unsuspected defect or a premature failure can be significant and that the lowest direct cost may not result in the lowest cost in use. In addition physicians tend to be close to decisions about purchasing the materials used in the care of their patients.

The message that Dr. Deming brings to physicians is that the costs of purchasing from quality suppliers can be reduced by creating long-term relationships with them. If a supplier knows his customers are going to be there for a long time, a relationship can be established that allows each to help the other increase the quality of the product or service produced. These same notions apply to the schools. What if nursing, medical, and administrative schools were to take this notion so seriously that they regularly refocussed their curricula to enable each graduate to be fully "fit for use," to borrow Juran and Gryna's (19) concept, at the time of employment in health care? How much less cost would there be to the system?

5. Improve Continuously and Forever

What are the methods or systems currently used to improve clinical care? we have an organized method? Is it coherent? Continuing medical education can be a valuable contribution, but what is being done to improve the processes involving other professionals who must work with and, in many cases, support the physician in caring for patients?

Everything a physician does for a patient is mediated by a system. Just getting the patient into the office for a visit involves a system, and the performance of that system will affect the likelihood that the physician will meet with the patient at the moment it will do the most good. Prescribing a medication involves a system, and getting the medication into the patient is another system. Because patients often are the critical component of the system that implements a physician's clinical strategy, the physician's personal system for transmitting advice and information to the patient deserves attention; its effectiveness should be measured continually. Medical or surgical procedures involve elaborate systems including the rationale used to decide when the procedure is appropriate, its actual performance, and the organization of follow-up care. Every step of these processes represents a potential opportunity for improvement.

Quality improvement involves making systems better, that is, reducing the number of occasions when things go wrong as well as the chance that they can go wrong. This is done by the people who are part of the system. Working together they will know how the system can be improved. But to do so they must know who the users of the system are and what their needs and expectations are, and they must have permission from those responsible for the organizational setting to make continuous improvement a part of their job. This means creating a climate that fosters an interest in, "what can be improved?" rather than, "who is at fault?" Every year Toyota generates millions of suggestions for improvement from its work force, and most are implemented. What if we in health care did that?

6. Institute Training and Retraining on the Job

Training and retraining are basic to medicine. For the physician, education and retraining are an ongoing part of professional life. Observation, performance under supervision, and eventually the teaching of others are used by physicians to acquire and retain the knowledge necessary to perform at the highest level. But what about employees in the office and other professionals with whom physicians interact? Is there sufficient attention to their continual growth both in knowing their role in the process of care and how to improve it? In today's environment everyone must know how to improve the processes for which they are responsible and must cooperate with improving the many other processes with which they interact. Is everyone trained to do that?

A question worth considering — do your employees and the other professionals with whom you regularly work know how their actions and performance relate to the quality of the service provided by you, the physician? How have you helped them understand that?

7. Adopt and Institute Leadership

Dr. Deming has categorized the causes of poor quality in the many organizations for which he has consulted over the years. In his earlier work he said 85% of the problems are the responsibility of management and 15% are the fault of the employees. His more recent assessment, reflecting his increased involvement with service functions, is that the mix is 94% and 6%, respectively. It is not scientific, of course, but in the context of the entire concept it makes sense.

The workers do not decide to buy second-rate components from suppliers; the employees do not decide to ship material that does not meet specifications just so the supervisor's quota can be met and the bonus earned. Investments in training for employees, decisions about the quality of supervision, and the willingness to listen to employees suggestions and make improvements are responsibilities of management; all have big impacts on the quality of the final product or service. In relation to health care it should be clear that physicians are part of management and must fulfill the responsibilities assigned to that role.

8. Drive Out Fear

This principle follows directly from the preceding principle, especially with respect to physician involvement in the quality improvement process. Improvement occurs when there is a willingness among people to speak up when they make a mistake, offer suggestions when they see ways their work could be done better, and consult with people in other units on whom they depend for the flow of their work. All too often however, these things do not occur because of fear of criticism, ridicule, or even the security of one's job. Physicians sit on all sides of this balance, preferring not to acknowledge mistakes, blaming others when things go wrong, and reluctant to propose improvements that impact on the territory of others (or their own). Fear in one form or another can compromise the energies for improvement in any health care setting.

9. Break Down Barriers Between Staff

When a person in one department is overheard complaining about the quality of the work done by someone in another department, that is a sure sign a barrier exists. Such a comment should be addressed only to the person whose work is found unsatisfactory. "That's her job, not mine" also indicates barriers. Physicians are not immune. They need to participate in the kind of communication that eliminates barriers and allows each person in the care process to know whether his or her performance complements the next person's nd vice versa. Everyone must be willing to listen to learn how to improve or her own process and willing to speak up so others can improve theirs.

10. Eliminate Slogans, Exhortations, and Targets for the Work Force

Posters that say things like "Reduce Accidents" or "Improve Quality" communicate nothing. People who see them are offended because they imply that those people do not care whether accidents happen or are unconcerned about quality. Instead of slogans, solid information is needed about what management is doing to make things work better, such as supporting a team trying to understand the causes of medication errors, infections, or delays in the multitude of things in the medical care process that represent quality patient care only if they are done on time.

11. Eliminate Numerical Quotas for Workers and Numerical Goals for Managers

It is important to find constructive ways to use numbers. Numbers are the vehicle by which measurement occurs, and measurement is essential to understanding the current level of quality and how it might be improved. The caution arises when numbers are used both to reward and punish employees, managers, or professionals.

Medicine is beginning to produce various numbers that may create perverse incentives. Using information on hospital readmissions to understand why they occur and whether there are ways to prevent the morbidity they imply need not be threatening. Using essentially the same data to score the performance of an individual hospital or physician may cause the development of attitudes in which an indicated hospitalization would not occur because of concern that the monthly quota of readmissions has been used up.

The per case reimbursement systems such as Medicare's Diagnosis Related Groups (DRGs) also invite misuse of numbers, in this case expressed in monetary terms. When everyone is committed to improvement, numbers become powerful. In the absence of commitment they can significantly limit the improvement of quality and even be counterproductive.

12. Remove Barriers that Rob People of Pride in Workmanship

No reward can exceed the knowledge that the work you do is valued. Being able to take pride in one's accomplishments helps motivate even higher levels of achievement. No incentive compensation program can match that sense of pride. Physicians are in the best position to provide personal acknowledgment of the important contributions made by those who care for patients or support the care process. Allowing people to make suggestions and participate in finding solutions that lead to higher quality helps them be proud of what they do.

13. Institute a Vigorous Program of Education and Self-Improvement

Informed people are more likely to contribute constructively to the improvement process. Dr. Deming says you never know when a pertinent idea will be sparked by an individual's knowledge about an unrelated discipline. Every organization should promote the interests of all its people in expanding their horizons and gaining new knowledge and skills. A hospital or health care setting in which everyone is continually learning and in which a clear sense of what is to be done for the benefit of its patients exists has enormous energies for continual innovation and improvement — strong predictors of success and survival in an uncertain time.

14. Put Everybody in the Organization to Work on the Transformation

It is appropriate that this is the last of Dr. Deming's points because it borrows from all the others and is the call to action. Everyone must be involved in the process of improvement. Each process involves interactions among subprocesses and the people who run them. Physicians cannot be successful with their improvement efforts unless the nurses participate in those efforts, the record room can only do so much without the support of the medical staff, and so on. Unless everyone is involved no one can succeed.

In addition, everybody needs to be involved in the transformation because improvements come mostly in small steps. The most effective improvement processes will be those where everyone is working to make a small improvement, secure it so it does not backslide, and then make another improvement.

At first progress will seem slow and the newest technology will be more showy and maybe have a bigger short-term effect. A comparison of the American and Japanese auto industries is pertinent here. Businesses in both countries adopted essentially the same technologic improvements over 30 years or so; the Americans even had a head start. But the ultimate difference in their products was the 2% or 3% gain in annual quality and productivity the Japanese were able to achieve through devotion to all the little things. Put everyone to work on the transformation. It makes the difference.

CONTRASTING STORIES

The initial orientation to the Hospital Corporation of America quality improvement process is a 2-day workshop. Once the basic concepts have been introduced the participants are organized into small teams, and each team is asked to apply the new methods to design a quality improvement for a specific case which, while hypothetical in the details, draws on the experiences regularly encountered by people practicing or working in hospitals.

One of the cases regularly used relates to medication errors occurring in hospitals. Summary data are provided on the number of errors reported by the nursing departments over several months. The team is asked to develop a process to discover the causes of these medication errors, to propose a way to deal with whatever they find to be the most significant cause, and to devise a method to measure the effect of the improvement.

At one of these workshops a participant on the team assigned to this case had a background in hospital risk management. After the team had presented its report, he indicated disappointment in the design of the case. He said that some errors were inevitable and the rate of errors in this case was already as low as it was reasonable to expect.

However, the experience of the managers of a major U.S. electronics manufacturing firm contrast this view. In one of their domestic divisions a machine for soldering components to printed circuit boards was producing defective solder welds about 0.04% of the time and that rate was viewed as too high by the managers of the process. Various attempts were made to adjust the machine so that it would perform at a better rate, but these attempts were not successful and the managers asked for budget approval to buy a new machine. They said there was no way to prevent this machine from making defective welds.

The new equipment was expensive, and the request was carefully scrutinized by those responsible for approving capital expenditures; they finally agreed to make the purchase. The order was placed and the availability of the old machine was advertised to other divisions of the company at a bargain price.

This company had a division in another country, and this other division had begun to practice continuous quality improvement. During a visit to the United States the managers of this foreign division learned that the soldering machine was available as surplus. They looked it over and felt it might have potential. Because the price was right they decided to take a chance and had it shipped home.

Once the machine had been installed in the new site the managers and employees responsible for this equipment began to apply the process of continuous quality improvement to its operation; gradually the rate of defective connections began to decline. Their approach was to study every aspect of the process by which the connections were being soldered and to increase their understanding of the interactions of all the components of this process. They searched for the root causes of variation in the quality of the welds.

By modifying the frame and the clearance to the heat source, improving the quality and consistency of the raw materials used to make the solder, carefully assessing the actions of employees in the operation of the machine, improving training, allowing only a limited number of employees to perform certain critical tasks, changing the design of the circuit board, and making changes to the process only when it had been demonstrated that the thing being changed was responsible for defective welds, the rate of defectively soldered joints declined from 0.04% to 0.004% in 18 months and to 0.0003%

after 5 years. A 99% improvement in the rate of defective welds had been achieved.

Meanwhile the U.S. division purchased the new machine. Once the installation bugs had been worked out they were again able to produce soldered welds with a defect rate of 0.04%. Attempts to improve that rate were not successful. How long that condition may have continued will never be known because company-wide adoption of a quality improvement process patterned after the system now well established in the foreign division eventually allowed a comparable intervention to occur and gradually reduced the defect rate of this machine as well.

COMMENT

Without a quality improvement process there is a tendency to accept rates of defects or errors that may be far above what would be achievable with the quality improvement process in place. The similarity in the attitudes of our student and of the managers of the American division of the electronics firm is striking. Both were willing to assume that the current process was doing the best that was possible. Whether the application of a quality improvement process will produce a conclusion to the medication errors story comparable to that of the soldering machine example remains to be seen. However, until a systematic search for the root causes of medication errors comparable to the exhaustive examination of the reasons for soldering defects has been done, it is not acceptable to suggest that we are doing the best we can. In fact it is almost guaranteed that we are not.

PROCESSES

The quality improvement process incorporates the notion that the production of any service or product involves the operation of processes (20,21). Usually a series of processes follow each other in a sequence leading to the output that is perceived by the end user. Medical services are no exception to this concept as they typically involve a series of discreet steps that in sum constitute patient care. A process is composed of five elements: 1) Suppliers provide 2) inputs on which an 3) action produces 4) outputs for 5) customers.

An example of a process encountered in everyday medical practice follows:

Process	Fill a prescription
Supplier	Physician
Inputs	Prescription for medication
Action	Pharmacy fills prescription
Outputs	Medication
Customer	Patient

Many processes incorporate a series of subprocesses, each of which has five elements. In the pharmacy, for example, there is a process for ordering drugs, another for stocking them on the shelves, another for keeping records of each prescription filled, and so forth. These subprocesses interact in customer and supplier relationships, and all affect the quality of the service for the final external customer, the patient.

In the physician's diagnostic process there is a subprocess for performing laboratory tests and another for taking roentgenograms. In both cases the physician is the direct customer of the subprocess and the quality of his service depends on the quality of the outputs he receives from these subprocesses. The action components of these two processes are the responsibility of the technicians and the pathologist or radiologist.

THE ROLES OF CUSTOMERS

Having determined that improvement occurs in the action phase of the process, what are the roles of the customers and suppliers? Because quality is defined in terms of the needs and expectations of customers, the customer role is not difficult to discern. The more clearly and completely the customer can state his or her needs and expectations, the better the operator of the action phase can plan and manage the improvement process. It is essential that methods be established for acquiring knowledge about customer expectations and how well they are being met on a regular basis.

When the number of customers is large, for example, patients, a survey may be necessary. If the number is small, however, such as the physicians in a group practice who are the customers of the laboratory, more direct methods would be possible. The objective is to have the most complete and current understanding of customer needs when considering improvements.

External and Internal Customers

In determining how to relate to customers, it is useful to distinguish between external and internal customers. Traditionally we think of customers just in terms of the end users of the product or service. Drivers of cars are customers of automobile companies and patients are customers of the medical care system. However, when the production of the service is viewed as a series of subprocesses, each with its own "customer(s)," the term takes on new meaning. Although understanding the views of the ultimate end user is essential to the overall management of an organization and its quality improvement process, the design of specific improvements is more directly related to how well the people responsible for the action component of each subprocess are informed about the level of quality they are producing for the next subprocess (22).

In the above example the physician is the internal customer of the laboratory; it is the physician's view about how well the laboratory serves the physician's patient care process that will influence improvements in the laboratory. Every interaction between the various functions in an organization involves a customer, the quality of whose work is affected by the quality of the previous (sub)process (23).

THE ROLE OF THE SUPPLIER

The supplier provides the input for the process. The actions that are part of the process will be as efficacious as the quality of the incoming input permits. The prior care giver, for example, a nursing home, plays a major role in creating the conditions for success of the next care giver, perhaps a hospital. When the hospital supplies the processes that precede those offered by a nursing home, the roles are reversed and the hospital is the "supplier." Thinking this way about prior care givers shows the importance of making "partners" of your "suppliers."

The role of the quality improvement supplier is not passive; the supplier does not wait for someone to complain and then look for a fault in the process. Instead, the supplier seeks information from customers. When the supplier laboratory learns that physicians are not pleased about the turnaround time for stat laboratory tests, the supplier laboratory can work with the physicians to make improvements. Close coordination of internal customer feedback with information about the capabilities of the preceding process will lead to optimum improvement.

This discussion reinforces the need for the commitment to improvement to precede all else. The events suggested here will not occur unless all the people who participate have a single purpose — the continuous improvement of quality.

HOW MANY CUSTOMERS ARE THERE?

There might be a tendency to infer from the preceding discussion that each process has a single class of supplier or customer. Although some customers may be more directly involved than others, most processes have various customers. The external customers of a single patient encounter, in addition to the patient, could include any or all of the following: the patient's family, the referring physician, the hospital, the third party payer, the patient's employer, or the managed care agent. Each has different and legitimate needs and expectations in relation to the quality of physician service, and the total quality of the service involves a summation of the extent to which these needs and expectations are met.

There may also be several internal customers of subprocesses. With services such as physical therapy or dietetics, which involve direct interaction with the patient, both the patient and physician are customers as well as the scheduling clerk and the billing office. Often two functions play both roles in relation to each other. In terms of the clarity and accuracy of the order to the pharmacy or laboratory, the physician is the supplier. The pharmacy should be aggressive in interacting with a physician whose orders are regularly not interpretable; hospital nurses should behave similarly. The physician becomes a customer of the pharmacy only after a clear and understandable order has been delivered. Understanding all of the subprocesses and sub-subprocesses to the most fundamental level, including the identification of the suppliers and customers of each, can be enlightening. At a minimum it makes improvement feasible.

TEAMS AND TOOLS

The actual operation of the quality improvement process is done largely by the people responsible for and knowledgeable about the process under consideration. This means quality improvement work must occur in groups or improvement teams (24). It follows that progress is directly related to the ability of people to function in groups created to improve something.

A lot of information about helping groups function effectively is available, but many American organizations have not taken advantage of the knowledge. A modest amount of training in the group process followed by a period of conscious application of the technique in a real setting can overcome many of the traditional failings of meetings. Clear purpose, firm agendas, specific time assignments to each item, on-site documentation of the meeting as it occurs, and the use of established group techniques such as brainstorming, nominal group technique, force field analysis, and rank ordering allow meetings to proceed briskly with everyone participating and decisions being produced with minimum wasted energy. A certain amount of training is necessary and first attempts will not be perfect, but those who regularly attend meetings where these methods are used become enthusiastic about how much is accomplished.

Quality improvement is an information-driven process. Jumping to conclusions without facts results in high percentages of wrong decisions with the accompanying wasted cost and impact on morale. Before a team can think about ways to improve a process, a careful and methodical analysis of the current process needs to be done. This involves a clear description of how the process actually operates, as opposed to how we think it operates or how it should operate. It requires the identification of things that might cause the process to not produce the desired output and then a count of the number of times various causes actually appear. It is only a beginning to learn that the output fails to meet expectations. The knowledge needed to make an improvement relates to the cause of the defect — the *root* cause.

Quality improvement also requires an understanding of how the output of the process varies over time. Variation is inherent in every process. Improvement is directly related to our ability to develop knowledge about these variations. Once an improvement is made, information is needed to know the effect of the change and the new level and variability of output that the process has achieved.

To use information productively in a group process it needs to be communicated effectively. Visual displays of information are preferred, and the quality improvement process has spawned or refined several tools for data display that are both simple and proven over many years of application in various settings. These tools help teams address the issues raised above (25,26).

The fact that the tools are simple and direct allows them to be used by everyone in an organization; this alone is an expression of their power. The following is a brief introduction to tools that would be unfamiliar to people not yet engaged in quality improvement. In addition to the tools discussed here, several other well-known methods for graphic presentation of data are used in the quality improvement process such as histograms, bar charts, and scattergrams. The techniques specifically adapted to the quality improvement process include:

Cause and Effect Diagram

The cause and effect diagram is used to display a large variety of information about a particular issue in a condensed and organized way (27). At the end of an arrow the effect is noted. Each major antecedent cause of that effect is represented by a branch line attached to the arrow line. The diagram represents an effort at logical thinking. It helps in understanding the measurement dimensions involved in an effort to learn about the causes associated with the effect under study.

The creation of a cause and effect diagram can be an individual or a group effort. Often it serves a team as a way of organizing all of its ideas about the causes of an undesired event, (medication errors, late or inaccurate laboratory results) or all of the ways an improvement could be achieved (error free medications, timely and accurate laboratory results). Figure 1 shows a cause and effect diagram for reasons a delay may occur in the initiation of antibiotic therapy for a patient diagnosed in the physician's office as septic.

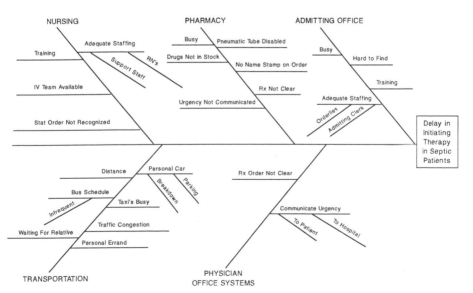

Figure 1. Delay in antibiotic therapy.

Pareto Diagram

A Pareto diagram provides a quick understanding of the relative importance of the variables in a data set (28). It is a rank-ordered histogram with an indicator of the accumulated percentage across the items ranked. It is often used to display data showing the reasons for defects or inadequacies in a process.

The Pareto diagram in Figure 2 shows the reasons for operating room delays in a hospital and the number of times each has occurred. It is typical of a Pareto diagram that the first few reasons represent a large proportion of the total reasons for the problem; these are referred to as the "vital few" compared with the "many others." In this case the first three reasons represent over 80% of the reasons for delay and an improvement effort addressing one of these is likely to make a bigger difference than one addressing any of the lesser reasons.

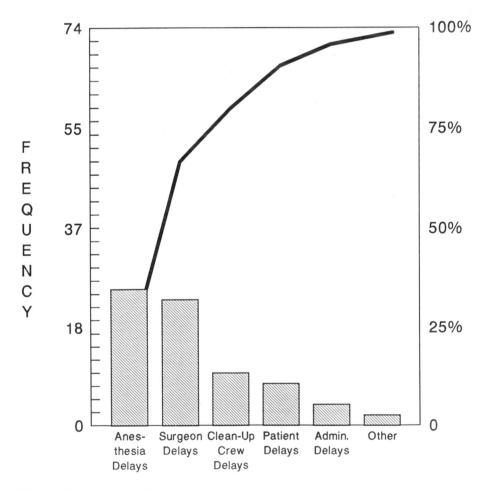

Figure 2. Pareto diagram: Reasons for operating room delays.

Flow Chart

There is a quality improvement cliche to the effect that a process cannot be improved until it is defined (29). Simply defining the process with a group of people who know best how it works can lead to immediate improvements, especially where everyone has a different idea of the process. The physician's office personnel who answer the calls of patients who phone to describe their symptoms and obtain advice about whether to come in is an example.

More often the advantage of defining the process is to see where and how the subprocesses intersect and where there are loops back that occur when the input from one process to the next is not complete or correct. The process for ordering a new medication in the hospital is presumed to be simple: the physician writes the order, it is copied by the clerk, it is delivered by a courier, the pharmacist reads it and prepares the medicine, which is then delivered back to the floor and given to the patient. It works that way sometimes. Figure 3 shows additional levels of the process that come into play when the order is not clear to the pharmacist or when the pharmacist and the floor nurse disagree in interpreting the prescription. These complications are part of the real process.

In medical care the time it takes for processes to function is often critical to the quality of the service. Understanding the process at a level of detail that defines the delays, discovers where they occur, and in turn prompts inquiry about whether a different process could reduce the delay can be rewarding. Thinking about and documenting processes will allow many opportunities for improvement to surface.

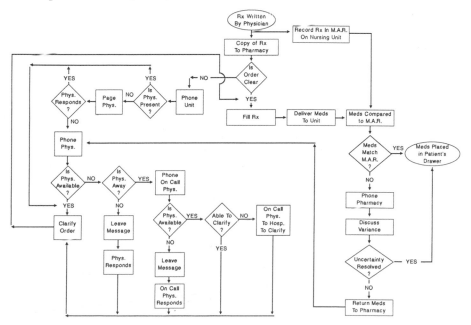

Figure 3. Pharmacy and nursing process when prescription is unclear.

Run Chart

The ability to understand how a process is performing over time is critical to its continuous improvement. Key quality characteristics are those aspects of system output that are significant to the customers of the process and that can be measured on a continuing basis. Data reflecting performance in relation to a key quality characteristic can be plotted on a run chart, permitting easy observation of the level and variability of the output over time (30).

Because data are often expensive to obtain, it is important to identify characteristics of the process that are most important to customers as well as indicative of variations in the quality of the process output. Examples of these quality characteristics include medication errors as a percent of total medications delivered, rate of repeat roentgenograms, minutes between significant events such as time from the physician's order to the completion of the task, number of patient complaints per month, and so forth.

The run chart in Figure 4 shows how trends in medication errors might appear and how valuable it is to have data over longer periods so that trends will become evident. A technical interpretation of this chart would conclude that there is something different between the colder months and the warmer ones. A job of the quality improvement process would be to discover what causes that difference.

Interpretation of a run chart improves with instruction and experience. The most important advice is to not overinterpret the data; variation is expected. So long as variation is without any apparent pattern it is not appropriate to ascribe meaning to high or low individual points. During the early phases of an improvement opportunity run charts help in understanding the extent of variation and identifying perceptible trends or cycles in the performance

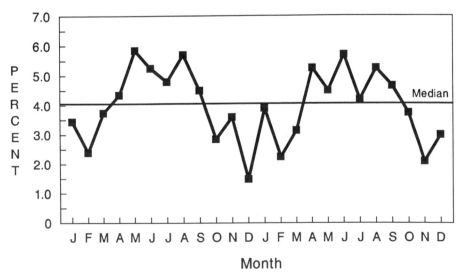

Figure 4. Run chart: Medical errors per 100 patients in City General Hospital.

of the process. Later, the same chart can document whether a change in the process has had an impact.

Control Charts

Quality improvement has its roots in the concepts of statistical process control. The control chart is the graphic component of the statistical process control method (31-33). It is the only tool that introduces a modicum of complexity. It is a statistical instrument and a certain amount of training is needed to understand how to apply the several variations of control charts and to interpret the information they display. These charts are similar to run charts in that the data reflects the performance of the system over time in relation to a key quality characteristic. Again, the display will reveal trends and cycles. An additional feature of the control chart is that it provides information about the predictability of the process. The control limits shown on a control chart reflect the historical variability of the process, and for a process that operates predictably (and with a distribution that is not highly skewed), more than 99% of the points will be within the limits. So long as the points remain scattered within the control limits the variation is almost certainly caused by the variability inherent in the routine operation of the process. If a point exceeds the limit, chances are very good that a special event has occurred to cause performance to change abruptly. Knowing whether variation results from a "special cause" or from routine events is important in determining what action management should take to reduce variation and improve the quality of the process.

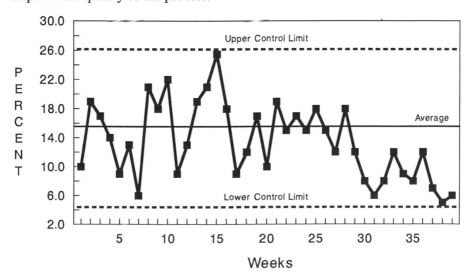

Figure 5. Control chart: Weekly percent of late appointments in the office practice of Jack Jones, MD.

Figure 5 illustrates the application of the control chart to patient waiting time in a physician's office. The quality characteristic being charted is the weekly percent of patients who wait more than 30 minutes beyond their appointment time to see the physician. The control limits reflect the historical variability of the system, which is typified by the first 20 points of the chart. Despite what appears to be significant variation, no point exceeds the control limit, and it is reasonable to conclude from this particular chart that the variation is inherent in the process of running this office. Neither high nor low points are indicative of an unusual event; they simply reflect how the elements of the office routine come together over each weekly period.

The balance of the chart is illustrative of data that would appear as changes are made in the routine process, first to reduce extreme variation and then to lower the rate at which patients are required to wait.

These quality improvement tools need data to be applied. Successful quality improvement teams will be those that can creatively and inexpensively obtain the data necessary to describe variations in process performance in relation to customer needs and expectations. In most cases it is the people who operate the processes who will be both the designers *and* the collectors of the information they need to understand the processes they operate.

CONCLUSIONS

We have suggested that there is a new opportunity for leaders in health care today who wish to make improvements in the quality of what they do. A rich theory base and applications literature are available, but require careful thought before being applied to health care. When these theories are applied, however, significant improvements are possible. These new methods require skill in conceptualizing what is done every day in slightly different terms, working with those who are a part of the daily processes of care, understanding the power of a statistical way of thinking about improvement, and most important of all, being committed to the continuous improvement of everything that is done for patients and other customers of the health care system today.

Acknowledgments: The authors thank the editors for their support and insight, the three reviewers for their thoughtful suggestions, and Kellie Campbell, secretary to the Hospital Corporation of America Quality Resource Group, for patiently keeping us organized.

References

1. Deming WE. *Out of the Crisis*. Cambridge, Massachusetts: MIT;1986:18-21.

2. Shores AR. *Survival of the Fittest*. Milwaukee: ASQC Quality Press;1988:85.

3. Mizuno S. *Company-Wide Total Quality Control*. Tokyo, Japan: Asian Productivity Organization;1988:16-7.

4. Feigenbaum AV. *Total Quality Control*. New York: McGraw Hill;1988:12-4.

5. Mizuno S. *Company-Wide Total Quality Control*. Tokyo, Japan: Asian Productivity Organization;1988:27-8.

6. Shores AR. *Survival of the Fittest*. Milwaukee: ASQC Quality Press;1988:247.

7. Deming WE. *Out of the Crisis*. Cambridge, Massachusetts: MIT;1986:309-10.

8. Walton M. *The Deming Management Method*. New York: Doss, Mead & Co.;1986:40-51.

9. Feigenbaum AV. *Total Quality Control.* New York: McGraw Hill;1988:15-7.
10. Ishikawa K. *What is Total Quality Control.* Englewood Cliffs, New Jersey: Prentice-Hall Inc.;1985:14-9.
11. Feigenbaum AV. *Total Quality Control.* New York: McGraw Hill;1988:149-50.
12. Ishikawa K. *What is Total Quality Control.* Englewood Cliffs, New Jersey: Prentice-Hall Inc.;1985:19-23.
13. Shores AR. *Survival of the Fittest.* Milwaukee: ASQC Quality Press;1988:2-3.
14. Walton M. *The Deming Management Method.* New York: Doss, Mead & Co.;1986:17-9.
15. Walton M. *The Deming Management Method.* New York: Doss, Mead & Co.;1986:10-6.
16. Deming WE. *Out of the Crisis.* Cambridge, Massachusetts: MIT;1986:121, 175.
17. Deming WE. *Out of the Crisis.* Cambridge, Massachusetts: MIT;1986:23-92.
18. Deming WE. *Out of the Crisis.* Cambridge, Massachusetts: MIT;1986:20.
19. Juran MM, Gryna FM. *Juran's Quality Control Handbook.* 4th edition. New York:McGraw Hill;1988:2.8-2.11.
20. Deming WE. *Out of the Crisis.* Cambridge, Massachusetts: MIT;1986:87-8.
21. Shores AR. *Survival of the Fittest.* Milwaukee: ASQC Quality Press; 1988:215.
22. Mizuno S. *Company-Wide Total Quality Control.* Tokyo, Japan: Asian Productivity Organization;1988:252.
23. Imai M. *Kaizen: The Key to Japan's Competitive Success.* New York: Random House;1986:51-2.
24. Sholtes PR. *The Team Handbook.* Madison, Wisconsin; Joiner Associates;1988:1.13-1.20
25. Mizuno S. *Company-Wide Total Quality Control.* Tokyo, Japan: Asian Productivity Organization;1988:154-6.
26. Walton M. *The Deming Management Method.* New York: Doss, Mead & Co.;1986:96-118.
27. Ishikawa K. *What is Total Quality Control.* Englewood Cliffs, New Jersey: Prentice-Hall Inc.;1985:18-9.
28. Ishikawa K. *What is Total Quality Control.* Englewood Cliffs, New Jersey: Prentice-Hall Inc.;1985:42-9.
29. Juran JM. *Juran on Planning for Quality.* New York: The Free Press;1988:18-23.
30. Wheeler DJ, Chambers DS. *Understanding Statistical Process Control.* Knoxville, Tennessee: Statistical Process Controls, Inc.;1986:99-102.
31. Stewart WA. *Statistical Method from the Viewpoint of Quality Control.* New York: Dover Publications;1986:1-79.
32. Ishikawa K. *What is Total Quality Control.* Englewood Cliffs, New Jersey: Prentice-Hall Inc.;1985:70-85.
33. Wheeler DJ, Chambers DS. *Understanding Statistical Process Control.* Knoxville, Tennessee: Statistical Process Controls, Inc.;1986:62-97.

Additional Readings

Deming WE. *Quality, Productivity and Competitive Position.* Cambridge, Massachusetts: MIT;1982.

Garvin DA. *Managing Quality.* New York: Free Press;1987.

Gitlow HS, Shelly J. *The Deming Guide to Quality and Competitive Position.* Englewood Cliffs, New Jersey: Prentice-Hall Inc.;1987.

Juran JM. *Managerial Breakthrough.* New York: McGraw Hill;1964.

Scherkenbach WW. *The Deming Route to Quality and Productivity,* Rockville, Maryland: Mercury Press;1986.

Wadsworth HM, Stephens KS, Godfrey AB. *Modern Methods for Quality Control and Improvement.* New York: John Wiley & Sons;1986.

COMMENTARY

For most of this book, the editors have assembled top authorities in the technical aspects of quality of care measurement. In contrast, Batalden and Buchanan's chapter introduces a management philosophy that integrates quality into the daily operation of an organization. Using the management approach pioneered by Deming, Buchanan and Batalden concisely yet thoroughly outline Deming's theories and demonstrate how they are beginning to be used in their institution, the Hospital Corporation of America. Unfortunately, in our view, only a few other health care institutions, notably Harvard Community Health Plan, have attempted the ambitious yet ultimately cost-saving program outlined in this chapter (1). Other industries have successfully implemented the Deming approach to quality management. Many readers are familiar with the tremendous financial success the Japanese enjoy. In the United States, the Ford Motor Company attributes its record earnings to adoption of the Deming quality management philosophy. We hope, as more health care organizations adopt the Deming philosophy, peer review journals will publish data documenting the efficiency (from an integrated quality and cost perspective) of this critical approach to health care management.

As is true with any management philosophy, the Deming approach cannot be explained simply with scientifically proven data. One of us (N.G.) felt that participating as an observer in the Hospital Corporation of America quality management process represented the best means of tying together potentially abstract theories into management action. Administrators at two different institutions described how they and their employees have begun to work with the Deming management approach. All managers in the hospital attended Quality 101, a 3-day course with an overall objective of helping the manager understand several key principles. First and foremost the customer is king; service improvement begins with identifying who your customers are and what their needs are. In addition, the customer is not only the end user of a particular service. There are intermediate customers as well. For example, many individuals are involved in the ordering, taking, and reading of a mammogram. The last critical principle learned in this course is that data and not "gut facts" should guide the manager toward slow, but continuous improvement in the entire service or care provided to specific customers. This implies that attention is devoted to all employees, all facets of the service in an effort to improve the entire process; not to focus in on the aberrancies.

After the entire management of the institution (imagine essentially shutting down a hospital so that everyone, not just an isolated individual, could learn a new management philosophy based on quality) attended this course, participants were asked to submit three ideas for a quality improvement program. The only criteria were that they be important yet not overly complex to execute. The latter was included as the hospital was just beginning to change management style from a traditional authoritarian style to one that involved all employees as part of the management process (though only managers attend the course, all employees are trained in Deming's quality management philosophy).

The Quality Improvement Process is guided by the Quality Management Council, made up of the senior management of the institution; meetings are held on a weekly basis until the group decides it has completed its task. How do committee members realize that they have completed the project; only when they have completed the PDCA cycle: Plan, Do, Check (with data not just gut facts), and Act (disseminate the results throughout the institution). At the first meeting, committee members decide the objectives or "opportunity statement" for the group. Meetings are expected to start on time and one of the committee members keeps the discussion to the pre-set (decided at the previous meeting) time. Meetings cannot last more than 1 hour. In addition to the timekeeper and other committee members, there is a recorder of minutes and a leader and facilitator (an outside individual who participates only when the group has difficulty completing its agenda). All positions rotate except for that of the facilitator and leader. After 45 minutes of discussing a pre-set agenda, the members evaluate the meeting (on a scale of 1 to 10 and subjective comments) and plan the agenda for the next meeting.

A quality improvement program on patient discharge represents an example of a topic recently completed at Quincy City Hospital, a hospital owned by the city of Quincy, Massachusetts, but managed by Hospital Corporation of America. The associate administrator of the hospital, Ms. Ellen Zane, was the leader of this group. The opportunity statement (project objective) for this quality improvement program was

> Within the last several years the Quincy City Hospital has been experiencing difficulty discharging and placing many of its Medicare patients into community placements once they are no longer at a hospital level of care and once they can be no longer cared for at home.
>
> The result of these Medicare patients remaining in the hospital post their acute illness is twofold. Firstly, their extended hospital stay creates a financial burden for the hospital as reimbursement for the continuing care of such patients is minimal. Secondly, admissions of other acute patients may be impacted because necessary beds are occupied by this population.
>
> It is necessary for the hospital to develop systems and strategies to improve the rapidity with which Medicare patients are discharged and placed within the community. (From a mimeo provided by Ellen Zane, associate administrator at Quincy City Hospital.)

After development of the opportunity statement, the committee members constructed a flow chart that documented the process of care for patient discharge. The team then worked to document the barriers to patient discharge. They used a fishbone chart to clarify the issue. Though the list of barriers appears clear cut, anyone experienced with group process can attest that the development of such a list requires tremendous effort to get a list that is both accurate and comprehensive yet receives group consensus. Very often each committee member initially has a differing conception of, for example, barriers to patient discharge. The achievement of consensus in such a project goes a long way to achieving the objectives enunciated in the opportunity statement.

With the completion of the fishbone chart, the team then collected data from which it developed a what, who, when, and why chart. This chart summarized what the team would do as a consequence of its planning process. The team next checked the actions that were taken on a pilot basis with further collection of data. This second set of data led to a reexamination of the pilot actions taken. Final recommendations were presented to the quality improvement council for dissemination throughout the institution. This final step is currently underway.

Is the Deming approach to quality management too mechanical and long-winded? Absolutely not. The enthusiasm and participation of each employee were impressive; the knowledge each committee member brought to bear on the meeting both in terms of the problem and quality improvement principles — words like hypothesis, Pareto chart, and variance evaluation swept through the room with precise technical responses sent back in response.

The broader and more difficult question with regard to the Deming approach to quality management is whether all constituents of the health care team, in particular the physicians, are willing to wholeheartedly work with Deming's principles. With adequate preparation — of the type which managers working for Hospital Corporation of America and Harvard Community Health Plan currently undergo — the answer is a qualified yes. However, it is helpful to point out salient characteristics of physician behavior that work both for and against the Deming approach. In so doing it will become clear why the physician is the most challenging professional to convert to the Deming philosophy, in particular, as compared with the nurse, clerk, or other essential team members.

The physician is historically and traditionally perceived to be the leader of the health care team (2). This can be both a strength and weakness. It can be a strength if the physician perceives a team to be in existence; this implies an element of negotiation even if the physician leader often tends to be authoritarian. The physician as leader concept can be a weakness when, as is often the case, neither the physician nor the clerk, for example, perceive a team to be in existence. It is easiest to create a team relationship with a physician when he or she is on salary (almost 50% of all physicians in the United States). With societal demands for physician accountability rising and increased salary pressure on physicians, team relationships between physicians in private practice and nonphysicians may be easier to develop in the future.

The role of the physician leader has been problematic not only because of his or her role vis-à-vis other members of the health care team but also because of the quality of the peer relationships. Historically, physicians have often been in economic competition with their peers as a result of the incentives inherent in the current fee-for-service system (4). In addition they have had difficulty confronting clinical deficiencies in their peers. Once a physician in good standing, always a physician in good standing. The Deming management philosophy demands that all team members articulate concerns, which when backed up with "actionable" data, are dealt with by all team members. Physician attitudes represent a critical potential barrier to patient discharge. Changing these attitudes requires effective peer relationships.

Does the Deming philosophy represent "cookbook" medicine? It is clear to me that such is not the case. The authors instead are urging the continual improvement of all the processes that affect the care of patients based on the application of the best scientific thinking. However, the maxims outlined by Batalden and Buchanan could be perceived as such by physicians. Physicians have had historical difficulty with protocols or any management approach that limits their clinical freedom of action (4). "Administrators who try to contain costs... are commonly perceived by physicians as impediments to progress and good clinical medicine, while they in turn are likely to view their physicians as extravagant and unmindful spenders" (5). Current efforts at utilization and peer review are often, understandably, met by physicians by a "how can I beat the system" attitude. Such an approach immediately dooms to failure any effort at implementing the Deming approach, emphasizing slow but continuous improvement in all aspects of the health care organizational process.

This commentary and Batalden and Buchanan's chapter will not sell physicians on the Deming approach. Rather it is meant to make interested readers aware of a management philosophy that can tie the technical aspects of quality of care measurement into daily management practice. We hope readers will be open to the philosophy, and some may even pursue further study in this management approach that has been so successful for many nonhealth care industries.

Though physicians memorize mounds of data, they often make clinical decisions on the basis of "gut facts." Unfortunately, most physicians in clinical practice do not learn the basics of statistics and thus often mistrust the application of scientific studies to the individual clinical setting. "My patient is different" represents a common physician refrain to a query from a peer review organization.

Physicians have been traditionally suspicious of organizational efforts to improve clinical care (6). This partly emanates from the American tradition of solo practice. It is also reinforced by our medical training and exposure to malpractice, which emphasizes that an individual physician bears responsibility for the entire care of the patient or maloccurrence. In fact, health care is too complex for one individual to be responsible for the factors affecting a patient's well-being. The passage of Medicare and Medicaid and the trend toward physicians on salary will facilitate an increased level of comfort between physicians and organizational behavior (7).

Can clinicians — nurses, physicians, and so forth — feel comfortable in an environment where they are only a part, albeit a critical one, of a team? In my opinion, clinicans do not have the luxury of this choice anymore. Health care delivery is too complex, costly, and effective to be left solely to the discretion of the clinician members of the team. We need to involve all members of the health care team, whether they be located in private offices or tertiary care hospitals, if medical care delivery is to truly aim at continuous improvement in the quality of care delivered to our ultimate health care customer — the patient. (The Editors)

References

1. Berwick DM. Continuous improvement as an ideal in health care. *N Engl J Med.* 320:1;53-6.
2. Shorter E. *Bedside Manners. The Troubled History of Doctors and Patients.* New York: Simon and Schuster; 1985.
3. Starr P. *The Social Transformation of American Medicine.* New York: Basic Books; 1983.
4. Anderson OW, Gevitz N. The general hospital: a social and historical perspective. In: David Mechanic, ed. *Handbook of Health, Health Care and the Health Professions.* New York: Free Press; 1983:311.
5. Friedson E. *Doctoring Together: A Study of Professional Social Control.* New York: Elsevier; 1975.
6. Friedson E. *Professional Power: A Study of the Institutionalization of Formal Knowledge.* Chicago: University of Chicago Press; 1986.
7. Colombotos J, Kirchner C. *Physicians and Social Change.* New York: Oxford University Press; 1986:115-62.

Chapter 6

Management Information Systems and Quality

DONALD M. STEINWACHS, PhD
JONATHAN P. WEINER, DR. PH
SAM SHAPIRO

INTRODUCTION

The attainment of high-quality health care is a universally accepted goal. Yet, the development of techniques for monitoring and assuring quality of care has not kept pace with other advances in medical technology. A comprehensive strategy for monitoring quality of care in an ongoing and efficient manner is needed. Automated management information systems (MISs) are widely used throughout health care systems and have the potential for achieving these goals. This potential, however, has not been tested (1).

Many of the concerns with quality reflect uncertainties regarding the consequences of changes in the health care system, both negative and positive (2). Questions are raised about the quality of care under alternative organizational and financing approaches, for example, preferred provider organizations (PPOs), and health maintenance organizations (HMOs), which offer care at lower cost or on a capitation basis; new types of managed care programs that use criteria to review the appropriateness of hospitalizations and specialty services as a basis for determining if payment should be made by the insurer; and primary care providers who are paid to function as gatekeepers and receive financial incentives to control the use of specialty services and hospitalizations by their patients. All these changes, and the process of change itself, raise concerns that the quality of care may be changing too (3).

Public attention is being drawn increasingly to indicators of quality, including mortality rates in hospitals, rates of inappropriate surgery, and malpractice claims. Although the demand is increasing, there are few mechanisms that provide information to the parties involved. The Joint

Commission on Accreditation of Health Care Organizations (JCAHO) sets standards for review and documentation, and until recently, almost exclusively emphasized structural and process indicators of quality. However, consumers and those parties paying the majority of their bills (that is, government and employers) want to know whether potential adverse outcomes can be prevented, and whether or not a patient receiving services will return to a level of functioning better than or equal to his or her status before treatment.

How can these concerns be addressed? How can data be tabulated efficiently to provide overall indicators of quality (that is, information predictive of the level of quality that may or may not be sufficient to draw conclusions)? What are the limitations of relying on existing data to measure quality? How will this information be used to improve care? These questions and others will be addressed from within the context of a discussion of the application of MISs to the task of monitoring, and ultimately, improving quality of care.

FRAMEWORK FOR EXAMINING QUALITY OF CARE

The basic framework for examining quality of care is drawn from Donabedian's (4) conceptualization of three dimensions: structure, process, and outcome. Structure includes the more stable characteristics of health care, including the organization of services, facilities, and personnel. Process encompasses all aspects of the patient's interaction with the provider and system of care, ranging from scheduling an appointment to diagnosis and treatment. Outcome of care refers to "the change in the patient's current and future health status that can be attributed to antecedent health care" (4). In the case of the latter dimension, the fundamental interest is in understanding the relationships that lead specific structures and processes to better outcomes.

This framework for examining quality does not define precisely what is meant by quality. Donabedian (4) indicates that the attribute we call quality reflects the extent to which health care achieves the most favorable balance of risks and benefits. In this definition he recognizes the importance of costs, and that patients and providers frequently must make tradeoffs.

There are other meanings of quality that share these elements. Recently Steffen (5) compared alternative definitions and suggested that the concept of quality should be defined as the capacity to achieve a desired set of goals. The issue in measuring quality is then to identify the goals of health care, determine what importance each of several goals has to the patient, provider, or society, and determine the extent to which these goals are being achieved. The measurement of quality is referred to as quality assessment. Generally, assessments are done using explicit criteria for judging quality that are expected to reflect the complex relationships of risks, benefits, and costs, and the potentially conflicting goals of patients, providers, and society. Quality assurance involves quality assessment as one step in a process that monitors quality of care indicators; conducts quality assessments where indicators suggest potential problems may exist; makes recommendations for improving care based on the assessment; and continues to monitor the problems into the future. In general, the MIS data sources used in monitoring quality provide indicators of quality, that is, information that may be predictive of the level of quality, but may not be sufficient by itself to draw strong conclusions.

Strategies for Monitoring Quality of Care

There are three established strategies for monitoring quality of care: case finding; provider profiles; and population-based measures of quality. The potential application of MISs to each strategy is discussed below.

Case Finding.   Case finding has a long tradition of practice in American quality assurance. This includes hospital mortality committees, tissue committees, and more recently risk management committees. Case finding methods are generally based on formal or informal criteria that identify patients at increased risk for having received suboptimal or inadequate care. Generally, cases are selected if they represent adverse experiences, for example, death or complications, to determine if the outcome is a result of poor quality care. If it is, then efforts are made to identify the cause and potential remedies.

There are few examples of case finding in ambulatory care. Moreover, their foci are less likely to be immediately life threatening. For example, at the Harvard Community Health Plan (HMO), an automated medical record system known as COSTAR (COmputer STored Ambulatory Record) has been used to flag cases in which a streptococcal infection has been diagnosed but the patient has not received appropriate medication (6).

Provider Profiles.   Creating provider profiles generally involves, collating statistics on individual providers to document patterns of practice, and comparing these data with some norm to identify exceptional patterns. Statistics on practice patterns may include hospital admission rates, average length of stay, ambulatory visit rates, specialty referral rates, use of ancillary procedures, and prescribing rates. Generally, provider profiles are used by many payers to identify high outliers for further utilization review, and low-use providers for inclusion in managed care networks (for example PPOs). MIS-based applications of provider profiles have principally been concerned with provider productivity and provider-generated costs.

There have been few applications of provider profiles to assess quality. In part, this has been due to the difficulty of adjusting provider practice patterns for differences in patient case mix. The Health Care Financing Administration (HCFA) has recently developed and released hospital-specific mortality rates based on Medicare data using a selected mix of discharge diagnoses. In ambulatory care, recent advances in case mix measurement may make provider profiles more meaningful (7; Weiner JP, Starfield BH, Steinwachs DM, Mumford LM. An ambulatory care case mix system for use under capitation. Presented at the Group Health Institute, Chicago, May 1988). As case mix measurement methods improve, provider profiles will become more useful in monitoring quality.

Population-Based Measures. Population-based approaches to examine health outcomes have a long history, beginning with the routine collection of death records to identify potentially preventable deaths. Only recently has population-based information become available on medical care (8). Kessner and colleagues (9) pioneered a tracer condition method for assessing quality that uses integrated information on process and outcomes of care for a selected set of diagnoses meeting criteria as tracer conditions. Since then, many other quality-of-care studies have used sample surveys, information systems, medical records, and other sources to develop population-based measures of quality (10). Yet, examples in which these approaches have been incorporated into ongoing quality assurance programs (11,12) are difficult to find.

Population-based approaches to quality of care differ from case finding and provider profiles in that information is presented on individuals who use services and those who do not. For example, the care of hypertensive patients who are diagnosed and are being seen routinely may meet all criteria for receiving high-quality care, yet the proportion of the population diagnosed and under care could be well below established estimates of the prevalence of this condition. Under such a scenario, case finding and provider profiles would indicate high-quality care, whereas a population-based approach would identify the problem of undertreatment, suggesting deficiencies in access and screening.

Quality of Care Issues

Quality of care encompasses a broad set of concerns with the structure, process, and outcome of health care. In the remainder of this chapter, attention will be directed at issues for which the application of data from an MIS is likely to be particularly useful; these include assessing adequacy of arrangements for access to care; adequacy of preventive care and problem identification; appropriateness of diagnostic and treatment procedures; continuity of care for chronic diseases; and occurrence of potentially preventable adverse outcomes of health care.

Access to Care. Access encompasses concerns with the appropriateness and timeliness of care being sought and received. Poor access to care may contribute to failures to receive routine preventive care, delays in the diagnosis and treatment of conditions, and ultimately, could be expected to contribute to poorer health outcomes. The adequacy of access can be measured in both relative and absolute terms. Relative measures include comparisons of visit rates across patient populations (for example, served by different providers) to determine if comparable groups have different rates of use or different levels of access. Utilization measures may target specific types of use, for example, the proportion of children with complete immunizations, or the proportion of adult women with a Papanicolaou test conforming to recommended guidelines (13).

Preventive Care. The Health Objectives for the United States (14) and the soon-to-be-published recommendations on routine preventive care by the U.S. Preventive Services Task Force indicate the growing role and importance of preventive care. Preventive care spans all age groups and includes primary prevention of disease and disability through inoculation and behavior change (for example, smoking cessation), as well as secondary prevention through the early detection and treatment of major chronic diseases (for example, hypertension, diabetes, cervical cancer). Preventive care involving specific services (for example, immunization) can be monitored using an MIS if the appropriate information is collected at each visit. In contrast, preventive care involving events not likely to be included in reporting systems, such as counseling on health risks, is more difficult to monitor without special efforts to collect this information.

Appropriate Diagnosis and Treatment.   Diagnosis and treatment are established areas for quality assessment. Criteria have been developed and applied by both local and national groups for quality review of many common acute and chronic conditions (15). Although many of these standards have been published, there is no central clearinghouse on criteria, and no group has assumed responsibility for periodic updating.

Criteria are usually developed to establish minimal standards of care for specific conditions. Most are based on data available in the patient's medical record. However, information on the patient's outcome status, not readily available in the chart, is being increasingly required. In general, an MIS will provide little or no information on health outcomes, unless complications and additional service utilization follow. Thus, other data sources will be needed, including special follow-up surveys or examinations. Even so, the MIS may facilitate collecting data. For example, the data system can be used to select individuals who have had a specific health problem (for example, essential hypertension) who should be included in an outcome assessment.

Continuity of Care for Chronic Diseases.   An increasing proportion of health care is concerned with the long-term management of chronic conditions. These conditions place special demands on the patient to comply with treatments over extended periods, and on the provider to assure continuity of treatment. Past experience has shown that significant numbers of patients will not return for periodic assessment when needed, yet few providers have ongoing systems for identifying breakdowns in follow-up.

One role for an MIS is to flag patients who have not returned for care, or who did not receive appropriate follow-up care. McDonald (16) has tested approaches for developing physician reminders based on an MIS that has been shown to be successful. The MIS should also be useful in identifying characteristics of patients that are associated with greater risk for not returning for care.

Adverse Outcomes.   The occurrence of a preventable adverse health outcome clearly indicates deficiencies in quality. Examples of such outcomes are the "sentinel events" developed by Rutstein and colleagues (17) and recently updated by the Centers for Disease Control. Three categories of sentinel events are identified: unnecessary disease, unnecessary disability, and unnecessary or untimely death. Unnecessary diseases include many of the infectious disorders and preventable causes of cancer, lung disease, and injury. Unnecessary disabilities include those arising from malnutrition and infectious diseases. Unnecessary and untimely deaths cut across many categories of disease. These sentinel events can be identified based on *International Classification of Diseases, Ninth Revision, Clinical Modification* (*ICD-9-CM*) coding of death certificates, hospital discharge data, and ambulatory encounter data. Thus, a population with complete utilization data can be routinely screened for the occurrence of sentinel events using an MIS.

Other health outcomes fall into a less clearly defined area; that is, they are often preventable. Medicare's professional review organizations (PROs) review such categories of potentially preventable hospitalizations, including admissions for diabetic ketoacidosis and readmissions for complications of surgery and medical treatments. An MIS that includes information on hospitalizations can provide the basis for identifying admissions that may be preventable. In many instances, determining whether admissions could have been avoided generally requires access to the medical record, possibly other sources of data, and a clinical reviewer. Thus, the MIS screening of cases is a first step in making a determination regarding quality of care.

Poorer health outcomes may not always result in death or hospitalization, and may not be easily identifiable unless special efforts are made to systematically collect information. Although research is in progress to test strategies for routinely collecting patient outcome information in ambulatory care, it is uncertain how affordable and valuable these methods will be in routine practice (Ware JE. Personal communication;1988).

MANAGEMENT INFORMATION SYSTEMS

The content of an MIS will vary across different settings. In the following discussion, the emphasis will be on ambulatory care, and to a limited extent, inpatient care.

The data recorded at each ambulatory encounter would be expected to be guided by the national recommendations for a minimal data set in ambulatory care. This set includes information on the patient, provider, diagnoses, and problems addressed at the visit; procedures done, and disposition status (18). Also it will be assumed that limited information is recorded on inpatient care, consistent with national recommendations for hospital discharge abstracts (19) or the more recent requirements by Medicare for uniform inpatient billing. Information on long-term care, including nursing home and home health care, will not be discussed, although these are of increasing importance as the population ages.

Recommended Structure of an Ambulatory Care MIS

The basic components of an ambulatory care MIS that are needed to support quality assurance applications include an enrollment and registration file; a provider file; and a utilization or claims file.

Enrollment and Registration.   Every enrollee in an insurance plan and each patient seen by a provider must be uniquely identified and described, based on minimal demographic information. Generally a unique numerical identifier is assigned (for example, social security number or medical record number). Moreover, minimal information on each person would be expected to include name, address, source(s) of payment, date of birth, sex, and primary physician (if applicable). Other information can be added to the enrollment and registration file, including marital status and clinical information that should be easily retrievable on a patient, for example, allergic reactions.

Provider File.   Every provider in the practice setting or participating in the health plan needs to be identified and described. Generally, a unique provider identification number (for example, tax number) is used to facilitate recording and processing. Minimal information on each provider would include name, specialty, and location of practice.

Utilization or Claims File.   For every patient encounter with a provider, information should be captured to record where and when the visit occurred, with whom, and for what purpose(s), including what services were provided. In a fee-for-service setting, these data are the crux of the claims transaction. In any environment, data recorded are determined by administrative requirements for billing and management reporting. However, the minimum data set would include patient identifier; provider identifier; date of encounter; place of encounter; diagnosis (one or more); laboratory and radiology services performed or ordered; surgical procedures performed or ordered; and billed charge for each service (may not be applicable within the prepaid setting).

This minimal set provides a basis for identifying patients seen with specific conditions (usually based on *ICD-9-CM* coded diagnoses) and the test and procedures done (usually captured in terms of Current Procedural Terminology codes).

The minimal data should be augmented, to the extent possible, to provide modest additional information, including preventive services (performed or ordered); medications prescribed; and disposition status (for example, referral, follow-up visit). This list could be extended even further to include information that would generally be captured in a medical record, whether it is a traditional hardcopy record or an automated system. These items would include presenting problem(s); physical examination findings; test results; and treatment plans.

In most instances, this information goes beyond what is readily collected by routine information systems designed to support billing and administrative needs. These data begin to meet clinical needs for patient care information and respond to pressures to include information potentially useful in examining quality.

In addition to information on ambulatory encounters, the utilization file should include minimal information on all hospital admissions or discharges. The national recommendations for the uniform hospital abstract and the current Medicare requirements define a minimal data set. This set includes patient age, sex, race, principal source of payment, and place of residence; physician identity (attending and surgeon); diagnoses, principal and secondary conditions; procedures performed; disposition status (for example, discharged home, dead, transferred); charges billed; and Diagnosis Related Group (DRG) category. Again, these data can be supplemented to provide greater detail on the circumstances leading to admission and the care received during hospitalization.

Essential Capabilities of an MIS

Beyond the data they incorporate, there are several aspects of system design and function that are particularly crucial when considering the applicability of an MIS to quality of care monitoring. These areas concern data accuracy and include: the reliability of diagnostic information; the completeness of the utilization information; and the accuracy and completeness of enrollment data.

Reliability of Diagnostic Information. The reliability of diagnostic information entered into an MIS is of pivotal concern when considering quality of care applications. In the 1970s, the Institute of Medicine assessed the accuracy of coded diagnostic data captured through uniform hospital discharge abstracting (20) and in the Medicare hospital claims files (21). More recently, the diagnostic coding used in DRG assignments was analyzed for a representative national sample of discharges (22). In both studies, rates of agreement varied substantially by type of condition, level of specificity at which the condition was coded, and size of hospital. Although the reliability of coding is probably improving as diagnosis becomes central to the payment process, reliability remains an important consideration when designing MIS-based quality monitoring systems.

There are two approaches commonly taken in the ambulatory setting to improve the reliability of coded diagnoses. Some practices use an encounter form with precoded diagnoses and require that providers check-off all applicable categories. Where there is no appropriate category, there may be a category for "other," or provisions to enter a diagnosis in text format. To minimize the number of precoded diagnoses, broad categories with no provision for modifiers, for example, chronic, recurrent, rule-out, are often used. To the extent this is done, accuracy of coding may be improved, but the specificity of the diagnostic information may be reduced.

Another approach that can provide more precise diagnostic information is to allow the provider to write all diagnoses in text form, and then use a computerized system for assigning diagnostic codes. This requires that the provider's diagnostic statement be entered verbatim and that a computerized dictionary be developed to assign a code to the statement. Experience has shown this can be done with reasonable efficiency, and it is possible to retain the provider's exact description (23). No matter what approach is taken, the accuracy and specificity of diagnostic information are central to most quality of care applications.

Completeness of Utilization Data. An MIS may not incorporate information on all ambulatory or inpatient services. This may be due to limits on coverage (particularly under indemnity insurance plans) that result in no information on services that are excluded from the benefit package. Also, experience has shown that even when comprehensive services are provided (for example, in HMOs), individuals may seek selected services elsewhere, paying either out-of-pocket or making claims on a secondary insurance policy. These missing information problems are not easily rectified. However, the magnitude and characteristics of the missing utilization data can generally be estimated by such techniques as surveys of the insured population.

Another and more correctable problem is that an MIS may not be designed to capture information on all inpatient and ambulatory care delivered. For example, in HMOs, specialty referrals to out-of-plan physicians, emergency room visits, and specialized hospitalizations are sometimes excluded. This can be remedied by adding these items routinely to the data set. However, this may not be a simple task, as information may have to be abstracted from bills and entered into the MIS database.

The utilization data found within the MISs of indemnity insurers, HMOs, PPOs, and other insurance arrangements are in a separate class from those of provider organizations. Although the insurer's system should capture data on services without regard to the point of delivery, a particular provider (for example, a hospital or group practice) is concerned only with services provided by that entity. When using this latter type of MIS to assess utilization patterns of a patient, gaps in completeness will be substantial for persons relying on several sources of care. For example, individuals may use one source for primary care and other sources for specialty care. Also, individuals may change providers over time without the knowledge of the providers.

Failure to recognize the limitations of the utilization information in an MIS may lead to suggestions that quality of care problems exist where there are none and vice-versa. These limitations need to be understood to effectively use an MIS in examining quality of care issues. Indeed, the completeness of utilization data may be sufficiently limited so that the MIS is not useful for monitoring applications.

Accuracy of Enrollment Data.   Enrollment or patient registration data provide the basis for linking demographic and insurance information to an individual's utilization records. Moreover, these data provide the basis for identifying a population at risk for using services, making is possible to calculate rates of use and proportions of the population receiving service during a specified period.

One data problem in this area relates to family insurance contracts purchased by or for a head-of-household. Under many insurance policies only the contract holder (for example, the employee) is identified instead of all persons within his or her family. Family members who use services are known, but there is no information on nonutilizing individuals. Some insurers are attempting to overcome this important limitation in enrollment information by asking employers to identify all family members at enrollment. This is generally not a problem for HMOs, which require information on individual enrollees to disburse a capitation payment to a contracting provider, whether or not the beneficiary uses services.

APPLYING AN MIS TO MONITORING QUALITY

Overview of Potential Measures

The indicators that a quality assurance system uses to monitor quality are central to that system. The measures incorporated into an automated monitoring system are initially limited to those based on data available within the MIS. This factor is the principal weakness of such an approach, yet within the constraint of available data, a broad range of quality indicators can be monitored. As increased use is made of MISs in monitoring, it can be expected that new items of information will be added to extend this monitoring capability.

Table 1 presents an overview of measures that potentially could be developed using an MIS. The measures are principally relevant to populations that have comprehensive coverage for inpatient and ambulatory care, and have an MIS that includes data on the entire utilization and claims experience. Table 1 organizes measures into five categories: overall access, preventive care, diagnosis, treatment, and outcomes of care. Within each category, general measures are proposed for monitoring, and specific examples of each are given. The interpretation of a specific measure as an indicator of quality may be based on a comparison with national practice guideline recommendations, standards of care developed locally, epidemiologic data, trends over time, or a combination of these factors.

For preventive care, there are national recommendations that are commonly used to assess the adequacy of pediatric and adult preventive services. In contrast, access will generally be monitored by examining trends over time, and in conjunction with other measures that indicate whether appropriate care is being received (for example, whether recommended standards for preventive care are being met). Other quality indicators may rely on comparisons with community or national data sources. For example, the proportion of a population diagnosed and under treatment for specific chronic diseases may be compared with epidemiologic estimates of disease prevalence developed through research studies, nationally or in specific communities. This comparison leads to an estimate of the extent to which individuals with a chronic disease have not been diagnosed and treated. Table 1 is not intended to be comprehensive of all possible measures, but indicates the breadth of measures possible and the basis for interpreting the measures as indicators of quality.

For several quality indicators outlined in Table 1, examples of actual applications are presented and discussed in the next section. Through these examples we will describe approaches for tabulating and presenting data relevant for making judgments; potential limitations; and approaches for resolving uncertainties due to these limitations.

TABLE 1. Monitoring Quality of Care Based on Measures Derived from an MIS

Quality of Care Issue	Measures	Example	Criteria
Access	Proportion of population receiving care during the year, classified by age and sex	% of children under age 2 seen for at least one well-care visit	National
		% of children seen in emergency rooms for any reason, for trauma, and for medical problems	Trends
Preventive	Proportion of population in specific age and sex groups receiving recommended tests or procedures	% of children by group having recommended immunizations in previous year	National recommendation
		% of women age 50 and over having mammography in past year	National recommendation
		% of deliveries with prenatal care beginning in first trimester	National recommendation
Diagnosis	% of population diagnosed (and under care) for specific chronic conditions by age and sex	% of adults diagnosed at one or more visits as having essential hypertension by age and sex	Epidemiologic data on prevalence of hypertension
	Average number of specific diagnostic tests per person per year	Average number of computed tomography scans per person per year	Trends and comparison data
Treatment	*Medications:* Average number of new prescriptions per person per year	Average number of new prescriptions for antibiotics per person per year	Trends and comparison data
	Surgery: Rate of surgical procedures per year; total, inpatient, and ambulatory (if applicable)	Cesarian section rate for all deliveries	Trends and comparison data
	Tests for monitoring: % of patients receiving specific monitoring tests during episode or over a defined period	% of hypertensives on diuretic medication having a serum potassium in previous year	Standards of care
	Follow-up care: % of patients receiving follow-up care in episode or over a defined period	% of hypertensives failing to return for care for 6 months or more	Standards of care
		% of children with repeated episodes of otitis media receiving audiometry	Standards of care

(Table 1. continued)

Quality of Care Issue	Measures	Example	Criteria
	Hospitalization: Rate of hospitalization, total and excluding obstetrics	Hospital days per 1,000 persons per year	Comparison data and trends
Outcomes	Hospital readmissions within 3 months of discharge	% of readmissions for same condition	Comparison data and trends
		% of readmissions identifying a complication	
	Occurrence of sentinel events	Flag potentially avoidable occurrence of sentinel events, such as advanced cervical cancer, diabetic ketoacidosis, surgical misadventures	Standards of care and comparison data

Access to Care

Utilization of services is an important indicator of access. If access is high, utilization will also be high, whereas reduced access will result in lower rates of use. The quality issue concerns assuring an adequate degree of access.

Incentives to provide or obtain care may be too open and contribute to inappropriate or excessive utilization. Many of the appropriateness review techniques applied in utilization management are specifically concerned with controlling access to inpatient services as a means to control costs (24). This issue is also of concern in ambulatory care (25).

At the other extreme, access may be too restrictive, either because the patient may not be able to afford services or because other barriers discourage utilization. Inadequate access to ambulatory care may reduce some costs in the short run, but can be expected to contribute to higher rates of emergency care and inpatient admissions when needed ambulatory care is not received (25,26). Certainly, patients may become dissatisfied with poor access and decide to change providers or insurance arrangements.

One approach for assessing changes in access to care is to examine trends in the proportion of the population being seen by a provider at least once a year, and among those receiving care, the average number of visits and inpatient days. An example of this type of assessment using an MIS was done to examine changes in access to psychiatric care in an HMO after an increase in the psychiatric visit copay rose from $2 to $10 per visit for the first 15 visits of the year (27). Also, during this period the enrollment was growing and the staffing of the department was increasing at a roughly comparable rate. Table 2 shows that despite the growth in enrollment, the number of new patients seen in psychiatry declined in the year of the copayment increase, and the number of continuing patients remained constant. Number of visits increased, reflecting a higher rate of use among existing patients.

TABLE 2. Effect of an Increase in Copayment on Utilization of Psychiatric Care in an HMO*

Patients	Before Copayment Increase				After Copayment Increase			
	1973		1974		1975		1976	
Total patients seen	1,121	(+18%)	1,317	(−7%)	1,221	(+10%)	1,348	
New patients	553	(+44%)	798	(−12%)	702	(+6%)	744	
Continuing patients	568	(−9%)	519	(0%)	519	(+16%)	604	
Mean visits per person served	5.4	(+5%)	5.7	(+7%)	6.1	(−3%)	5.9	
Average enrollment	15,175	(+19%)	18,042	(+5%)	18,875	(+4%)	19,608	

*Numbers in parentheses show percentage of change between years.
Reprinted with permission. Hankin JR, Steinwachs DM, Elkes C. The impact on utilization of a copayment increase for ambulatory psychiatry care. *Med Care*. 1980;**18**:807.

One cannot determine from these trends whether what occurred was beneficial or not. In this example, the MIS provides information to measure the magnitude of the effect on access. In this case, the data suggest that new patients are being discouraged from utilizing mental health services. Determining the impact on a quality of care would require special investigations to measure need for care and the effects of changes in access to care on outcomes. A judgment would have to be made whether the magnitude of effects on access to care observed justify an investment in special inquiries.

Preventive Care

Monitoring routine preventive care using an MIS requires collecting data on specific screening tests, immunizations, and diagnostic procedures. In concept this is feasible, but it is not always done routinely. Recent efforts by Stuart to assess the adequacy of Papanicolaou testing among recipients of Medicaid Aid to Families with Dependent Children show one approach (Stuart M. Practice variation in ambulatory care: utilization cost and quality for Medicaid users. Dissertation submitted to the Johns Hopkins University School of Hygiene and Public Health, 1988). In Table 3, the proportion of women (in each of two age groups) who received a Papanicolaou test during 1 year is shown. These proportions are then related to the regular source of care, that is, the provider to whom most visits during the year were made. The percent of women having Papanicolaou tests was higher in community health centers; hospital outpatient departments, private physicians, and those with undetermined sources of care were lower and more similar. Note that these percentages are only for women who have received some care during the year. Including the nonutilizers would provide population-based rates that would be lower than the ones shown. These figures suggest that many women are not receiving regular Papanicolaou tests.

TABLE 3. Proportion of Female Medicaid Eligibles Receiving a Papanicolaou Test Classified by Type of Regular Care Source

Regular Source of Care*	Number of Users†	Percent Having Papanicolaou Test in Year	
		Ages 12-17	Ages 18-44
Hospital outpatient department	8712	15.6	28.8
Private physician	6736	12.1	32.5
Community health center	1602	36.6	62.6
Undetermined	7203	20.5	40.2

*Regular source identified as source of care to which most ambulatory visits occurred during the year. Source undetermined if no source has a majority of visits.

†Users include all Baltimore City Aid to Families with Dependent Children Medicaid eligibles continuously enrolled July 1984 to June 1985 and having at least one paid claim for ambulatory physician services.

Reprinted with permission. Stuart M. Practice variation in ambulatory care: utilization cost and quality for Medicaid users. Dissertation submitted to the Johns Hopkins University School of Hygiene and Public Health, 1988.

Diagnosis and Treatment

The use of an MIS to assess the adequacy of diagnosis and treatment has received limited application, largely because in most MIS data sets, there is little information by which to judge the appropriateness of the diagnostic process. Generally no history or test result findings from physical examination are directly available. Moreover, the diagnostic statement on the visit record may be only a tentative or rule-out diagnosis. The frequent inability to distinguish tentative from confirmed diagnoses represents one limitation of *ICD-9-CM* coding. Only in automated medical record systems (28) or enriched encounter systems (29) has it been possible to undertake a systematic examination of the diagnostic process, and this has not been done extensively.

Opportunities to assess the adequacy of treatment are more promising, but also depend on the accuracy of the diagnostic information recorded. In a fully automated medical record system, the dependency on diagnosis alone may be overcome by using laboratory findings to augment or replace diagnostic information. For an MIS, this is generally not possible. Even so, experience suggests that an MIS can provide useful information for monitoring treatment and follow-up care.

The principal method developed for using an MIS to examine the process of care for acute conditions is the episode of care. An episode of care includes all the services received as a result of a specific episode of illness. Note that not all episodes of illness will have an episode of care (that is, if no care is received) and the timeframes of each may not coincide (that is, the episode of illness is expected to begin before the episode of care, and follow-up care may be received after the illness episode is over).

Criteria can be used with MIS data to link services that are part of a single episode. Criteria can be based on identifying visits that have the same or related diagnosis and that have occurred within a specified time interval. It has been shown that the choice of the episode time interval will have some effect on the results. In Table 4 the effect of using different time intervals to link visits for 10 different conditions is shown. Based on MIS data from the Maxicare HMO in Los Angeles, this table shows a decline in incidence (per 100,000 adults) and increase in average visits per episode as the time interval is increased from 3 to 6 weeks. The choice of time interval should be based on the natural history of the condition and patterns of medical care. This can be tested by comparing it with episodes based on medical record review (30).

In another population using MIS-based data, intervals for episodes were created for children with otitis media. For purulent otitis, visits had to occur within 3 weeks of each other to be considered part of a single episode of care. If the condition was serous otitis media, time interval of 6 weeks between visits was allowed. These intervals were developed in consultation with pediatricians and were designed to take into account the natural history of the disorder and the providers' patterns of practice. To validate the criteria, a comparison was made between episodes based on MIS data and episodes based on chart review.

The classification of otitis media episodes as purulent, serous, or mixed (that is, involving both serous and purulent) was based on the MIS diagnostic information. In comparing the MIS episodes classification to one based on the medical record, the rate of agreement was high (over 85%) (31).

Otitis media provides an example of a common acute condition where treatment patterns might be analyzed once episodes of care are developed from an MIS. In studies done at the Columbia Medical Plan (HMO), the Plan's physicians developed quality of care criteria for diagnosis, treatment, follow-up, and outcomes of care (32). The MIS-defined episodes of care were used to compare patterns of care with criteria for use of prescribed medications, follow-up visit, audiometry testing, and referral to an otorhinolaryngologist (ENT) specialist. Criteria indicated that children with frequent recurrent

TABLE 4. Incidence and Visit Rates: The Effects of Alternative Definitions of an Episode of Care*

Disease	Incidence (per 100,000)		Average Visits Per Episode	
	3 Week	6 Week	3 Week	6 Week
Gastroenteritis	3,399	3,299	1.15	1.20
Otitis	4,846	4,410	1.54	1.70
Acute pharangitis	5,538	5,427	1.10	1.13
Influenza	4,048	4,011	1.07	1.08
Asthma	1,394	1,212	1.55	1.81
Urinary tract infections	5,314	5,020	1.26	1.34
Eczema	6,317	6,193	1.10	1.14
Sebaceous disease	4,876	3,735	1.23	1.64
Vertebraic pain	5,223	4,734	1.38	1.56

*The time noted was used to determine whether two visits with related diagnoses were to be considered part of the same episode of care. Data from Maxicare HMO (sample based on 27,000 continuously enrolled adults 18 and over).

Reprinted with permission. Steinwachs DM. An application of the GMENAC physician requirement model to empirical data derived from three HMOs. Final report to the Bureau of Health Professions, DHHS under contract no. HRA-232-81-0035, Hyattsville, Maryland, February 1983.

TABLE 5. Relationship of Follow-up Visits to Number of Otitis Media Episodes in the Previous 12 Months

Episodes in 12 months	Number of Individuals	Proportion with		
		Follow-up	Audiometry Visit	ENT Referral
		%		
1	172	39	3	5
2	112	35	5	6
3	52	40	8	6
4+	48*	48	2	12

*Twenty-nine individuals had four episodes; 13 had five episodes; 5 had six episodes; and 1 had seven episodes.

Reprinted with permission. Steinwachs DM, Yaffe R. An approach to the review of utilization and quality of ambulatory care. Joint Meetings on the Operations Research Society of America and The Institute of Management Sciences, San Juan, Puerto Rico, 1974.

episodes should be seen for follow-up care, tested for hearing deficits, and referred for specialty evaluation.

In Table 5, the relationship of number of episodes in a year to receipt of care is shown. There is only a modest increase in follow-up, audiometry testing, and referral across the three levels. From the perspective of quality monitoring, this illustrates the capability to develop episode data and apply it against criteria-setting guidelines for follow-up and treatment.

Chronic Care Management

Two approaches have been applied to the description of patterns of care for chronic conditions. One is based on the episode concept in which there are a series of episodes over time. An alternative is to examine the pattern of care over specified time intervals, for example, 1 year. Both approaches will be illustrated and can be useful depending on the specific quality issue.

Chronic conditions such as hypertension may be underdiagnosed due to problems in access to care or failures to routinely screen patients at risk. To assess the extent to which there may be failures in diagnosis, the proportion of enrolled patients diagnosed with a chronic condition (for example, hypertension) can be compared with epidemiologic data on expected prevalence (9). In Table 6, the diagnosed prevalence of essential hypertension is shown for all adult enrollees in an HMO. Two criteria were applied to measure diagnosed prevalence: the presence of a diagnosis of hypertension at one or more visits and the receipt of an antihypertensive medication. If prescription data had not been available, a criteria could have been used requiring at least two visits with the diagnosis. This would minimize the potential classification of individuals with labile elevated pressure as having essential hypertension. The diagnosed prevalence shown is somewhat lower than would be expected from epidemiologic estimates of prevalence among younger adults. This suggests that more attention may need to be paid to early diagnosis among this group.

Table 6 also shows the percentages of diagnosed and treated adults who received at least one filled prescription for an antihypertensive medication during the year. Although the percentage is reasonably high, one would expect it to be closer to 100% because few hypertensive patients would be expected to be taken off therapy. These data suggest that 10% to 15% of patients do not maintain continuity of treatment.

The ability to identify hypertensive patients and determine if they are continuing to receive care depends largely on routinely collected diagnostic information. To assess the adequacy of this information, a comparison of judgments based on the MIS and the medical record was made (31). In a sample of 151 cases, 93% of contacts were defined as hypertension visits, based on MIS data; 93% of the time, the chart agreed. In contrast, 82% of the visits identified in the medical record as explicitly involving the care of hypertension were identified using MIS data. Overall, these rates of agreement are acceptable for most statistical applications to monitor the level of continuity and trends over time.

If prescripton data are not routinely collected in the MIS, then reliance has to be placed on the diagnosis recorded at a visit. Continuity of treatment may be indicated by having a return visit for the care of the condition or a prescription refill for a medication used to treat the condition. In Table 7, an example is shown of an MIS-derived tabulation that identifies hypertensive patients seen in a hospital outpatient department (33). The report identifies characteristics of hypertensive patients who do not keep a follow-up appointment (based on date of next scheduled appointment recorded on encounter form), and who fail to reschedule and return at a later date. As shown, higher no-show rates are found among males, younger adults, and those not covered by Medicaid or Medicare insurance. Shorter and longer appointment intervals are associated with higher no-show rates. The shorter

TABLE 6. Prevalence of Hypertension and Percent of Patients Continuing on Hypertensive Medications

Enrollees' Age and Sex	Percent Diagnosed and Given Prescription Anytime* (n=9117)	Percent Given Prescription or Refill during Year
Age 17 and over	3.4	82
Male	3.2	80
Female	3.6	84
Age 17-44	1.4	74
Male	1.5	72
Female	1.3	76
Age 45-64	9.5	86
Male	8.6	88
Female	10.4	85
Age 65 and over	25.6	85
Male	25.9	73
Female	25.4	91

*Tabulation limited to continuously enrolled adults during July 1974 to June 1975; diagnosis and antihypertensive medication could have occurred in prior year or current year.
Reprinted with permission. Steinwachs DM, Mushlin AI. The Johns Hopkins Ambulatory Care Coding Scheme. *Health Serv Res.* 1987;13:36-49.

TABLE 7. Characteristics of Hypertensives Failing to Keep Appointments and Lost to Follow-up

	Percent of Patients Having Index Visit	Percent of No Shows	Percent Lost to Clinic Follow-up*
Total, *n*=2137	100	33	14
Sex			
Male	29	40	19
Female	71	30	12
Age			
Under 45 years	20	38	18
45-64	39	31	11
65+	22	23	9
Unknown	19	42	21
Source of payment			
Medicaid	43	31	12
Medicare	27	25	10
Other and self-pay	30	44	21
Appointment interval			
Under 1 month	14	53	41
1-2 months	50	31	11
3-6 months	28	25	11
Over 6 months	8	33	16

*Those not having at least one additional record visit within 6 months of the index visit.
Reprinted with permission. Steinwachs DM. Measuring provider continuity in ambulatory care: an assessment of alternative approaches. *Med Care*. 1979;17:551-65.

intervals are generally given to new patients. Rates of lost to follow-up parallel the no-show rates.

The information shown in Table 7 identifies hypertensive patients at increased risk for poor continuity. Previous research has shown that interventions with these patients can reduce noncompliance and increase blood pressure control (34). At a minimum, special efforts should be made to minimize the effects of financial access barriers and to remind patients of appointments.

These applications illustrate approaches for monitoring the care of major chronic conditions that can be undertaken with routine MIS data. Where apparent deficiencies are identified, recourse to the medical record or other data sources may be needed to identify specific solutions to problems.

Adverse Health Outcomes

Until recently, the principal use of an MIS to examine outcomes has been related to mortality. Wennberg and Gittlesohn (35) have examined variations in surgical rates and their relationship to mortality. Studies have related the number of surgical procedures to mortality and found that for some procedures, increasing volumes are related to declining mortality (36). The HCFA has produced national data on case mix adjusted hospital mortality rates (40) and Blumberg (38) has proposed a risk-adjusted method for examining surgical mortality. These are examples of approaches for identifying excess mortality and potential quality of care problems. It is still too early to know how effectively this information can be used to identify deficiencies in quality. It does appear that it should be useful for identifying providers whose mortality experience is substantially different than the average.

Hospital admissions for sentinel events have been used as indicators of deficiencies in quality. Also, hospital readmissions have been used as a measure that should be sensitive to variations in the quality of inpatient care (39). The episodes of care can be used to measure readmissions. An episode is created around an index admission, including care both before and after discharge. Readmissions occurring within the episode have been examined and related to specific changes in hospital payment (40), raising concerns that per case payment (for example, DRG payment) may contribute to higher rates of readmission.

Very promising work using insurance claims data in Canada has shown that computer-applied criteria can be developed to identify readmissions that result from complications (41). Criteria have been applied to screen hospital discharge data to identify patients who have been readmitted as a result of complications after surgery. These have been validated through medical record reviews. Using criteria such as these will make it possible to determine whether there are institutional, geographic, and insurance related differences in complication rates. They provide a basis for ongoing monitoring of readmissions that would be considered potentially preventable.

Although advances are being made in this area, it is recognized that more comprehensive approaches to outcome assessment than those based on current MIS capability will be needed to systematically monitor quality. This might be achieved by augmenting MIS encounter and hospitalization data with outcome information obtained through patient surveys at defined intervals after an inpatient or ambulatory episode. This would provide self-reported measures of health status that could be used to measure recovery and health outcomes.

CONCLUSIONS

The technology for applying an MIS to monitor quality has been developing for some time but remains largely untested in routine applications. However, there are many demands for this to change. Public concern with the quality of health care is rising as previous arrangements for health care, which were stable for many years, are modified. When PPOs are developed, everyone wants assurance that the preferred providers are not only less expensive but will provide high-quality care. As the HMO industry has grown and evolved, competition with existing insurance and practice arrangements is not only in terms of cost, but claims of "better" quality care (42).

The findings of variations in surgical rates have also raised comparable questions regarding differences in health care expenditures and outcomes across geographic areas in this country. Recent efforts to explain some of these variations by assessing the appropriateness of the procedure have shown that appropriateness, one aspect of quality, does not explain large differences in procedure rates (43). Thus, considerable work needs to be done to develop our capabilities to measure differences in system-level quality that contribute to differences in utilization and cost of health care.

Although many of the larger questions concerning differences in quality of care across communities and provider organizations are still unanswered, a broad base of experience now exists for measuring quality at the individual patient level (10). In most cases, these patient level measures can be aggregated to develop population-based measures. Such measures can be used to describe and compare aspects of the quality of care across different systems. For example, the proportion of populations receiving indicated preventive care can be compared across systems or communities, as can the adequacy of care for individuals with specific conditions.

Even more important, these patient-oriented measures have relevance for the providers and administrators who are directly responsible for patient care. The approaches described for applying an MIS to monitor quality of care indicators can be applied by HMOs, PPOs, and insurers to measure changes over time and to compare the care provided with accepted standards. Potential deficiencies would be expected to be remedied. Although these concepts may be widely accepted, they are not widely applied.

There are several considerations that have limited more rapid acceptance and application of MIS-based quality assurance methods. Until recently, few insurers have routinely required coded diagnostic information on ambulatory visits, thus the opportunity to apply these approaches has not been present. Second, many have been uncertain regarding the utility of claims data for examining quality. It is expected that this will be changing as more experience is gained in the application of MISs. Third, at one time many might have doubted that anyone was interested in this type of information, whereas concern with the cost of care appeared to dominate other issues. However, information related to quality is attracting interest by the public, employers, and insurers. Although these groups do not share a common perspective, all recognize that the quality and the cost of care are intertwined, and efforts to address one must consider the consequences for the other. We know much more about how to measure and monitor costs than quality. Indeed, the development of MISs in health care has been principally motivated by needs for better fiscal and resource information to support management. Now that pressures are growing for improved quality management, efforts are beginning to expand the scope and content of MISs to address basic quality issues. As this progresses, the potential for quality of care monitoring based on MISs can be expected to emerge as a new resource to improve American health care.

Acknowledgments: This work was supported in part by a grant from the CIGNA Foundation.

References

1. Steinwachs DM. Management information systems: new challenges to meet changing needs. *Med Care.* 1985;**23**:607-22.
2. Brook RH, Lohr KN. Monitoring quality of care in the Medicare program: two proposed systems. *JAMA.* 1987;**258**:3138-41.
3. Blendon RJ. The public's view of the future of health care. *JAMA.* 1988;**259**:3587-93.
4. Donabedian A. *The Definition of Quality and Approaches to Its Assessment.* Ann Arbor, Michigan: Health Administration Press; 1980.
5. Steffen GE. Quality medical care: a definition. *JAMA.* 1988;**260**:56-61.
6. Barnett GO, Winickoff RN, Dorsey JL, Morgan MM, Lurie RS. Quality assurance through automated monitoring and concurrent feedback using a computer-based medical information system. *Med Care.* 1978;**16**:962-70.
7. Smithline N, Arbitman D, eds. *Ambulatory Case Mix Classification Systems.* A special issue of *J Ambulatory Case Mgm,* Vol 11, August 1988.
8. Shapiro S. End result measurements of quality of medical care. *Milbank Mem Fund Q.* 1967;**45**:7-30.
9. Kessner DM, Kalk CE, Singer J. Assessing health quality — the case for tracers. *N Engl J Med.* 1973;**288**:189-94.
10. Donabedian A. The quality of care: how can it be assessed? *JAMA.* 1988;**260**:1743-8.
11. Williamson JW. Formulating priorities for quality assurance activity: description of a method and its application. *JAMA.* 1978;**239**:631-7.
12. Palmer RH. The challenge and prospects for quality assessment and assurance in ambulatory care. *Inquiry.* 1988;**25**:119-31.
13. Aday L, Andersen R, Fleming G. *Health Care in the U.S.: Equitable for Whom?* Beverly Hills, California; Sage Publications; 1980.
14. U.S. DHHS. *Promoting Health and Preventing Diseases: Objectives for the Nation.* Washington, DC: U.S. Government Printing Office, 1980.
15. Weiner J, Steinwachs DM, Powe N. *The Development of a Quality Assurance System Based on Insurance Claims Data.* Final Report to the CIGNA Foundation by The Johns Hopkins University Health Services Research and Development Center, Baltimore, Maryland, 1989.
16. McDonald CJ. Protocol-based computer reminders, the quality of care, and the non-perfectability of man. *N Engl J Med.* 1976;**295**:1351-5.
17. Rutstein DD, Berenberg W, Chalmers TC, Child CG 3d, Fishman AP, Perrin EB. Measuring the quality of medical care: a clinical method. *N Engl J Med.* 1976;**294**:582-8.
18. U.S. DHHS. *Ambulatory Medical Care: Minimum Data Set. A report of the United States National Committee on Vital and Health Statistics.* Publication No (PHS)81:1161; 1981.
19. U.S. NCHS. *Uniform Hospital Abstract: Minimum Basic Data Set. (Vital and Health Statistics,* Series 4, No. 14). Public Health Service. Washington, DC: U.S. Government Printing Office; 1972.
20. Institute of Medicine. *Reliability of National Hospital Discharge Survey Data.* Washington, DC: National Academy of Sciences; 1980.
21. Institute of Medicine. *Reliability of Medicare Hospital Discharge Records.* Washington, DC: National Academy of Sciences; 1977.
22. Hsia DC, Krushat WM, Fagan AB, Tebbutt JA, Kusserow RP. Accuracy of diagnostic coding for Medicare patients under the prospective-payment system. *N Engl J Med.* 1988;**318**:352-5.
23. Steinwachs DM, Mushlin AI. The Johns Hopkins ambulatory care coding scheme. *Health Serv Res.* 1978;**13**:36-49.
24. Gertman PM, Restuccia JD. The appropriateness evaluation protocol: a technique for assessing unnecessary days of hospital care. *Med Care.* 1981;**19**:855-71.
25. Steinwachs DM, Yaffe R. Assessing the timeliness of ambulatory medical care. *Am J Public Health.* 1978;**68**:547-56.
26. Louis DZ, Gonnella JS, Zelezuik C. *An Approach to the Prevention of Late Hospital Admissions in Stemming the Rising Costs of Medical Care: Answers and Antidotes.* Battle Creek, Michigan: W.K. Kellogg Foundation; March 1988: 147-57.
27. Hankin JR, Steinwachs DM, Elkes C. The impact on utilization of a copayment increase for ambulatory psychiatric care. *Med Care.* 1980;**18**:807-15.
28. Barnett GO, Winickoff RN, Morgan MM, Zielstorff RD. A computer-based monitoring system for follow-up of elevated blood pressure. *Med Care.* 1983;**21**:400-9.
29. Whiting-O'Keefe QE, Simborg DW, Epstein WV, Warger A. A computerized summary medical record system can provide more information than the standard medical record. *JAMA.* 1985;**254**:1185-92.

30. Kessler LG, Steinwachs DM, Hankin JR. Episodes of psychiatric utilization. *Mea Care.* 1980;**18**:1219-27.

31. Steinwachs DM, Yaffe R. An approach to the review of utilization and quality of ambulatory care. Joint Meetings of the Operations Research Society of America and The Institute of Management Sciences, San Juan, Puerto Rico, 1974.

32. Mushlin AI, Appel FA. Testing an outcome-based quality assurance strategy in primary care. *Med Care.* 1980; **18**(Suppl):1-100.

33. Steinwachs DM. Measuring provider continuity in ambulatory care: an assessment of alternative approaches. *Med Care.* 1979;**17**:551-65.

34. Levine DM, Green LW, Deeds SG, Chwalow J, Russell RP, Finlay J. Health education for hypertensive patients. *JAMA.* 1979;**241**:1700-3.

35. Wennberg J, Gittlesohn A. Variations in medical care among small areas. *Sci Am.* 1982;**246**:120-34.

36. Bunker JP, Luft HS, Enthoven A. Should surgery be regionalized? *Surg Clin North Am.* 1982;**62**:657-68.

37. Jencks SF, Williams DK, Kay TL. Assessing hospital-associated deaths from discharge data: the role of length ofstay and comorbidities. *JAMA.* 1988;**260**:2240-6.

38. Blumberg MS. Risk adjusting health outcomes: a methodologic review. *Med Care Rev.* 1986;**43**:351-93.

39. Anderson GF, Steinberg EP. Hospital readmissions in the Medicare population. *N Engl J Med.* 1984;**311**:1349-53.

40. Rupp A, Steinwachs DM, Salkever DS. The effect of hospital payment methods on the pattern and cost of mental health care. *Hosp Community Psychiatry.* 1984;**35**:456-9.

41. Roos LL Jr, Cageorge SM, Austen E, Lohr KN. Using computers to identify complications after surgery. *Am J Public Health.* 1985;**75**:1288-95.

42. Weiner JP. Assuring quality of care in HMOs: past lessons, present challenges, future directions. *GHAA J.* 1986;**7**(1):10-27.

43. Chassin MR, Kosecoff J, Park RE, et al. Does inappropriate use explain geographic variations in the use of health care services? A study of three procedures. *JAMA.* 1987;**258**:2533-7.

COMMENTARY

Steinwachs and colleagues expertly summarize the pertinent issues confronting increased use of MISs in the measure of quality. Until the recent explosion in managed care, no incentive on the part of third party payers to use their mountains of MIS-based data to measure quality existed. This lack of incentive contributed to the scientific problems inherent in the use of MISs to measure quality. Accuracy of coded information and uncertainty as to the types of required information represent formidable obstacles to effective use of MISs to measure quality.

Steinwachs and colleagues skillfully summarize the significant progress that has been made to address these scientific and organizational barriers. Of critical importance from an organizational point of view is that the cost of measuring quality from an MIS will be significantly less than other comparable measures. This and the fact that much of the information will be used for utilization management will heighten the importance of MIS-based quality of care information. In summary, the MIS will assume significant importance in the measurement of both an overall plan's (health insurance or managed care operation) quality of care "score" and, more importantly, from a physician's point of view the individual practitioner's performance not just on cost but on quality of care provided to his or her panel of patients.

Surprisingly, the continued emphasis on cost cutting will facilitate the use of MISs to measure quality in various ways. From a pure utilization management point of view the inclusion of protocol-based methodology to measure excess utilization of a particular procedure can also be used by interested parties to examine problems of access to care. Aetna Life and Casualty has already begun to incorporate protocol-based clinical algorithms in its utilization review operations. The clinical sophistication of these algorithms will permit the data to be used for both quality and cost evaluations.

With respect to provider profiles, Steinwachs and colleagues appropriately point out that MIS-based provider profiles have until recently only been concerned with physician cost productivity. As the industrial model of quality assurance begins to seep beyond the Harvard Community Health Plan, among a few others, health care insurers and managed care organizations will realize that increased quality (increased quantity does not mean increased quality) will lead to decreased costs. This, together with the public's demand for such information, will heighten the use of provider-based measures of quality. Are we going to see the public release of physician-specific measures of quality? Not in the short term. In the long term this will occur, particularly if the organizations representing the medical community do not involve themselves in the setting of standards of physician performance that can be obtained from the MIS. Although the actual physician-specific data should be confidential, it is reasonable for the public to have access to and be able to comment on the standards that public and private payers use in the measurement of physician quality.

Table 1 provides an excellent framework from which to understand both the multidimensional character of quality and the types of information one can obtain from an MIS. The information summarized can be used for various purposes. Steinwachs and colleagues are providing a menu of approaches from which organizations, health care providers, and the public can choose those quality of care variables best suited to their needs.

The future for the use of MISs in quality measurement is very bright. The recent work of Wennberg and associates (1), which documents the clinical utility of the MIS, is very exciting. In this study, claims-based information is used to document complications of prostatectomy, many of which are not included in medical textbooks. Wennberg and colleagues have taken this research one step further and are integrating this clinical information obtained through the MIS into videodiscs (Wennberg J. Presentation at CIGNA Corporation, July 1988). The patient can then view this material in deciding whether or not to go ahead with the prostatectomy. Advances in clinical understanding derived from an MIS can then be utilized not only to improve quality from both an MIS and patient satisfaction point of view, but to involve the patient in decisions affecting his or her welfare. As physicians and other health care providers intimately know, the patient should be the ultimate customer. (The Editors)

Reference

1. Wennberg, Roos N, Sola L, et al. Use of claims data systems to evaluate health care outcomes: mortality and reoperation following prostatectomy. *JAMA* 1987;**257**:936-46.

Chapter 7

Measuring the Quality of Office Practice

SHELDON GREENFIELD, MD

INTRODUCTION

Efforts to judge the quality of medical care have produced a substantial amount of research. However, because most of the scientific attention has been focused on the evaluation of hospital care, there are few techniques for evaluating office practice (1-5). Valid and reliable methods for assessing the quality of care provided for hospitalized patients by individual physicians, groups of physicians, or health care institutions are inappropriate or have limited application to care provided for outpatients in office practices. Consistent results linking what physicians do in practice to changes in patients' health status are lacking.

There are pressing issues that underscore the need for methods that accurately reflect the quality of office practice. Medical care in general is becoming increasingly office-based. Cost-containment pressures and advances in technology have interacted to increase the number of procedures done in the office or outpatient setting. Hospitals are becoming the site of care for only the sickest patients. Whether or not hospital care should have been delivered at all (that is, the "appropriateness" of hospital care) may be a direct consequence of what physicians do or do not do in office practice.

The current restructuring of the delivery systems in which medical care is provided (for example, individual practice associations [IPAs], preferred provider organizations [PPOs], health maintenance organizations [HMOs]) creates an urgency to identify "what works" — what features of the care provided by physicians in office practice lead to care of the highest quality and ought to be preserved in this restructuring, and what features provide an opportunity to configure health care systems proactively as a function of the determinants of quality care provision?

What are the elements of high-quality office-based care and how should they be measured and evaluated? Researchers, medical educators, and policymakers have dichotomized medical care into two parts — technical care and interpersonal care — each of which can be judged by its process or outcomes. Evaluating the technical process of care involves assessing whether and to what extent an individual physician met the standards of practice for diagnosing and treating a patient with a specific health problem. Evaluating the *outcomes* of technical care requires that quality be judged using the patient's health status (physiologic or functional). Evaluating the *process* of interpersonal care involves assessing the dynamics of the physician-patient relationship. Evaluation of the *outcomes* of interpersonal care has not been well researched. Whether outcomes of interpersonal care should be assessed separately from outcomes of technical care is an important issue, particularly in office-based practice, where high-quality technical care may be subverted by a patient with whom the physician may not have optimal rapport.

Methods for measuring the processes and outcomes of technical and interpersonal office-based care are limited but available. Once these measures are obtained, how should they be used to judge the quality of care? What, for example, defines high-quality care in terms of patients' functional status and quality of life? What proportion of hypertensive patients in a physician's practice should be controlled for that physician to be judged as providing adequate care? How should the performance of an individual physician or group of physicians be judged? Should physicians' performance be compared with some absolute standard set by peers? Should he or she be compared with other physicians in the same specialty caring for the same types of patients? What factors, such as case mix, should be controlled for when making these comparisons?

This chapter outlines approaches to quality of care assessment that can be used to evaluate office-based practice, including new approaches that are in developmental stages; and discusses ways to improve the quality of care provided by individual physicians through the use of information from quality of care evaluations. It is critical that physicians accept evaluation as part of routine office practice for the purpose of self-improvement. If the goal of quality of care assessment is to improve patient care and patients' health, then approaches to this assessment that are not used by physicians in daily practice will be expensive failures that the health care system cannot afford.

APPROACHES TO THE ASSESSMENT OF OFFICE PRACTICE

The most time-honored method for evaluating the quality of care provided by physicians involves comparing the information in the medical records of patients with a specific disease condition with standards set by a group of physicians expert in treating the disease. The limited information in most medical records maintained in office practices hinders this traditional assessment method. Further, because the care provided in hospitals tends to be more homogeneous due to the predominance of a single disease with a more acute course, standards are more easily arrived at for hospital-based care than for outpatient care, in which patients may have several, comorbid conditions that interact to affect appropriate management.

Accurate evaluation of the quality of office-based care using traditional approaches requires a method that will tolerate the limited information in office practice medical records and yet reflects the dynamic and changing nature of disease management for patients with several conditions. Using less traditional methods, it may be possible to obtain the most comprehensive evaluation of the quality of office practice by measuring patients' reports of their health outcomes. Measures of patients' functional status and other patient reports of health have recently shown potential use for assessing quality of care (6,7). Algorithms have shown promise as a technique representing an advance over traditional methods for evaluating the technical process of care in offices (1,2,8,9). This discussion begins with the evaluation of the process of care, focusing on algorithms, and concludes with the evaluation of the outcomes of care, focusing on patients' functional status and quality of life.

Algorithms and the Evaluation of Office Practice

Why Algorithms?   For the sake of the discussion in this chapter, there are no definitional differences between the terms "algorithm" and "criteria map." The former is usually used in the context of prospective clinical decision making and the latter in the context of retrospective evaluation of physician performance. The short answer to the question posed is that algorithms or criteria maps, give the most faithful representation of the care provided by physicians to individual patients with a specific disease. Unlike other methods of evaluating the quality of care provided by physicians, the branching format of algorithms individualizes or tailors the standards of care, approximating the decisions a physician would have made in caring for a patient with a given disease (1,10). Figure 1 shows an algorithm developed to evaluate office-based care for patients with chronic obstructive pulmonary disease. This algorithm was developed by a group of academic and practicing physicians (8). It begins with the patient's symptom state — whether the patient had any, some, or all of the following symptoms: dyspnea, wheezing, chest tightness, or cough. Patients are then divided into two groups: those with infection and those with heart failure. Different care and therefore different standards are specified for each group. Physicians treating patients with chronic obstructive pulmonary disease who have heart failure as the cause of their symptoms would be held to different guidelines from physicians treating patients with infection superimposed on chronic obstructive pulmonary disease. Although this distinction may appear trivial, traditional methods of quality of care assessment do not usually discriminate the unique needs of one subgroup of patients from another. For example, for a patient with chronic obstructive pulmonary disease and dyspnea, wheezing, or cough, both congestive heart failure and pulmonary infection would have to be ruled out for the care to be judged as adequate. In contrast, after the algorithm shown in Figure 1, physicians' care would not be judged inappropriate if they failed to admit

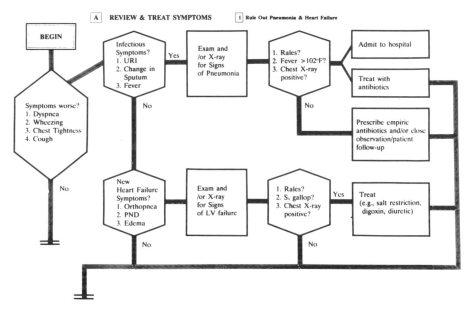

Figure 1. Criteria map for chronic obstructive pulmonary disease. URI = urinary tract infection; PND = paroxysmal nocturnal dyspnea; LV = left ventricular. Reprinted with permission. Stulbarg MS, Gerbert B, Kemeny M, et al. Outpatient treatment of chronic obstructive pulmonary disease — a practitioner's guide. *West J Med.* 1985;**142**:842-6.

a patient with symptoms of dyspnea, wheezing, chest tightness, or cough with further symptoms of infection (upper respiratory infection, change in sputum, or fever) if he or she did not have rales, high fever, or a chest roentgenogram that showed signs of pneumonia. As with traditional methods, all cases in which physicians failed to admit a patient with symptomatic chronic obstructive pulmonary disease *and* signs of lower respiratory infection including rales, high fever, or chest roentgenogram confirmation of pneumonia, would be reviewed for exceptional circumstances before being declared inadequate care.

The principal value of algorithms over traditional methods for assessing the quality of office-based practice is that they clarify the patient populations to which the standards of care apply, so that the important decisions and the specific contingencies that led up to those decisions can be evaluated accurately. Two additional values of algorithms over traditional methods for evaluating office-based practice are related to the branching format of algorithms. First, this format allows for maximum use of the limited information in the medical records in most physicians' offices. This information, although not comprehensive, may document the highly specific, heuristic thinking of physicians in practice and may consequently be all that is needed to make accurate evaluations of care. Second, in outpatient medicine, where often the studies of clinical efficacy often do not support one clearly superior approach to diagnosis or management over another, algorithms allow for the choice between several options in the evaluation of care. The maximum possible flexibility is therefore allowed for when evaluating the quality of an individual physician's performance.

TABLE 1. Differences Between Prospective and Retrospective Algorithms

Prospective Algorithms	Retrospective Algorithms
Directive, care not yet delivered	*Reactive*, care already delivered
Logically complete; must include rare diagnosis, remote events	Logically incomplete; used as initial screen; deviations reviewed individually
Narrower range of options at important decision points	More extensive range of options at important decision points
Independent of medical records	Dependent on information in medical records

A final point must be addressed: The very notion of a detailed algorithm has sometimes been a source of irritation to clinicians. Often called the "cookbook" approach to medicine, algorithms can be viewed as reductionist, controlling, and simplistic, overlooking the complexity and "art" of care needed to manage patients optimally. It must be acknowledged that algorithms were originally conceived as prospective guidelines for teaching clinical decision making to nurse practitioners and physicians' assistants (11). In this context, it was necessary that these guidelines be as complete as possible to make the course of management clear for even the most complex and unusual clinical circumstances; algorithms were therefore directive and highly specific. Further, because the care could be directed prospectively, fewer options needed to be specified at important decision points. In contrast, when algorithms are used retrospectively to evaluate care already delivered, their character changes markedly. Used for this purpose, algorithms are not directive, but reactive, developed to reflect the multiple acceptable variations that may define adequate medical care. Other inherent differences between algorithms used prospectively and retrospectively in evaluations of care are shown in Table 1. In the end, rather than being the "cookbook" approach to medical care, algorithms and their multiple derivatives may provide a fairer evaluation of physicians' performance than other approaches that ignore medical decision making.

Do Algorithms Work?   The validity of most methods for evaluating quality of care generally has not been rigorously tested. To determine whether care was evaluated accurately using algorithms or other methods, it would be necessary to determine whether care assessed as inadequate resulted in poor patient outcomes more often than care assessed as adequate. Such a study was done for hospital-based care (12). In this study, the evaluations of care using algorithms predicted the outcomes of care for emergency room patients presenting with chest pain better than the evaluations of the same care using traditional criteria.

A more common approach for determining the validity of any method for quality of care assessment is to subject the standards to expert judgment. The consensus of a panel of physicians expert in treating the disease or condition being evaluated is accepted as evidence of the "face" validity of the standards. In a study (9) of the evaluation of care for patients with urinary tract infections, algorithms were judged to be a more accurate reflection of care than standards in traditional list format.

Now is the time to question the validity of any method for evaluating the quality of care. This is especially important for methods that are less well developed, such as those for evaluating office-based care. If physicians' performance is to be compared against practice standards and assessed as adequate or inadequate, and physicians are to be held accountable for inadequate care, what is the best way to formulate those standards to yield the most accurate results? How do we discriminate accurate from inaccurate results from quality of care evaluations? The most optimal way is to compare those results with patient outcomes. Some studies are beginning in this direction. The National Study of Medical Outcomes (7), for example, provides an opportunity to link what physicians do in practice with the outcomes experienced by chronically ill patients over a 2-year period. Fowler and associates (6) have linked patient outcomes to the performance of prostatectomy under varying clinical circumstances. However, no one has used patient outcomes to validate retrospective evaluations of office-based care using algorithms or any other quality assessment method. Such studies are both timely and necessary if we are to make judgments about the quality of any medical care with reasonable certainty.

How Are Algorithms Generated?   Regardless of its validity, no method for evaluating quality of medical care will be valuable unless it can be used by physicians in daily practice. To be useful to clinicians, quality assessment methods must be practical, reflect practice accurately, rely on information that is easy to get, and, most importantly, be relatively easy to generate and modify in response to changes in clinical thinking. Does the specialized architecture of an algorithm prevent its development by the average practicing clinician? No, although it helps to have had experience. However, with some guidance provided by available materials or courses in algorithm generation (such as that currently taught at the Harvard Community Health Plan), enough experience can be gained to put together an algorithm that reflects the standards of a given office practice. Algorithms that have been generated in this fashion have appeared in the literature (2,8 13).

The goal in generating an algorithm is to outline the major pathways or important decisions for highly specific subclasses of patients to yield enough data to evaluate care for most patients with a given health problem. The first stage is to identify a health problem that is common in a practice and that, if the practice includes more than one physician, all agree is a problem. The health problems that are the best candidates for algorithms are those that have the greatest probability for variations in individual physician's performance, those that are suspected targets for improving care, and those for which consensus regarding the standards of practice around important decisions can be reasonably attained.

After such a health problem is identified, the physician or group of physicians providing care for this problem in the practice should delineate the major decisions involved in the diagnosis and management of the problem. Once these decisions are identified, the subcategories of patients to which they apply should be specified. For example, using the algorithm shown in Figure 1, if a patient presents with an exacerbation of chronic obstructive pulmonary disease, the physician must determine whether heart failure or infection was the cause of the deterioration. The algorithm would therefore branch immediately into two major sections: that dealing with the work-up and management of heart failure and that dealing with the work-up and management of infection.

Another example of the development of an algorithm can be drawn from a study by Palmer and colleagues (2). The criteria for follow-up of abnormal serum glucose levels were as follows: "among previously diagnosed diabetics with a serum glucose of greater or equal to 300 mg/dL, treatment should be adjusted to restore glucose control, unless lack of control was attributed to temporary stress or infection or to persistent patient inability to comply with treatment or was disproved by other laboratory evidence such as a normal repeat serum glucose or a normal glycohemoglobin value. If treatment was changed, a follow-up serum glucose was required" (2). These contingency statements define a piece of an algorithm for the management of diabetes. Drawn diagrammatically, they would appear as Figure 2.

The details for constructing an algorithm cannot be discussed adequately here. As noted above, there are materials and courses available to provide support in the generation of algorithms for the evaluation of the quality of care. It is important to note, however, that once the algorithm is drafted,

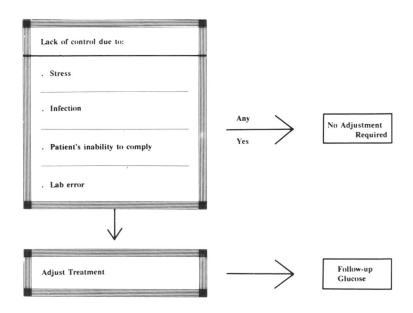

Figure 2. Criteria map for diabetic patients with serum glucose greater than 300 mg/dL. Reprinted with permission. Palmer RH, Strain R, Maurer J, et al. Quality assurance in eight adult medicine group practices. *Med Care*. 1984;**22**:632-43.

the standards of care that it enumerates must be agreed on by at least those physicians who are members of the practice and preferably, reviewed by some external physicians also expert in delivering care for the health problem being evaluated. There are various techniques for obtaining consensus regarding standards of care from groups of physicians (14). These techniques are as easily applied to standards in algorithmic format as to standards in other quality assessment formats.

How Should Data from Quality of Care Evaluations Be Used?   There are many studies in which information regarding costs of care or variations in patterns of care has been fed back to physicians. These studies have been summarized in an excellent comprehensive review by Eisenberg (15). However, there are few examples in the literature that document productive ways for using data from quality of care assessments using any technique, much less algorithms. An outstanding example of feedback of quality of care information shows the potential for this type of evaluation to change the quality of patient care. In the context of eight general medicine provider groups in two academic hospitals and six neighborhood health centers, Palmer and colleagues (2) developed algorithms for four medical care tasks — follow-up of low hematocrits, cancer screening for women, monitoring of patients on digoxin, and follow-up of abnormal serum glucose levels. Criteria for each of these tasks were ratified by physicians at each of the health care settings. After the evaluation, cases deviating from the algorithm were reviewed by a physician representative to identify exceptional circumstances that would explain these deviations. Information regarding the performance of individual physicians was then made available to those physicians. Various actions were taken after this feedback to improve patient care, including revisions in the system for follow-up of abnormal laboratory results, changes in the interprovider referral policy, recall of specific patients for additional care, changes in laboratory reporting system, and changes in the algorithm itself. Although the improvements in care were modest, this study serves as a model for the dynamic use of quality of care assessment information in a program of quality assurance. Future studies must deal more directly with three critical issues: physician involvement in all aspects of quality of care evaluation from criteria setting to the consequences of negative performance; presentation of information in a more timely way (for example, using on-line entry of patient information on the same day that care is provided) such that patient care can be more immediately influenced; and incentives for change, both internal and external, to the health care delivery system. These incentives must be part of any quality assessment process if it is to improve patient care.

Algorithms and Appropriateness Guidelines.   We are beginning to see many of the elements of algorithms used to modify various approaches to quality of care assessment. In the development of appropriateness standards, for example, guidelines are beginning to reflect the essential character of algorithms. Contingency "if-then" criteria are appearing with greater frequency (16-18). Subcategories of patients are being defined more specifically. In fact, appropriateness can be considered in the context of algorithms. Embedded in a section of an algorithm for patients with angina such as the one in Figure 3

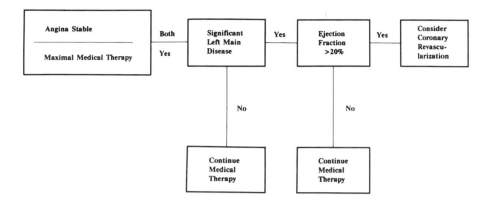

Figure 3. Algorithm for unstable angina. Reprinted with permission. Winslow CM, Kosecoff JB, Chassin MR. The appropriateness of performing coronary artery bypass surgery. *JAMA.* 1988;260:505-9.

is an appropriate guideline for the decision to undertake coronary revascularization (17).

Algorithms can therefore be structured to indicate the circumstances under which a procedure would be judged inappropriate and which alternative strategies could be recommended. This kind of algorithmic guideline could stand alone or be placed in a more comprehensive algorithm for patients with angina, identifying the many decisions that could lead to coronary bypass surgery. Cost-containment pressures combined with the high morbidity and mortality associated with certain procedures have singled out such procedures for studies of the appropriateness of their use using "appropriateness guidelines." These guidelines evaluate a single decision. Algorithms, in contrast, broaden the scope of the evaluation to include all the decisions, including diagnostic tests, referrals, medications, return visits, as well as procedures and hospitalizations. In this way, the algorithm makes a more comprehensive characterization of the quality of care provided for an illness by an individual physician, group of physicians, or health care delivery system.

Algorithms and Cost Containment. The evaluation of cost-containment strategies can also be incorporated in the general structure of an algorithm. Where a less expensive test, procedure, or general diagnostic or management strategy can be substituted for a more expensive one, the algorithm can be structured to include such alternatives, weighing their utility in the context of all decisions identified in the algorithm. As for appropriateness guidelines, cost-containment strategies can be structured in algorithmic format, and can be considered individually or in the context of a more comprehensive algorithm.

Medication monitoring is another aspect of office-based quality of care that emphasizes cost-containment and can be considered in algorithmic format. Abundant evidence shows that physicians have difficulty getting good drug information, may prescribe drugs that interact with others, may prescribe too many medications, may not be aware of side-effects, or may be unwilling to use drugs with which they are unfamiliar (19). Various strategies designed to help physicians monitor patients' medications have been developed and tested (20,21). Whether highlighted as a special set of problems or included as part of a broader approach, medication monitoring is important to the comprehensive assessment of the quality of office-based practice and can be easily integrated into decision-oriented algorithmic format.

Methodologic Issues in Quality of Care Assessment Using Algorithms. There are some important unresolved methodologic issues in the assessment of care. Some of these issues are unique to algorithms; others represent problems for quality of care assessment in general. First, what is the appropriate "unit of analysis" in which data should be presented? Should it be presented by an individual physician's group of patients, across physicians or practices, across systems of care, or across geographic regions? The answer to these questions is in part determined by the purpose to be served by the evaluation of quality. However this question has important methodologic implications. How many patients with a given condition for each physician, for example, are needed to give a reliable representation of the quality of that physician's care for that condition? How many conditions should be sampled to give a reliable overall estimate of the quality of care provided by an individual physician? How many patients are needed to reliably estimate the care provided by a specific health care system? Further research in the context of on-going quality assessment programs needs to be conducted to address the generalizability of "scores" derived from the measurement of the quality of care.

Second, how are the results of quality of care assessments to be interpreted? What thresholds of deviations from the algorithm define poor quality? Are some deviations more critical than others? There is some evidence supporting the need to "weight" various decisions identified in algorithms with respect to their importance in determining patient outcomes (12). Studies that begin to test the relationship between the decisions enumerated in algorithms and the outcomes experienced by patients are now timely and essential to the rational identification of areas for improvement in the care provided by physicians.

Limitations of Algorithms. No discussion of the nature and use of algorithms for assessing the quality of office-based care would be complete without some clear statement of their limitations for that purpose. First, as with traditional quality assessment methods, they depend on the medical record. Even the branching format of algorithms cannot compensate for sparsely documented care. Further, certain aspects of care are not routinely documented in the record. In the example from Palmer and colleagues (2), patients' ability to comply with treatment recommendations was built into the evaluation of care (Figure 2). Such information rarely appears in records of most office practices. Second, the criteria that form the basis of the algorithm are rarely supported by efficacy studies. The standards of care in any form of quality assessment are only as good as the science of medicine that they reflect. If we are to develop meaningful methods for identifying "quality" in the most positive sense, then the standards of care must be based on solid evidence that specific elements of the process of medical care lead to specific patient outcomes.

Finally, algorithms "decompose" patient care into individual elements for the purpose of identifying discrete deviations that constitute poor quality care, that is, deviations that would or should result in poor outcome. However, discrete deviations do not necessarily sum to a poor patient outcome, nor does the absence of deviations from an algorithm guarantee good patient health. In office-based practice, the relationship between process and outcome is not strong enough to rely entirely on any evaluation of process to assess quality of care. The use of patient outcomes to evaluate care addresses most of these limitations.

Outcomes and the Assessment of Office-Based Practice

The evaluation of the process of care alone does not capture the nature of disease management in the outpatient setting. As stated above, outcomes are necessary to complement process or to use to identify situations in which the process of care needs to be scrutinized more carefully. The use of patient outcomes in the evaluation of the quality of care allows for a more comprehensive comparison of the care provided by physicians across several patient groups and various aspects of care. In areas where the science of medicine falls short or where efficacy studies do not provide a clear route to diagnosis or treatment, the clinician must rely on individual judgment or instinct. When patient outcomes are used to measure the quality of care delivered, the evaluation of care can reflect good or bad clinical judgment rather than whether the physician chose certain specified strategies. In this sense, the ends justify reasonably bounded means.

Certain patient outcomes, such as functional status and quality of life, allow for maximum comprehensiveness in assessing quality of care. The interpersonal aspects of office-based care — *persuading* patients to take medication, return for follow-up, and undergo noxious outpatient procedures; *eliciting* patients' psychosocial problems or concerns or beliefs about care that may impair medical treatment; and *accounting* for patients' values when setting on a course of action — may have important consequences for patient care. The best measures of the process of patient care cannot adequately reflect the interpersonal dimension. This is best reflected in measures of patients' functioning and quality of life.

Evidence is building that patient outcomes provide valid and reliable estimations of the quality of individual physician's care. In the context of the National Study of Medical Outcomes (7,22), scores for patient outcomes (controlling for case mix) are being generated for individual physicians. Those scores will be used to compare the care provided in different health care delivery systems, in practices with a wide range of resource use, among different physician specialties, and in different geographic areas. Preliminary evidence from this study suggests that a generalized score can be obtained for an individual physician that is an accurate and stable estimation of that physician's care. Other investigators are also using patient functioning and quality of life to gauge the quality of care (6,23). However, these studies do not assess the performance of the individual physician. Further studies are needed to determine whether and to what extent these individual "patient outcome" scores must be adjusted (by patient characteristics, system of care characteristics, or physician characteristics) before fair comparisons of care can be made.

Are patient functioning and quality of life reasonable outcomes of the care provided by an individual physician? The most desirable evidence to address this question is not available, that is, that physicians differing on some known criterion of excellence ranked identically when patient outcomes were used to assess quality of care. Recent evidence suggests, however, that these measures, as they are being increasingly refined, are valid for discriminating between the care provided by individual physicians. Early studies used patients' functional status to predict use of health care services and mortality. More recent studies have shown that patients' functional status correlates with traditional physiologic outcome measures, such as forced expiratory volume in 1 second (FEV_1) (24), blood sugar, and blood pressure (25,26). A recent study shows the validity of a functional status measure. In a study of 9,385 patients in the offices of 362 physicians in three major U.S. cities, patients and their physicians were asked to indicate whether they (the patient) had specific medical conditions and symptomatic complaints (7). Patients were also asked to complete a 20-item functional status questionnaire. The results of the association between patients' reports of the presence of specific illnesses, physicians' confirmation of the presence of those illnesses, and patients' functional status are shown in Figure 4. The broken line represents "well patients" (those who denied having any chronic disease whose physicians confirmed that they were disease-free). Each disease condition is graphed according to its mean level of impact on physical function, role function, social function, mental health status, health perceptions, and reported pain. As evident, the more severe the disease, the greater the dysfunction. Further, each condition generates a unique signature.

The demonstrated association between patient functioning and physiology indicates that what the physician does (to manage blood sugar, to control blood pressure, to treat chronic obstructive pulmonary disease) has a direct impact on patient outcomes. These health status measures have achieved the level of validity required to include them, along with traditional outcome markers, in the monitoring of care for chronic diseases. They differentiate those with and without chronic disease. They fit the clinical patterns of disease. They show more dysfunction for the more severe disease conditions. The mean for each category of patient functioning (physical, role, social) for each disease condition could be used as the standard of care, below which physicians' performance would be subjected to additional scrutiny.

Measures of patient outcomes are available for use in quality of care assessment. Substantial work has been done on the development and testing of generic measures of patient functioning and quality of life (25-27). Feasible

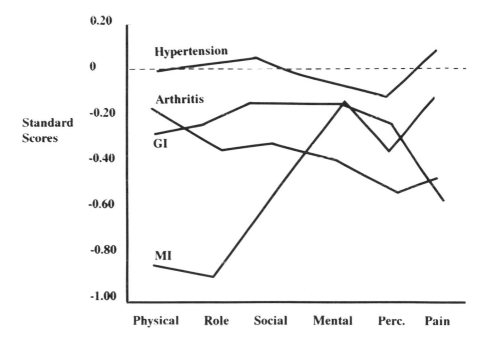

Figure 4. Health profiles for patients with four conditions. GI = gastrointestinal; MI = myocardial infarction.

methods now exist for measuring patient functioning and quality of life in the context of busy office practices (22). In individual office practices these measures could be used to evaluate the quality of the physician's performance and provide maximum opportunity for improving patient care through feedback.

How should patient functioning and quality of life outcomes be used in quality of care assessment? As with traditional methods of the process of care, the procedural steps for using patient outcomes to evaluate the quality of care include obtaining scores for individual physicians, setting standards below which care will be reviewed, and obtaining the consensus of groups of physicians regarding the standards to be used in defining quality. To obain interpretable quality assessment information using patient outcomes, the scores of individual physicians, groups of physicians, systems of care, and so forth, must be adjusted for the factors that may cause errors — variations not due to differences in the quality of care provided. Such factors include case mix, optimal time-window for making judgments about care, and the absence of "normal values" for outcome measures. These factors can be overcome. With respect to case mix, for example, there are several techniques for modifying scores, in order to render accurate judgments about the care provided. "Baseline" measures of patients' functioning can be used to adjust any scores obtained at some later period. Independent measures of the severity of patients' health conditions can be used to adjust "baseline" or "one-shot" measures of patients' functioning. The total disease burden of the patient (the aggregated comorbid conditions the patient has) can also be used to adjust patients' functional status. Recent evidence indicates that the conclusion drawn about the quality of patient care may be very sensitive to case mix adjustment (28-30). Further research is needed to identify and adjust for factors that cause inappropriate conclusions about an individual physician's performance judged using patient outcomes.

Limitations of Outcome Measures. There are three basic limitations to the use of patient functioning and quality of life as measures of the quality of medical care. First, they are nonspecific. They may reflect factors other than the medical care received by the patient. Second, they do not provide targeted information to improve patient care. Outcomes do not give behavioral feedback regarding the specific elements of physicians' performance that must be changed. Third, research has not shown that quality of life can be improved. There may be more to it than the delivery and receipt of high-quality medical care. These limitations do not discredit the use of patient outcomes in quality of care assessment. Rather, they suggest that patient outcomes must be used judiciously, nonpunitively, and in conjunction with other measures of the quality of care, including structure and process.

IMPROVING THE QUALITY OF OFFICE-BASED CARE

There is empirical evidence, summarized by Eisenberg (15), that if given detailed, accurate information reflecting the quality of care they provide, physicians can and do modify their behavior to improve patient care. He identifies specific programmatic features needed to maximize the effective use of quality assessment information including individualized information provided to each physician, normative information about their position relative to their peers, and provision of the information by a colleague in a position of clinical leadership.

Will algorithms, retrospective and prospective, and guidelines for appropriateness, cost strategies, and outcomes be used and incorporated into practice? There is considerable pressure to impose national standards or guidelines that deal with both cost and quality. No matter how expert and prestigious the developers, the process of handing down guidelines, outcome standards, algorithms, or any quality of care criteria will be met with natural and legitimate resistance by providers. For the 70% to 90% of decisions that are judged to be equivocal or possibly appropriate, physicians will and should reserve the right to develop, review, amend, or restructure quality of care standards according to local epidemiologic conditions. There are three reasons national normative standards need to be individualized: high prevalence of diseases such as the acquired immunodeficiency syndrome (AIDS) may alter the diagnostic evaluation for common problems; the presence of social conditions, such as a high proportion of lower socioeconomic class patients, may override usual diagnostic and treatment decisions; and the presence of physical and psychosocial comorbidities may have an effect on the threshold for action.

Those who advocate national guidelines should not consider a plea for individualizing standards as an attempt to undermine "normative" medicine. In our extensive algorithm and outcome research, most of the judgments made by "national" experts are supported by local physicians. The value of individualizing standards by including the opinions of local physicians in the standard-setting process far exceeds any dangers from compromising on high quality. After all, the willingness of physicians to engage in continuous quality of care evaluation and improvement programs stemming from a sense that they are actively shaping these programs is the key to the improvement of quality.

In conclusion, advances in the understanding and development of methods for assessing the quality of care have progressed to the point where it is possible to use them in office practice. To become part of routine practice, these methods must be feasible, must allow for behavioral feedback, and must be credible to practicing clinicians. Some combination of the use of algorithms, or any standards that include branching logic, to measure the process of care, along with measures of patient outcomes, constitute a configuration that holds the greatest potential for improving the quality of office-based care.

References

1. Greenfield S, Lewis CE, Kaplan SH, Davidson MB. Peer review by criteria mapping: criteria for diabetes mellitus. *Ann Intern Med.* 1975;**83**:761-70.
2. Palmer RH, Strain R, Maurer J, Bothrock JK, Thompson MS. Quality assurance in eight adult medicine group practices. *Med Care.* 1984;**22**:632-43.
3. Heller TA, Larson EB, LoGerfo JP. Quality of ambulatory care of the elderly: an analysis of five conditions. *J Am Geriatr Soc.* 1984;**32**:782-8.
4. Palmer RH. *Ambulatory Health Care Evaluation: Principles and Practice.* Chicago: American Hospital Association; 1983.
5. Brook RH, Williams KN, Rolph JE. Controlling the use and cost of medical services: the New Mexico Experimental Medical Care Review Organization — a four-year case study. *Med Care.* 1978; **16**(Suppl):1-76.
6. Fowler FJ Jr, Wennberg JE, Timothy RP, Barry MJ, Mulley AG Jr, Hanley D. Symptom status and quality of life following prostatectomy. *JAMA.* 1988;**259**:3018-22.
7. Stewart AL, Greenfield S, Hays RD, et al. Development of outcomes measures for patient with chronic conditions: functional status and well being. *JAMA.* 1989; In press.
8. Stulbarg MS, Gerbert B, Kemeny M, Boushey HA, Gullion DS. Outpatient treatment of chronic obstruction pulmo- nary disease — a practitioner's guide. *West J Med.* 1985;**142**:842-6.
9. Greenfield S, Kaplan SH, Nadler MA, Deigh-Hewertson R. Physician prefer- ence for criteria mapping in medical care evaluation. *J Fam Pract.* 1978;**6**:1079-86.
10. Greenfield S, Blanco DM, Elashoff RM, Ganz PA. Patterns of care related to age of breast cancer patients. *JAMA.* 1987;**257**:2766-70.
11. Greenfield S, Komaroff AL, Pass TM, Anderson H, Nessim S. Efficiency and cost of primary care by nurses and physician assistants. *N Engl J Med.* 1978;**298**:305-9.
12. Greenfield S, Cretin S, Worthman LG, Dorey FJ, Solomon NE, Goldberg GA. Comparison of a criteria map to a criteria list in quality of care assessment: the relation of each to outcome. *Med Care.* 1981;**19**:255-72.
13. Gerbert B, Greenfield S, Stulbarg M, et al. Clinical algorithms for medical care: development by practicing physicians. *Mobius.* 1983;**3**(4):10-6.
14. Park RE, Fink A, Brook RH, et al. Physician ratings of appropriate indica- tions for six medical and surgical procedures. *Am J Public Health.* 1986; **76**:766-72.
15. Eisenberg JM. *Doctors' Decisions and the Cost of Medical Care.* Ann Arbor, Michigan: Health Administration Press Perspectives; 1986

16. Chassin MR, Kosecoff J, Solomon DH, Brook RH. How coronary angiography is used: clinical determinants of appropriateness. *JAMA*. 1987;**258**:2543-7.

17. Winslow CM, Kosecoff JB, Chassin MR, Kanouse DE, Brook RH. The appropriateness of performing coronary artery bypass surgery. *JAMA*. 1988;**260**:505-9.

18. Winslow CM, Solomon DH, Chassin MR, Kosecoff J, Merrick NJ, Brook RH. The appropriateness of carotid endarterectomy. *N Engl J Med*. 1988; **318**:721-7.

19. Avorn J, Soumerai SB. A new approach to reducing suboptimal drug use. [Editorial]. *JAMA*. 1983;**250**:1752-3.

20. Avorn J, Soumerai SB. Improving drug therapy decisions through educational outreach: a randomized controlled trial of academically based "detailing." *N Engl J Med*. 1983;**308**:1457-63.

21. Schaffner W, Ray WA, Federspield CF, et al. Improving antibiotic prescribing in office practice. *JAMA* 1983;**250**:1728-32.

22. Stewart AL, Hays RD, Ware JE Jr. The MOS short-form general health survey: reliability and validity in a patient population. *Med Care*. 1988;**26**:724-35.

23. Croog SH, Levine S, Testa MA, et al. The effects of anti-hypertensive therapy on the quality of life. *N Engl J Med*. 1986; **314**:1657-64.

24. Kaplan RM, Atkins CJ, Timms R. Validity of a quality of well-being scales as an outcome measure in chronic obstructive pulmonary disease. *J Chronic Dis*. 1984; **37**:85-95.

25. Proceedings of the advances in health assessment. *J Chronic Dis*. 1986;**40** (Suppl 1):15-1935.

26. Kaplan SH. Patient reports of health status as predictors of physiologic health measures in chronic disease. *J Chronic Dis*. 1987;**40** (Suppl 1):27S-40S.

27. Kaplan SH, Greenfield S, Ware JE Jr. Assessing the effects of physician-patient interactions on the outcome of chronic disease. *Med Care*. 1989; In press.

28. Greenfield S, Aronow HU, Elashoff RM, Watanabe D. Flaws in mortality data: the hazards of ignoring comorbid disease. *JAMA*. 1988;**260**:2253-5.

29. Charlson ME, Pompei P, Ales HL, Mackenzie CR. A new method of classifying prognostic comorbidity in longitudinal studies: development and validation. *J Chronic Dis*. 1987;**40**:33-83.

30. Couch JB, Nash DB. Severity of illness measures: opportunities for clinicians. *Ann Intern Med*. 1988;**109**:771-3.

COMMENTARY

The ambulatory care sector represents the greatest challenges facing quality of care measurement. Most quality of care measurement efforts have focused on hospital-based care both for ease of access and because hospitals usually contain the sickest patients. Many pressures are encouraging researchers to study the outpatient sector. Health services are rapidly shifting from the hospital to the outpatient arena. As a consequence, the intensity of care is dramatically higher in the ambulatory sector particularly since the institution of diagnosis related groups (DRGs) in 1982.

The rise of managed care organizations (MCOs) has also heightened the importance of quality of care measurement in the ambulatory sector. The tie-in between MCOs and quality has occurred for several reasons. On the one hand, HMOs, PPOs, and other new forms of health care delivery promise to deliver total care to the patient, thus heightening the importance of outpatient delivery. Unfortunately, the promise has not been realized. Many MCOs not only do not emphasize prevention but have begun to institute deductibles and copayments similar to those seen in traditional health insurance packages. Furthermore, it is unclear whether the potential for increased preventive care in an HMO environment is possible in an increasingly competitive financial situation for all health care delivery organizations. Despite the financial problems of most MCOs, third party payers are still interested in enrolling beneficiaries into these programs. This desire to encourage or force individuals into MCOs that by definition limit beneficiary access to their physician of choice, has heightened third party payer interest in quality of care measurement. These measures must transcend the hospital sector; hence the importance and timeliness of Dr. Greenfield's thorough review of ambulatory quality of care measures.

How do HMOs stack up with traditional health insurance using some of the measures discussed in Dr. Greenfield's chapter. The most famous experiment that looked at this issue is the Health Insurance Experiment (1). Though this and many other studies indicate that managed care provides comparable quality service to health insurance, the conclusions are referrable only to staff model HMOs (1-3). No adequate studies have been published comparing, for example, IPAs with PPOs. Dr. Greenfield's current work, the Medical Outcome Study, promises to provide important information comparing various forms of managed care organizations against each other (Greenfield S. Presentation at a conference held at CIGNA Corporation, March 1988).

Delivery of care to the disadvantaged in MCOs represents a critical research topic. Published data indicate that low-income individuals do not fare as well in MCOs as their middle class counterparts (4). Despite these problems, cost constraints continue to encourage state and federal agencies to look to MCOs for fiscal relief. It will be important to carefully follow the use of MCOs for health care for the poor.

From a clinical point of view, Dr. Greenfield has appropriately devoted a great deal of attention to the use of algorithms in the measurement of quality. The American Medical Association has recently signed a contract with scientists at the RAND Corporation to jointly develop "practice parameters" (Announced at a meeting on physician practice patterns sponsored by the Physician Payment Review Commission, October 1988). Algorithms will be useful not only to measure clinical quality provided in different organizations but also to provide information on the quality of care provided by individual physicians. This in turn can be used by traditional insurance companies to limit payment to physicians providing inappropriate care and by MCOs to limit capitation payments to primary physician gatekeepers. Dr. Greenfield summarizes the issues that need to be resolved (weighting of variables and so forth) before this type of information can be ethically used for compensation of physicians. However, internal organizational constraints may force the use of these measures before health services research has answered all relevant questions. This possibility heightens the need for physician acceptance of measures utilized, a point Dr. Greenfield repeatedly makes.

Dr. Greenfield appropriately emphasizes the limitations of measurement of quality in the ambulatory care arena. We hope current federal research initiatives in MCOs and practice patterns will rapidly advance the field. Researchers are focusing a great deal of attention on outcomes. Three overall approaches are vying for attention. Jack Wennberg and colleagues have championed the small area variation analysis approach. That is, within small geographic areas (for example, within a city) significant variations in practice patterns exist for both inpatient and outpatient care. The RAND Corporation group led by Bob Brook has focused on untoward outcomes, particularly mortality. This measure, though critical, will have less relevance for the ambulatory sector compared with the hospital. At the same time it will be important to understand whether the volume of care for a particular diagnosis has quality of care implications. That is, it is known that the number of coronary artery bypass grafts performed in a specific institution does have implications for morbidity and mortality. Does the same volume phenomenon hold true for the care of, for example, hypertensive patients? The last approach to quality of care measurement in the ambulatory setting is advocated by several groups of researchers. Ware, Greenfield, Berwick, and others have focused on patient-derived information as providing a promising source of information relevant to the outpatient sector. Paul Ellwood has established a new organization, Quality Quest, which attempts to maximize information from the patient. Though we have distinguished between these three approaches — all of which have separate chapters devoted to them in this book — it is equally clear that they overlap and will benefit from advances in each other's approaches.

It is heartening to see the ferment currently occurring in the quality of care measurement arena. This is particularly important, because the marketplace that increasingly emphasizes restrictions on patient access to their physician of choice will not wait for reliable and valid quality measures. (The Editors)

References

1. Brook RH, Ware JE, Rogers WH, et al. Does free care improve adults health? Results from a randomized controlled trial. *N Engl J Med.* 1983;**309**;1426-34.
2. Luft HS. HMOs and the quality of care. *Inquiry.* 1988;**25**:147-56.
3. Cunningham F, Williamson J. How does the quality of health care in HMOs compare to that in other settings? An analytic literature review: 1958-1979. *Group Health Journal.* 1980;**1**(Winter):4-25.
4. Ware JE, et al. Comparison of health outcomes at a Health Maintenance Organization with those of Fee-for-Service care. *Lancet.* 1986;May 3:1017-22.

Chapter 8

The Joint Commission on Accreditation of Healthcare Organizations

JAMES B. COUCH, MD, JD

THE JOINT COMMISSION: AN OVERVIEW

The Joint Commission on Accreditation of Healthcare Organizations (JCAHO) is the first professional health care association to set standards for the voluntary accreditation of different types of health care organizations. The JCAHO operates under the assumption that quality health care can be promoted most effectively through the development, dissemination, revision, refinement, and enforcement of standards that are established by experts in the professional areas being evaluated.

The Joint Commission is not a governmental or quasi-governmental entity. It is composed of and governed by private health care professionals. The JCAHO cannot sanction noncompliant organizations, unlike a governmental agency that has the authority to protect and preserve the public health. Whatever authority or influence the JCAHO may possess is derived indirectly from its prestige and acceptance by other agencies with sanctioning authority (for example, state licensing bodies, the Medicare Program, the Office of the Inspector General, and so forth).

This chapter examines the evolution of the Joint Commission and how it operates, its influence in the voluntary accreditation of health care organizations, its expansion into additional areas affecting the quality of health care, its attempts to continue to play a prominent role in the rapidly changing health care industry, and how clinicians, especially internists, will be affected and may respond. The chapter provides the reader with some understanding of the JCAHO's evolving role in the evaluation of health care, which is currently occupying the time and resources of a growing number of agencies in the private and public sectors.

HISTORY OF THE JOINT COMMISSION

The Hospital Standardization Program

On December 20, 1917, the American College of Surgeons (ACS) formally established the Hospital Standardization Program. This constituted a one-page statement concerning minimum requirements for hospitals to meet to promote the delivery of high-quality medical care. In 1918 the College began an on-site inspection program for hospitals with more than 100 beds. The "Minimum Standards" concerned the organization of the medical staff; qualifications for membership; the need for medical staff bylaws; rules and regulations; and policies for monthly staff meetings, departmental medical care review, and the keeping of complete and competently staffed laboratory and radiologic facilities (1).

At the first annual inspection, only 89 of 692 hospitals met these minimum standards. Although the College made the numbers public, it burned the list of hospitals in the furnace of the Waldorf Astoria Hotel, New York, to keep it from the press. Some of the most prestigious hospitals in the country had failed to meet the most basic standards (1). Spurred on by the American medical community, compliance with these standards became a widely accepted indicator of hospitals' commitment to maintain and improve the quality of health care delivery.

Evolution of the Joint Commission

As the hospital standardization program became increasingly popular, a need developed for a broader base of support than what one national medical specialty association could sustain. By 1951, 3,000 hospitals had been surveyed and accredited. In 1951 the American College of Physicians (ACP), the American Hospital Association (AHA), the American Medical Association (AMA), and Canadian Medical Association (CMA) joined The American College of Surgeons (ACS) to establish the Joint Commission on Accreditation of Hospitals (JCAH). The Canadian Medical Association withdrew in 1959 and was replaced by the American Dental Association (ADA) in 1980. The JCAHO is governed by a Board of Commissioners composed of 21 representatives from the five member organizations. In 1981 a public commissioner was added to represent consumer concerns (1). In 1989 two additional consumer members were added.

The Joint Commission began its formal voluntary accreditation program, the Hospital Accreditation Program (HAP), in 1952. In time, the number of hospitals accredited through the HAP increased to 5,300 (84% of all hospitals). By the late 1960s, JCAH accreditation had achieved widespread acceptance. In 1965, Congress passed Public Law 89-97, the Medicare Act. Written into this law was a provision that hospitals accredited by the Joint Commission were "deemed" to be in compliance with most of the "Medicare Conditions of Participation for Hospitals" (2). In addition, an increasing number of public (for example, Medicaid) and private (for example, Blue Cross and Blue Shield) purchasers of health care have come to regard accreditation by the Joint Commission as a prerequisite for inclusion in their health benefit plans. This recognition extends to the decision by most state agencies to certify or license these health care institutions or organizations (1).

Over the past two decades, the Joint Commission has begun to extend its accreditation program to health care organizations other than hospitals. In the late 1960s and early 1970s, it developed survey and accreditation services for long-term care organizations, ambulatory care organizations, programs for the mentally retarded and developmentally disabled, psychiatric services, alcoholism programs, drug abuse programs, and community mental health service programs. The Accreditation Program for Hospice Care was added in 1983, the Home Care Program was added in 1986 (and became effective for surveys in 1988), and the Managed Care Program is scheduled for implementation in the middle of 1989. The expansion of the Joint Commission's scope of review made it ripe for a name change: It became the Joint Commission on Accreditation of Healthcare Organizations (JCAHO).

RECENT PUBLIC SECTOR DEVELOPMENTS

Despite the JCAHO's recognition, federal and state regulators recently have begun to evaluate health care organizations independent of their Joint Commission accreditation. Highly regulated states, such as New York, have elaborate Department of Health Regulations. The New York State Department of Health has taken the "Medical Staff" standards of the *Accreditation Manual for Hospitals* and codified them into state regulations required for continued licensure. States such as New York have taken these actions to put "teeth" into the JCAHO standards. These states have realized that periodic inspections by state agencies with authority to impose immediate, direct sanctions for significant noncompliance were necessary to effect the goals and objectives in the HAP.

In addition, federal programs have become involved in the past few years as their database on clinical outcomes has grown. The Health Care Financing Administration (HCFA), through its Health Standards Quality Bureau (HSQB), is beginning to play an increasingly important role, as are the office of the Inspector General in conjunction with HCFA and the Peer Review Organization (PRO) program. Through analysis of their clinical databases, these agencies are questioning whether certain hospitals with a documentable history of patient care deficiencies should continue to treat Medicare patients even when these hospitals are Joint Commission accredited. Although these agencies are not direct competitors of the JCAHO, their increasing prominence in the health care quality debate has diminished the dominance of the JCAHO in such matters.

THE DEVELOPMENT OF STANDARDS

Evolution

Joint Commission standards have become not so much specific prescriptions, but general guidelines for health care organizations concerning how to improve quality of care. Considerable flexibility in terms of compliance with JCAHO standards remains. "Standards" are developed for all the operational components of health care organizations. What actually constitutes quality of care is highly controversial. Standards may be developed and designed to reflect certain structural and procedural attributes of health care organizations, which, by professional consensus, are generally associated with high-quality health care delivery.

Compliance with current Joint Commission standards merely shows a health care organization's *potential* for providing high-quality health care. As covered in detail below, the Joint Commission's "Agenda for Change" for the 1990s will require health care organizations to demonstrate not only their *potential for* but their actual *provision of* care within "acceptable" clinical outcome ranges (3). However, the JCAHO does not intend to abandon those principles or standards that require careful recording of the *process* that documents *how* organizations continuously attempt to *improve* clinical performance. In effect, how an organization uses clinical performance information to improve itself, as opposed to where the information places the organization on an evaluative scale at a specific point in time, will be the major determinant of the accreditation awarded (3).

Approval Process for Proposed Standards

The JCAHO follows a fairly strict procedure when developing new standards or accreditation surveys. The first step, after the initial drafting of proposed standards achieved through an interaction of JCAHO staff and expert task forces, is review by a Professional and Technical Advisory Committee (PTAC). These committees are made up of representatives of organizations committed to and responsible for the type of health care delivery for which the standards are being developed. Once approved by the PTAC, the standards are sent for initial review by the Standards and Survey Procedures Committee (SSP) of the Board of Commissioners (4).

After review by the SSP Committee, the proposed standards are circulated for comprehensive field review. Field review involves sending proposed standards to hospitals, medical associations, and other health care organizations for evaluation and comments. After revisions from the field review process are made, the proposed standards are resubmitted to the PTAC and SSP committees for approval. Once approved at these levels, the proposed standards are submitted to the Joint Commission's Board of Commissioners for adoption and subsequent implementation in later editions of the various accreditation manuals (4,5).

THE MONITORING AND EVALUATION PROCESS

The current (late 1980s) approach by the JCAHO to assess and facilitate improvement of the quality of health care services delivery is the "monitoring and evaluation" process. This approach evolved from the principles in the "Quality Assurance" chapter of the *Accreditation Manual for Hospitals* first appearing in 1979, which in turn evolved from a medical audit process previously promoted by the Joint Commission. This audit process had required accredited organizations to engage in and document the completion of ongoing empirical audits of the appropriateness of different aspects of medical care as documentable in patient charts. However, too many organizations became preoccupied with the process of performing a certain number of empirical audits. As a result, the ultimate goal of these audits, that is, to improve care quality, become lost in organizations' efforts to meet periodic audit "quotas."

The monitoring and evaluation process has 10 steps: assigning responsibility for monitoring and evaluating activities; delineating the scope of care provided by the organization; identifying the most important aspects of the care the organization provides; identifying indicators (and appropriate clinical criteria) that can be used to monitor these important aspects of care; establishing thresholds for the indicators (for example, particular mortality or morbidity rates) at which further evaluation of the care is triggered; collecting and organizing the data for each indicator; evaluating the care when the thresholds are reached to identify problems or opportunities to improve the care; taking action to correct identified problems or to improve care; assessing the effectiveness of the action and documenting the improvement in care; and communicating relevant information to other individuals, departments, or services, and to the whole organization's quality assurance program (6).

THE SURVEY AND ACCREDITATION PROCESS

The survey and accreditation process is aptly described as the Joint Commission's major product. This process is summarized in the JCAHO publication, *An Introduction to the Joint Commission* (4).

... The primary purposes of a survey are to assess the extent of an organization's compliance with the Joint Commission standards that apply to the services it provides and to help the organization achieve improved compliance. There are six standards manuals: the *Accreditation Manual for Hospitals (AMH)*, the *Ambulatory Health Care Standards Manual*, the *Consolidated Standards Manual*, the *Hospice Standards Manual*, the *Long Term Care Standards Manual (LTCSM)*, and *Standards for the Accreditation of Home Care*.

...Accreditation surveys are designed to enable the surveyors to assess the extent of an organization's compliance with Joint Commission standards. This is accomplished through one or more of the following means:

- Documentation of compliance provided by organization staff;
- On-site observations by Joint Commission surveyors; and
- Verbal information concerning the implementation of standards, or examples of their implementation, that will enable a judgment of compliance to be made.

...For some accreditation programs, the standards manual serves as the survey report form. In the manuals, each chapter is in outline form, and each standard and required characteristic is followed by a five-point rating scale, which indicates the scores surveyors use to rate substantial compliance, significant compliance, partial compliance, minimal compliance, or noncompliance.

...The Joint Commission recognizes that new or revised standards may require extended time for full and effective implementation. Accordingly, a system called "implementation monitoring" is used to track organizational progress toward compliance. Organizations that are found to be in less than significant compliance with these standards will receive recommendations in the accreditation report. However, these recommendations do not affect an organization's accreditation status. Implementation monitoring enables the Joint Commission to provide additional assistance to health care organizations in interpreting and meeting standards requirements. The process also affords organizations an opportunity to determine their own progress towards full compliance with new standards.

Once the survey report form has been completed, the surveyors return their findings to the Joint Commission in Chicago. Following detailed analysis of the survey findings, a determination is made concerning the accreditation status of the organization.

...An accreditation decision is made on the basis of the survey findings and any other relevant information. The major factors that affect accreditation decisions include evidence of overall compliance with standards, progressive advancement toward more complete compliance, and the absence of any serious areas of noncompliance with standards regarding such areas as assuring patient safety or maintaining acceptable quality of care.

...If an organization is granted accreditation with contingencies, the organization enjoys full accreditation status, but it must act to remove the contingency within a set period of time, as determined by the Joint Commission. The Joint Commission determines the method and the time frame for removal of any contingencies.

...A contingency can be removed when the organization demonstrates compliance with the standards in question. Such compliance is demonstrated when an organization submits an acceptable written report on its progress or when the Joint Commission conducts a survey visit that focuses on the areas of previous noncompliance. The Joint Commission determines whether a progress report, a focused survey, or both will be necessary to address identified contingencies. If a contingency is not corrected within a prescribed period of time, an organization may lose its accreditation.

...If, after reviewing all pertinent material and information, the committee decides to deny accreditation to the organization, the organization has a right to appeal the decision before it becomes final. The appeals procedures, which include access to a hearing and, ultimately, review by the Board of Commissioners, are outlined in each of the standards manuals.

Before a recommendation for nonaccreditation is made, representatives of the surveyed organization are given the opportunity to discuss areas of noncompliance that caused accreditation to be denied. Those representatives are then given an opportunity to document compliance and to meet with representatives of the Joint Commission. If an organization does not take advantage of these opportunities or is unsuccessful in persuading the Joint Commission of its efforts to comply, the organization may be notified of its nonaccreditation (7). This nonaccredited status remains in effect for

6 months, at which time the organization may be resurveyed. This 6-month waiting period may be waived by the president of JCAHO if the organization can document sufficient progress in correcting vital deficiencies in a shorter period (7).

According to Donald Avant, JCAHO's vice president for accreditation surveys, about 8% to 10% of hospitals surveyed get "tentative nonaccreditation" notices from the JCAHO, indicating a hospital will not receive accreditation unless it presents evidence that it has corrected a quality of care problem (8). Beginning in 1989, such hospitals will be charged for the additional resources expended by the JCAHO to assist in their achieving compliance (8).

The accreditation status of organizations may be determined by the public, although the specific findings of surveyors leading to that status generally may be protected from disclosure, even from many governmental agencies (7).

EXTENSIONS OF THE ACCREDITATION PROGRAM

Ambulatory Care Organizations

The Joint Commission's Accreditation Program for Ambulatory Health Care was established to encourage the provision of quality patient care through a peer-based consultative and educational survey process. The Accreditation Program for Ambulatory Health Care (AHC) accredits over 300 programs, including 166 hospital-sponsored programs; 95 government-sponsored programs; 40 Indian health service clinics; 38 Veterans Administration outpatient clinics; 9 U.S. Navy clinics; 7 U.S. Air Force clinics; 1 U.S. Coast Guard clinic; 40 ambulatory surgery centers; 23 community health centers; 12 college health centers; 7 group practices; and 1 urgent care center. The standards development and survey and accreditation process for AHC is essentially the same as the one outlined previously. The Joint Commission serves as an educational and service organization to these groups as it does to the 5,300 hospitals it accredits (9).

Hospice Care

The Joint Commission currently accredits all types of hospice providers, including independent hospice programs; hospital-based programs; home health agency-based programs; and programs that are a service of other health care organizations. The peer review process in hospice programs in unique in several ways: Many of the surveyors are the original leaders in the development of hospices in the United States; hospice surveyors routinely accompany a hospice team member to the home to observe assessment and care, and talk to the patient and family members about the receipt of care; and the hospice standards require the demonstration of continuity of care across different care settings (9).

The Home Care Project

The Joint Commission accredits approximately 1,000 hospital-based and hospital-affiliated home care organizations. These home care agencies are accredited based on their compliance with the standards in the "Home Care Services" chapter in the 1986 edition of the *Accreditation Manual for Hospitals.* The Joint Commission initiated a 2-year project in January 1986 to develop standards for the delivery of home care services by both facility-based and community-based organizations.

The proposed scope of the standards will address acute intervention provided on a short-term or long-term basis; high technology services such as intravenous therapy and chemotherapy; hourly services provided by nurses, homemakers, and home health aides; and durable medical equipment provided in conjunction with patient care.

This new accreditation process became available in 1988. Accreditation will be available to community- or hospital-based organizations, as well as home care services that offer only one service or a continuum of home care. The home care standards used in the survey represent a consensus of home care providers nationwide (9).

Psychiatric and Substance Abuse Facilities

The Joint Commission accredits various programs and services that offer inpatient, outpatient, residential, and partial day treatment to patients of all ages. These programs and services include alcoholic and drug abuse programs; community mental health service programs; forensic psychiatric services; programs for the mentally retarded and developmentally disabled; and psychiatric services.

More than 1,200 facilities, programs, and services are accredited by the Joint Commission under the nationally recognized standards published in the *Consolidated Standards Manual for Child, Adolescent and Adult Psychiatric, Alcoholism and Facilities Serving the Mentally Retarded/Developmentally Disabled* (9).

Long-Term Care

More than 1,400 long-term care facilities are accredited by the Joint Commission. The Joint Commission surveys and accredits long-term care facilities under the nationally recognized standards published in the *Long Term Care Standards Manual.* The Joint Commission also publishes the *Directory of Joint Commission Accredited Long Term Care Facilities*, which may be used as a reference tool for health care professionals and as a resource directory for consumers concerned about quality long-term care (9).

To bolster the JCAHO's current lack of growth in this important problem area, *The Long Term Care Standards Manual* has recently been completely revised for surveys beginning in 1989. The standards development and approval process, as well as the survey and accreditation process, closely emulates that of the Hospital Accreditation Program (HAP) and the other accreditation programs of the Joint Commission.

Managed Care Organizations

Within the last 2 years, the Joint Commission has begun the development of a formalized accreditation program for managed care organizations (MCOs). The Joint Commission has already signed a contract with the 38 "PruCare" managed care plans of the Prudential Insurance Company. In addition, they have received the endorsement of the 96 managed care plans of the Blue Cross/Blue Shield Association of America whose member plans operate 96 managed care plans. In general, the proposed credentialing for MCOs will integrate the 10-step monitoring and evaluation process into the specific components of these distinctive delivery systems. At the time of this writing, the specific proposed timetable called for publication of the new managed care standards in June 1989. MCOs could apply to be accredited within several months thereafter.

Third Party Evaluation

The Joint Commission also pursues engagements with third parties to conduct evaluations of prepaid health plans. This has been achieved successfully for both Ohio's and Minnesota's Medicaid health maintenance organization (HMO) plans. A proposal to provide this service has also been submitted to the Department of Health Services of Hawaii.

Movement Into Risk Management

In 1989 new standards related to clinical aspects of risk management will appear in the "Governing Body," "Management and Administrative Services," "Quality Assurance," and "Medical Staff" chapters of the *Accreditation Manual for Hospitals*. A glossary definition (10) of the term "risk management" has also been approved for the 1989 edition of the *Accreditation Manual for Hospitals*:

> The standards pertaining to risk management in this manual address only those risk management functions relating to clinical and administrative activities designed to identify, evaluate, and reduce the risk of patient injury associated with care. The full scope of risk management functions encompasses activities in health care organizations that are intended to conserve financial resources from loss. These functions include a broad range of administrative activities intended to reduce losses associated with patient, employee, or visitor injuries; property losses or damages; and other sources of potential

organizational liability. Many of these activities are beyond the scope of Joint Commission standards.

Perhaps the most significant aspect of these 1989 Risk Management Standards is that they require the medical staff to identify potential risks in clinical components of patient care and safety; develop risk evaluation criteria to pinpoint areas of patient risk; correct identified problems in clinical care; and develop a system to prevent future risk management problems (11).

THE AGENDA FOR CHANGE

The Changing Health Care Environment

Previously, there has been an implicit assumption of high quality in the health care system, based largely upon public trust in physicians and health care institutions. Now, as awareness grows that there is wide variability in utilization rates, practice patterns, and clinical results, the public — through government, business, insurers, consumers and other interest groups — is seeking information concerning how much of this variation reflects actual quality differences (3).

The Joint Commission's Response

The Joint Commission has been the major national organization setting standards for medical quality since its inception in 1951. However, during the past few years, its dominance in this area (perhaps even its leadership position) has been challenged by a growing number of public and private agencies. The recent tumultuous changes in health care financing and delivery have pushed the JCAHO to adopt a new plan for its future in order to retain its relevance in the rapidly changing, data-driven health care industry of the 1990s. In its "Agenda for Change," the JCAHO by the early 1990s will begin to expect accredited organizations not only to demonstrate their *potential* to improve medical care, as documented in their peer review materials, but to *actually* demonstrate this improvement through clinical outcome assessment systems (3).

Scope of the Program

Five components comprise the research and development activities related to the Agenda for Change: identification and selection of clinical indicators; identification and selection of organizational and management indicators; development of risk adjustment methods; establishment of an ongoing monitoring and evaluation process; and modification of survey and accreditation procedures (3).

Clinical Indicators of Performance

According to the JCAHO, "an indicator is a defined, measurable dimension of the quality or appropriateness of an important aspect of patient care" (3). Indicators describe measurable care processes, clinical events, complications, or outcomes, about which data can be collected. In the context of the Agenda for Change, clinical indicators will serve as measures of clinical outcomes, such as death, hospital-acquired infection, severe adverse drug reactions, and return to the operating room from the recovery room. Other clinical indicators may relate to changes in health status, patient satisfaction, "quality of life," and other less adverse events or changes. These indicators will permit thresholds to be established; if the experience of an organization at any point is beyond that threshold, the need for internal evaluation and improvement will be triggered (3).

In the past, JCAHO accreditations have focused on organizational structures and processes. This focus, to the exclusion of clinical outcome assessment, would render the Commission ineffective in the 1990s. As explained more fully in Chapter 1 by Drs. Goldfield and Nash, the major purchasers of care are beginning to demand that providers vying for spots on employee health benefit plans demonstrate their superiority through severity of illness adjusted clinical outcome assessment systems similar to those explained by Dr. Iezzoni in Chapter 3. The Agenda for Change, then, may be viewed as an initiative by the JCAHO to help surveyed organizations continuously assess where they stand and need to improve relative to comparable organizations' severity-adjusted clinical outcomes.

The Joint Commission is using expert clinical task forces and pilot testing in selected health care organizations to determine the best available clinical indicators to use in quality assurance programs of accredited organizations. At the time of this writing, the anesthesia, obstetrical, and hospital-wide clinical indicator task forces had developed their initial set of clinical indicators for pilot testing. Chairmen for the expert task forces in cardiovascular medicine, oncology, trauma care, general surgery, mental health care, and long-term care had been selected and began their development of clinical indicators in early 1989.

Risk Adjustment Methods

To permit equitable comparisons of clinical outcomes among surveyed organizations, adjustment for the average severity of illness of patients treated is required (3). Severity of illness adjustment is also important to set evaluation thresholds at levels that minimize the production of false-positive and false-negative results in the initial screening process for potential quality of care problems meriting further investigation. The clinical indicator expert task forces are also being asked to identify patient covariates associated with each clinical indicator that may affect severity of illness and thresholds for clinical indicators.

A thorough analysis of the various risk adjustment, case complexity, or severity indexing systems is beyond the scope of this chapter. For such an analysis, please see Chapter 3. There are also additional sources of information concerning the various systems and methods by which to evaluate them (12-14).

Management Indicators of Excellence

With assistance from an expert task force, the Joint Commission has identified key dimensions of organizational function that exert the greatest influence on quality of care. The 12 principles, which are intended to apply to all health care settings, include mission; culture; strategic programs and resource plans; organizational change; the role of the governing body management, and clinical leadership; leadership qualification, development, and assessment; resources; clinical competence of independent practitioners; recruitment, development, evaluation, and retention policies and practices; evaluation and improvement of patient care; organizational integration and coordination; and continuity and comprehensiveness of care (15). At the time of this writing these organizational indicators were undergoing field review. Once finalized, these indicators may provide a template for reviewing current accreditation standards and for developing a more relevant "streamlined" set of standards (3).

Based on the products of the management indicators task force, and the results of the recent survey (16) of hospital chief executives, board chairmen, and medical staff president, a new proposed chapter in the accreditation manual called "Hospital Leadership" is being developed. This chapter is intended to replace the current chapters on "Medical Staff," "Governing Body," and "Management and Administrative Services." Specifically, the new chapter is to include standards requiring hospitals to define their "mission," scope of services, organizational structure, and the roles and responsibilities of the various hospital leaders; the primary activities expected of governing body members, executives, and medical staff leaders necessary in the functioning hospital; formulation of the documents regarding coordination of the activities of these three groups of hospital leaders; and proof of open and continuous communication among all three groups and a method for conflict resolution (excerpts from an address by Dennis O'Leary, MD, at the American Medical Association's Hospital Medical Staff Section Annual Meeting, Chicago, June 24, 1988).

Database Management System Development

The Agenda for Change anticipates that the Joint Commission and accredited institutions will jointly participate in a continuous-flow monitoring system in which clinical *and* organizational data are periodically and regularly transmitted from the field, entered in a Joint Commission database, aggregated and analyzed, and then fed back to the organization (3).

At regular intervals throughout the accreditation period, accredited organizations would routinely collect these clinical and organizational data and submit them to the Joint Commission either in writing, by personal computer diskettes, by data tape, or perhaps even by modem. The frequency of data collection will be determined in light of cost, feasibility, and the need for timely analysis by the Joint Commission. It could be as often as quarterly (3).

The JCAHO would process this data, and provide timely feedback to the health care organization as additional input to its ongoing self-monitoring process. This would permit three general types of feedback: comparison of organizations' performance to internal expectations; comparison of organizations' performance to external expectations based on "national thresholds of acceptable performance" adjusted for local conditions; and comparison of organizations' standing in "norm references' summaries" relative to the distribution of indicator data from similar (but anonymous) peer group institutions (3).

IMPACT AND RESPONSE

Ambulatory Care Review

Clinicians devoting a substantial amount of their practice time to ambulatory care organizations should prepare for the Joint Commission's survey of these organizations. Clinicians participating in all types of ambulatory care organizations (including general medicine practice centers, HMOs, multispecialty groups, and so forth) will be affected. Clinicians practicing in these organizations should become aware of the requirements of the *Ambulatory Health Care Standards Manual*, and help prepare their organizations for these surveys.

Clinicians participating in the outpatient setting should participate in ongoing peer review, including outpatient chart review to ascertain aberrant practice patterns that may result in unexpected hospitalizations. Timely and appropriate completion of records, and appropriate use of laboratory tests, participating hospitals, consultants, and various technologies should be monitored continuously.

This review process could have a substantial impact on clinicians practicing in the outpatient setting. Monitoring and evaluating processes comparable to those used in the inpatient setting will be applied in the outpatient setting. This may have the effect of standardizing outpatient medical practice. It will be difficult to apply severity adjustment or other monitoring and evaluating systems in their current form to the outpatient setting. However, not only the JCAHO, but other regulatory agencies and purchasers, likely will attempt to do so in the 1990s.

Internists may establish themselves, if they have not already, as the logical managers of ambulatory care organizations because of their broad medical training and movement into managerial roles in group practice settings. Internists may provide specific expertise to the JCAHO concerning clinical and managerial indicators of excellence for ambulatory care organizations. They should help prepare their ambulatory care organizations for surveys by implementing and monitoring appropriate and responsive ambulatory care quality management systems. Specifically, they should be instrumental in the development and adoption of clinical care protocols to optimize the quality and cost-effectiveness of managing outpatients. Although the development and adoption of these protocols may not fulfill the standards alone, they should provide evidence to JCAHO of the commitment of internists' ambulatory care organizations to comply with the monitoring and evaluation process.

Hospice Care Review

To the extent that clinicians use hospices, they should know which ones are JCAHO accredited and what the criteria for accreditation are. Clinicians should be aware that a unique feature of the hospice accreditation survey is the assessment of continuity of care across different institutional settings, including the home and hospice settings. This involves interviewing not only health care professionals involved in providing care, but also the patients and families receiving it. As these settings become increasingly important in caregiving, clinicians may be restricted to sending their patients only to accredited hospices.

Internists will care for a disproportionate number of terminally ill patients in the future. The cost of keeping these patients in the inpatient setting may become prohibitive. However, these economic forces could result in the discharge of inpatients to hospice facilities not equipped to deal effectively with their acute, though terminal, conditions. Because internists are becoming increasingly familiar with the needs of terminally ill patients and their families, they should be able to play a leading role in the JCAHO's development and modification of standards concerning the continuing care of these patients. Through appropriate specialty organizations, task forces, and national conferences, internists should provide special expertise to hospices concerning medically appropriate management, including intake and disposition, of terminally ill patients.

Home Care Review

Whether they are hospital- or community-based, clinicians should know which home care organizations are JCAHO accredited and what the requirements of accreditation are. It is particularly important for them to be aware of the adequacy of staff and their qualifications to provide technically sophisticated services such as intravenous therapy, outpatient dialysis, home care artificial ventilation, and hyperalimentation. Accreditation should provide internists with some degree of assurance that such agencies are capable of providing acceptable quality care to their patients. Internists should play an integral role in helping the JCAHO extend its recent initiatives in accrediting home care programs, and subspecialists may help develop standards for home care therapy involving technologically sophisticated procedures.

It will become increasingly important for clinicians to send their patients only to facilities with some record of quality, as evidenced by JCAHO accreditation or some other equivalent certification. Failure to refer patients to such facilities may reflect badly on the clinical performance of such internists.

Psychiatric and Substance Abuse Facility Review

To the extent that internists use these facilities, they should know their JCAHO accreditation status. These facilities are some of the fastest growing of their kind in the health care industry. With the increasing demand for access to these facilities by nonpsychiatric physicians, clinicians should be aware of the extent of these facilities' commitment to and demonstration of high quality, as opposed to merely profitability.

Internists on the medical staff of such organizations should take an active role in the ongoing quality management and peer review responsibilities in preparing these facilities for accreditation. They should be particularly involved in making certain that adequate systems to ensure appropriate and effective medical management of patients are being used. Although not psychiatrists, internists may provide special expertise to the JCAHO. General internists may refer patients regularly to these facilities. They should be reliable sources for comparing patients' pre-entry and post-facility status, an important indicator of the performance of such programs.

Long-Term Care Review

The demand for long-term care will grow at unprecedented rates in the near future with the continued "graying" of the population and increasing efforts to reimburse more generously for this care. As reimbursement becomes more generous, long-term facilities will become more popular. These settings will play a major role in the health care industry. As these facilities grow, clinicians must be able to distinguish ones that have a documentable history of high quality and commitment to ongoing self-evaluation.

Internists (especially geriatricians) will play a disproportionately large role in referring patients to long-term care facilities. As with hospices, internists should be able to provide specific expertise to the JCAHO concerning the special needs of these patients and their families, which accredited facilities should fulfill. In addition, internists should be able to provide special expertise and impact concerning the ongoing medical management needs of patients with chronic conditions.

Managed Care Organization Review

Clinicians are becoming increasingly involved with all types of MCOs (HMOs, preferred provider organizations, [PPOs], individual practice associations [IPAs]). Although the JCAHO accreditation program for managed care is still new, it is growing rapidly. In the near future, it will be important for clinicians to know whether or not the MCO seeking their participation is JCAHO accredited or not. A growing number of purchasers of MCO services may limit their approved health benefit plan list to those groups with Joint Commission accreditation.

Even if JCAHO accreditation does not become a prerequisite for inclusion in employee health benefit plans, clinicians will enhance their own marketability by limiting their own participation to MCOs accredited either by the JCAHO or a competing group that accredits organizations (for example, Dr. Ellwood's Quality Quest, Inc., the American Medical Care Review Association, and so forth). MCOs are coming under increasing criticism and scrutiny. To the extent that internists wish to bolster their own claims that they are only associated with the "highest quality" plans, they should make accreditation by some group a prerequisite to their own participation.

Internists, particularly general internists, have played and should continue to play an even greater role in MCOs as both clinicians and managers. For that reason, internists should be able to contribute to the development of both clinical and managerial indicators of excellence in managed care systems. In addition, internists, by virtue of their considerable involvement in the care of internal medicine patients in managed care systems, should be instrumental in the production of appropriate clinical protocols to ensure high quality and cost-effective diagnostic and therapeutic management of these patients. As increasing data become available through mandated health data disclosure legislation, internists should become recognized as clinical performance evaluation specialists concerning the care provided in managed care systems. Such expertise should be invaluable as the JCAHO struggles to become a sophisticated medical management information system as opposed to one mainly driven by "expert consensus building."

Risk Management

The JCAHO will incorporate risk management standards into its accreditation surveys starting in 1989. It will be important for all clinicians to take an increasingly active role in the assessment and minimization of risk situations that could lead to patient injury and litigation. They must help prepare their organizations for accreditation surveys and document how their active involvement in this area improves the overall quality of health care delivery.

Internists may not be as involved in risk management programs as those in "inherently riskier" specialties (for example, anesthesiology or obstetrics). However, this lack of involvement must change. Procedure-oriented internists clearly need to be involved in establishing protocols to minimize the risk for injury from various invasive procedures. General internists need to be involved concerning both their use of these specialists and the management of their own patients. Areas of concern include (but are not limited to) proper documentation, provision of informed consent, and relations with patients, their families, and other physicians. By virtue of their broad general training and growing managerial experience, general internists may function best as medical risk management coordinators for both their departments and their institutions to help them meet these new standards and to minimize litigation risk.

Development of Clinical and Managerial Indicators

The JCAHO's development of clinical indicators should include most of the major medical specialties by the early 1990s. Admittedly, the Joint Commission is a consensus-driven body. As such, internists, *as individuals*, cannot have a major influence on the precise direction of the JCAHO. Nevertheless, the JCAHO cannot ignore the concerns and suggestions of large groups of physicians, especially when those groups are broad-based or act through the agency of a specialty organization, such as the American College of Physicians.

The Joint Commission invites an ongoing dialogue with all practicing physicians. If clinicians have developed their own set of clinical indicators to monitor important aspects of care, they should share these and their experiences with the JCAHO. Clinicians should stay abreast of the JCAHO's development of clinical indicators so that they can suggest modifications or adoption and usage at their institutions. Through members of the Organizational Indicators Task Force, clinicians with experience in managerial capacities may also provide input to the JCAHO concerning their impressions of what aspects of health care organizations are associated with the consistent delivery of high-quality health care.

Risk-Adjustment Methods

Clinicians should become familiar with risk-adjustment or severity indexing systems for evaluating clinical performance in the next few years (17). How well these systems work at their institutions is of vital interest to the JCAHO; clinicians should relate their experience with the various systems to the JCAHO. Clinicians will be substantially impacted by the use of severity adjustment systems used not only by the JCAHO, but also by many other public and private sector regulatory and purchasing agencies. (Please refer to Chapter 3 for details.)

Currently the JCAHO does not anticipate adopting any of the severity adjustment systems covered in Dr. Iezzoni's chapter. Clinicians, when acting as consensus groups through their organizations, may be able to influence the JCAHO concerning the range of specifications and patient covariates (for example, age, sex, complications, comorbidities, and so forth) to consider in designing severity adjustment systems.

Clinicians should become leaders in using risk adjustment methods in the next few years leading up to the JCAHO's implementation of their new accreditation program. They should be able to provide specific input to the JCAHO concerning what patient covariates are important in influencing clinical outcomes in the wide array of patients' clinical presentation.

Because of their broad-based training in internal medicine and involvement in their care of patients, which is subject to monitoring and evaluating systems, internists will be disproportionately impacted by severity adjustment systems. Thus, they should obtain as much information as possible about them. They will be used not only by the JCAHO, but by many other public and private regulatory and purchasing entities. As a starting point, they should refer to Dr. Iezzoni's chapter, and its specific supporting references and materials.

Data-Based System Development

Even clinicians without data systems backgrounds may provide feedback concerning their institution's ability to implement the "continuous flow monitoring system" anticipated by the JCAHO in the early 1990s. The movement into large-scale data-based management systems may be fraught with peril for the JCAHO, a heretofore consensus-driven body heavily dependent on "expert opinion." Achieving the kind of "continuous flow" medical management information system between the JCAHO and its thousands of surveyed organizations may take considerably longer than anticipated. Clinicians from states such as Maryland, Pennsylvania, Colorado, and Iowa (among others) with ongoing statewide medical management information systems may provide invaluable input to the JCAHO. They have experience concerning the logistics and obstacles involved in imposing this kind of sophisticated information system on a "professional consensus" culture such as the JCAHO. Clinicians from these states may also comment on the usefulness of the contemplated quarterly "norm-referenced" summaries comparing their institutions to others in their "peer group" and against "national" thresholds of acceptable performance.

Moreover, an increasing number of clinicians *do* have some background in medical systems development. They may provide specialized expertise to the JCAHO in this area. Because of their specialized medical training, internists could help the JCAHO design the most useful formats for standardized, comparative clinical performance reports. This is true even for internists without specialized medical systems development expertise.

Clinician input increases the chance of utilization of medical systems in the design of responsive educational programs to improve medical quality and cost-effectiveness. Data-based management systems similar to those contemplated by the JCAHO must be designed with ongoing input from clinicians, particularly internists, if the informational reports produced by them are to be used effectively.

CONCLUSIONS

The JCAHO has come a long way since the one-page American College of Surgeon's hospital standardization program first published in 1917. The JCAHO's current emphasis on monitoring and evaluating the quality and appropriateness of medical care is the foundation on which its developing clinical outcome assessment program, the Agenda for Change, is based. Grafted onto the JCAHO's consensus-driven foundation will be a sophisticated, interactive, nationwide medical management information system. Time will tell concerning whether this graft will take or not.

In addition to its Agenda for Change, the Joint Commission is expanding its accreditation work in its 5,300 hospitals, more than 300 ambulatory care organizations, approximately 1,000 hospital-based and -affiliated home care organizations, 1,400 long-term care facilities, 1,200 psychiatric and substance abuse facilities, and a steadily growing number of hospices, MCOs, and governmental agencies.

Clinicians in general, but especially specialists and subspecialists in internal medicine, may perform important functions in implementing the Joint Commission's recent medical quality management initiatives. Through their general and specific experiences in various types of health care organizations, they may improve the JCAHO's evaluation of these facilities. Clinicians should be able to provide particularly valuable input to the Joint Commission in the development of its clinical outcome assessment program (the Agenda for Change). Working through their national medical specialty societies, areas of input may include the refinement of clinical and managerial indicators of excellence, the evaluation of various risk adjustment methods, and the improvement of the usefulness of clinical performance reports produced by database management systems.

The Joint Commission is entering a new chapter of its history, as it attempts to remain a leading force in medical quality assessment and management. This area is increasingly giving way to the efforts of other agencies. To compete effectively with these agencies, the JCAHO must be able to change from an organization primarily driven by expert consensus to one highly sophisticated in the development and effective use of medical management information systems.

Currently, the JCAHO is still in the cocoon stage of its Agenda for Change. According to Mary Neubauer, RN, of Morristown Memorial Hospital in New Jersey, a pilot hospital as of the time of this writing, there is still no reportable experience on the merits of the clinical indicators being evaluated there. I believe the physician director of the Office of Quality Assurance of the AMA, John Kelly, MD, PhD, is convinced that physicians will look to the AMA as the ultimate arbiter of how to provide high-quality medical care. Although the Joint Commission may provide the blueprint, the AMA and the various national medical specialty societies in its House of Delegates, will provide the "bricks and mortar." In addition, the federal and state governments will probably enforce standards of care. For example, according to a *Wall Street Journal* investigation, between January 1986 and June 1988 at least 156 hospitals were threatened with sanctions or actually sanctioned for violations of federal quality standards, even though all these institutions remained JCAHO-accredited, some of them even up until the time they were shut down (18).

As pointed out in the *Wall Street Journal* article (18), the JCAHO may encounter conflicts when it comes to notifying regulatory agencies about surveyed organizations' deficiencies, even when those deficiencies may be severe enough to endanger the public health. As described earlier, the JCAHO is made up of five national health care associations that represent the interests of hospitals, physicians, and dentists. The JCAHO's 24-member Board of Commissioners is composed of representatives from these five organizations (plus three consumer representatives in 1989). The 21 nonconsumer commissioners are, in turn, appointed or elected by these five organizations' leaders (that is, their ruling bodies and Houses of Delegates). From this, it may be concluded that JCAHO policies are largely controlled (albeit indirectly) by these national medical and hospital associations. Such policies include those providing for the high degree of confidentiality afforded to JCAHO survey findings. These confidentiality policies may restrict access to survey findings even by various "high-level" governmental officials. As a result of recent public outcry, beginning in July 1989, the JCAHO intends to identify publicly those 8% to 10% of hospitals who receive "tentative nonaccreditation" notices (8,19).

The HCFA, through its Health Standards Quality Bureau, has an ongoing responsibility to report to Congress concerning the performance of the JCAHO. This is necessary for Congress to justify the continued use of health care organizations' JCAHO accreditation status to indicate sufficient compliance with the "Conditions for Participation" in the Medicare program. Nevertheless, according to the October 12, 1988 *Wall Street Journal* article (18), Congress has yet to receive both the 1986 and 1987 HCFA report on the JCAHO.

The HCFA is taking advantage of its ready access to a huge Medicare clinical claims database. Researchers there led by Henry Krakauer, MD, PhD, are attempting to correlate various physician practice patterns with severity-adjusted clinical outcomes in Medicare patients. Fruition of this effort in the next few years could upstage the JCAHO in its own efforts to set the stage for medical quality management in the 1990s and early 21st century. The same could be said for the increasing number of state data commissions, most notably that in Pennsylvania. Such commissions may achieve through the clout of purchasers by 1990, what it might take the JCAHO until 1995 to achieve in terms of influencing severity-adjusted clinical outcomes of patients in a favorable manner.

Nevertheless, the Joint Commission is making steady, though sometimes punctuated, progress in meeting its ambitious timetable. In less than 2 years, it has assembled and completed preliminary work with four clinical and managerial indicators task forces. It is developing its own system through determination of what patient covariates affect clinical outcomes the most consistently and reproducibly. It has named the chairmen of the six clinical indicator task forces beginning their work in 1989. It also is merging its current "Medical Staff," "Management and Administration Services," and "Governing Body" chapters into one "Hospital Leadership" chapter. This chapter's contents will reflect the importance of ongoing communication among and integration of the functions of these three bodies in the modern hospital.

It would seem that the largest obstacle for the JCAHO to overcome will be the development of the necessary data collection, analysis, and dissemination systems. Currently, this has proven to be the biggest impediment even for various data commissions operating on a considerably less imposing statewide basis. What the JCAHO is attempting to achieve through development of a system that would permit continually updated, quarterly "norm-referenced" summaries of organizational performance is indeed admirable. To achieve this goal even by 1995 would elevate the science of medical quality management to a level that would transcend all previous efforts. The path to that goal, however, is strewn with potholes, detours, and even roadblocks (logistical and political). Still, the JCAHO is the organization with the broadest-based representation of professional organizations involved in self-regulation of the quality of health care in the world. As members of the professional organizations the JCAHO represents, all clinicians have a strong stake in its success.

Acknowledgments: The author thanks Karen Mascot, whose typing and organizational skills are only exceeded by her patience in deciphering my penmanship.

References

1. Roberts JS, Coale JG, Redman RR. A history of the Joint Commission on Accreditation of Hospitals. *JAMA.* 1987;**258**:936-40.
2. U.S. Dept. of Health Education and Welfare. *Conditions of Participation for Hospitals.* Social Security Administration; 1966.
3. O'Leary DS. *The Joint Commission's Agenda for Change.* Chicago:JCAHO; 1987:1-10.
4. O'Leary DS. *An Introduction to the Joint Commission — Its Survey and Accreditation Processes, Standards, and Services.* Chicago:JCAHO; 1988:1-42.
5. *QHR Consultant Manual.* Boman; Chicago:JCAHO; 1988:11-2.
6. Excerpts from the proposed preamble to the "Quality Assurance" chapter in the *Accreditation Manual for Hospitals of the Joint Commission on the Accred-itation of Health Care Organizations.* Chicago:JCAHO; 1988 (with the author's parenthetical additions). For more detail, see Fromberg R. Medical staff monitoring and evaluating: departmental review. Chicago:JCAHO;1988.
7. *Accreditation Manual for Hospitals.* Chicago:JCAHO;1988:xx-xxii.
8. Burda D. JCAHO to charge for follow-up accreditation survey. *Mod Health Care.* 1988;September 9:10.
9. O'Leary DS. *Accreditation Program for Ambulatory Health Care.* Chicago:JCAHO;1988:262-71.
10. O'Leary DS. *Joint Commission Perspectives.* Chicago: JCAHO;1988:7-9.
11. Rozovsky FA. New JCAHO risk management standards: the potential impact on staff privileges. *Staff Privileges Report.* 1988;**1**(1):1,8.

12. Iezzoni LI, Ash AS, Moskowitz MA. *MedisGroups: A Clinical and Analytic Assessment.* Waltham, Massachusetts: Brandeis University Health Policy Research Consortium; 1987:1-57.

13. Thomas JW, Ashcraft MLF, Zimmerman J. *An Evaluation of Alternative Severity of Illness Measures for Use by University Hospitals.* Ann Arbor, Michigan:Department of Health Services Management and Policy, School of Public Health, University of Michigan; 1986.

14. Jencks SF, Dobson A. Refining case-mix adjustment—the research evidence. *N Engl J Med.* 1987;**317**:679-86.

15. *Organizational Principles: Field Review.* Chicago: JCAHO; August 1988.

16. *Report on the Joint Commission Survey of Relationships Among Governing Bodies, Management and Medical staff in U.S. Hospitals*; Chicago: JCAHO; 1988:1-14.

17. Couch JB, Nash DB. Severity of illness measures: opportunities for clinicians. *Ann Intern Med.* 1988;**109**:771-3.

18. Bogdanich W. Small comfort: prized by hospitals, accreditation hides perils patients face. *Wall Street Journal.* October 12, 1988.

19. Bogdanich W. Panel will name hospitals failing minimal standards. *Wall Street Journal.* January 16, 1989.

COMMENTARY

The JCAHO took root 71 years ago when the American College of Surgeons, acting as concerned consumers of hospital services, attempted to set minimum standards for quality of care. As physicians expanded their power base as the undisputed guardians of America's health, the profession's watchdog role over the quality of the physicians' workshop grew. Being the one organization that focused on health care institutional quality when nobody else had much to say about it, the Joint Commission acquired the aura of unquestioned authority: Quality was what the Joint Commission said it was. It became difficult for a single hospital, albeit a prestigious one, to forego its approval.

The Joint Commission continues to define its mission and draw its power from the consensus of an autonomous professional community. Attainment of consensus is a slow and frequently cumbersome process, but the Joint Commission's methods evolved less to foster flexibility or efficiency than to assure voluntary compliance through the power of its pronouncements. The political nature of its culture may have been defined on that early day when the names of the hospitals failing the first inspection were burned in the furnace of New York's Waldorf Astoria Hotel to keep the press from obtaining them. Adherence to standards has been sought privately and voluntarily, with the emphasis on structural capability to do things right rather than on whether the right things actually were being done. Today, its governing board is composed of 7 representatives of the hospital industry, 13 representatives of medical organizations, 1 dental representative, what has recently become 3 members from the public at large. Thus, despite all the discomfort it may cause the health care institutions it accredits, the Joint Commission remains primarily a provider organization, political in its culture and processes and more concerned about protecting the confidentiality of its professional constituents than informing the public.

Though some of its critics argue that it is too much governed by the same industry it seeks to regulate, JCAHO's philosophy is that it can be successful in improving health care organizations only if they are within its fold. Only osteopathic hospitals and facilities too small or too new to afford the expense of the surveys do not turn to the JCAHO for accreditation. It presently accredits about 85% of the nation's hospitals, surveying more than 1,500 each year. Of these, only 4 were denied accreditation in 1986 and 5 in 1987. But more than 98% of hospitals surveyed each year have "contingencies," areas lacking strict compliance with JCAHO standards.

Lest the potential for embarrassment outweigh the desirability of an accreditation process undertaken voluntarily, JCAHO sees the need to accompany pressure for improvement with assurances such as confidentiality and sufficient time to remedy any faults. A hospital with serious contingencies is notified of tentative nonaccreditation status and given 6 months to comply. In practice, it may not be surveyed again for as long as a year. Meanwhile, it retains its fully accredited status as far as the public is concerned. The JCAHO will disclose only the date of the last survey and "yes" or "no" as to whether the hospital is currently accredited. The only way for a physician or other citizen to learn about possible contingencies is from the state department of health in states where hospitals are required to submit their survey results as part of state inspection. If a hospital loses its accreditation, it can reapply again in 6 months on the same basis as a hospital that had never previously been considered. Because nearly all major facilities enjoy the benefits of accreditation at any given date, and refusal to accredit is so rare, it is difficult to determine whether the process does, indeed, have any effect on improving quality.

In contrast to JCAHO's approach, HCFA presents the public with seven volumes of hospital-specific risk-adjusted mortality data each year, gathered from Social Security records of Medicare patients. No judgment is rendered. In fact, the only commentaries issued with the data are the responses from the hospitals themselves. The range of "normal" hospitals is very wide, and the extent of information that can be gathered without further sophisticated statistical analyses is relatively scant; however, the data are openly available for public study and interpretation, and very good or very poor results can be discerned. PRO activity also is generally in the public domain. The reasons may have less to do with intent than with sunshine laws and the legal difficulties of denying to taxpayers information that they are paying their public servants to collect, but the result is that public awareness of hospital performance now has become a reality and a potential incentive to improve.

The New York State Department of Health, which has publicly denounced the collaborative and educational approach of the Joint Commission and no longer relies on its surveys, takes a giant step beyond simply informing the public. It undertakes a protective role by ferreting out hospitals with less than satisfactory performance and closing them down. In the view of the hospital industry, its vigor is sometimes excessive and can create an adversarial atmosphere. Although high-pressure tactics may improve the quality of care in some areas, problems may arise when hospital practices become needlessly defensive in response to threats of investigation or groundless censure.

Over the last decade, payers and the public have gained their own leverage as consumers of health care services and have gained greater access to objective information about health care quality nationwide. Computer systems have facilitated the gathering of large bodies of data and encouraged their use to guide decision making. Decisions based on external features and opinion, however authoritative they may be, no longer are unquestioned. Competing sources of information and public attacks on the Joint Commission as responding too slowly to quality problems and sacrificing public safety to parochial concerns of the organizations it accredits have weakened the Commission's public stature. Political and technological shifts of this magnitude generally have not been kind to industry leaders.

The Agenda for Change was announced in 1986 as the Joint Commission's bold new initiative. Publicly embracing the new technology, it proclaimed a shift to data-driven monitoring and institutional reorientation, to be accompanied by a revision of standards and survey procedures. Though the target date of 1990 is fast approaching, the data driven cultural style remains alien to the Commission's standard operating mode. To date, progress on the agenda for Change includes the development of indicators for pilot testing in three clinical areas, and three more task forces have just been convened. Seventeen pilot sites thus far have yielded only anecdotal reports of their progress. It is unclear whether the Commission is internally capable of managing the collection, risk adjustment, and analysis of the large bodies of data required to accomplish the sort of evaluation promised in the Agenda for Change.

In contrast, HCFA has succeeded in merging massive databases, developing new data sets, and marshalling resources far in excess of the Commission's budget. The HCFA mortality release, for all its failings, has evolved to a point of remarkable year-to-year consistency and a high degree of face validity. Some accredited hospitals whose quality problems have been disclosed independently can be easily identified by their high Medicare risk-adjusted mortality rates. HCFA's aggressive development and dissemination of outcome-based assessments of performance has made it a major force in the field, and even JCAHO is exploring the adaptation of HCFA's data to its own needs.

Other new challenges abound. Private vendors are marketing quality assurance tools that, while striving to support JCAHO requirements, are moving beyond the Commission's traditional concerns. Professional and hospital groups are working vigorously in the area of quality assurance, taking their lead from environmental pressures over which the Joint Commission has little control. New databases acquired by state data commissions and cost containment councils supported by payers, business groups, and providers' organizations are proliferating, each designed to screen performance in a different way. In a period of abundance of hospital beds, competition requires a sophistication in market differentiation for which a simple accreditation certificate is inherently inadequate. With limited time and resources, JCAHO can no longer write American health care's entire quality agenda.

Amidst the plethora of competing claims, the Joint Commission must redefine its mission and role in the light of its corporate triumphs and expertise. Its organizational orientation and insight are formidable, and its emphasis on institutional excellence is in keeping with the best modern thinking about quality control, continuous improvement, and the pursuit of excellence. The Commission can attempt to regain dominance over the entire field by mastering new technology and imposing its view of the proper flow of information on health care shareholders and stakeholders alike, or it can assume a new position in a spectrum of organizations, each assessing health care quality in its own way and from its own unique perspective. There is no reason the Commission must develop its own database, outcome indicators, or risk-adjustment methods. Defining acceptable bounds and processes and guiding health care providers in effectively closing the loop from insight to improved performance is a worthy goal well in keeping with the Commission's venerable mission, culture, and expertise. Its role may be to remain the embodiment of consensus building rather than move into high technology innovation.

Attempting political solutions to technical problems leads to O-rings that do not work, but technical solutions to political problems are equally futile. HCFA, with great resources and power, has focused on aspects of health care quality monitoring and evaluation that its administrators believe are within the scope of the organization's political mandate and capability. Other groups are claiming their piece of the action. JCAHO's ambitious initiative for change spans all these efforts and must either blend with them, eclipse them, or lose out in one or more of the critical endeavors of quality monitoring, evaluation, management, and improvement. Although the outcome will significantly affect providers, consumers, and payers, the choice remains with the Joint Commission's leadership and board. (Michael Pine, MD, MBA, President, Michael Pine and Associates, Inc., Chicago, IL 60615; (312) 643-1700)

Chapter 9

Malpractice, Clinical Risk Management, and Quality Assessment

LAURA MORLOCK, PhD
ORLEY H. LINDGREN, PhD
DON HARPER MILLS, MD, JD

INTRODUCTION

The past decade has been characterized by rapid to explosive growth in the frequency and size of payments for medical malpractice claims, as well as in premiums for professional liability insurance. The impact on physicians and health care institutions has been profound. Approximately 80% of medical malpractice claims — and virtually all of the most serious claims — result from adverse incidents in hospitals. These patterns have generated increasing interest among policymakers and the health care community in the potential of hospital-based clinical risk management programs directed toward malpractice claim control and prevention.

A primary objective of clinical risk management programs is to reduce the frequency of preventable adverse occurrences that lead to liability claims through activities designed to identify, evaluate, and decrease the risk for patient injury associated with clinical care (1-3). Other objectives are to decrease the number of claims and control the costs of claims that do emerge, through prompt identification and follow-up of maloccurrences and improved communications between providers and patients. Such programs also attempt to finance risk through the most economical methods (1).

Methods for clinical incident reporting or occurrence screening that result in "early warning systems" are essential. These methods consist of various strategies for identifying adverse patient occurrences, defined as incidents that under optimal conditions are not a normal consequence of a patient's disease or treatment (4). Adverse patient occurrences serve as "red flags" for undesired outcomes that warrant further review to determine if the care provided was appropriate.

In occurrence (clinical incident) reporting, criteria that define specific adverse patient outcomes must be reported by physicians or hospital staff, either at the time they are experienced or observed or shortly thereafter. In occurrence screening, adverse patient outcomes usually are identified through review of all or a percentage of medical charts, using a generic set of criteria (such as presence of nosocomial infection) that may be applied to all charts. In addition, specialty or service-specific criteria may be used for a more focused review. For over a decade efforts have been made to develop generic and focused criteria for these reporting and screening systems. There is a growing literature documenting and comparing the adverse patient outcome "yield rates" of various approaches, as well as the extent to which they provide early warning of incidents that result in malpractice claims.

These systems — whether based on clinical incident reporting, occurrence screening, or some combination — are important for two reasons: First, the identification of events through these strategies may facilitate early investigation and possible intervention to avert or diminish adverse consequences and potential liability exposure. Second, accumulation of information makes possible the creation of databases that may help identify strategies to prevent repeated maloccurrences (4). Increasingly, information from these systems also is used in medical staff privileging, credentialing, and other peer review activities in order to improve patient care. The active participation of physicians, including strong support from clinical leadership, is essential for these efforts to succeed.

This chapter reviews the current state of the art with regard to clinical risk management strategies. The first section discusses factors that have generated increasing interest in risk management efforts, with emphasis on continuing concerns with medical malpractice issues. The second section summarizes results from studies on the size and scope of the problem of physician-related patient injury. The third section compares alternative approaches used for the identification of adverse patient occurrences, followed by a section on the uses of such information in the management of individual claims and in the strengthening of peer review and quality assurance activities. The final section suggests areas of needed research and explores emerging issues in clinical risk management.

MEDICAL MALPRACTICE AS A NATIONAL CONCERN

Legal and Insurance Issues

Medical malpractice is defined as negligent care by a health services provider that causes injury to a patient. Legal actions charging medical malpractice may be brought against a physician, other health care personnel, a hospital or other type of health care facility, or others involved directly or indirectly in patient care. Claimants who believe they have been injured as the result of provider negligence usually seek compensation for medical treatment and rehabilitation, as well as lost wages if appropriate (economic damages). They also may request compensation for changes in the quality of life or for the amount of pain they have experienced as a result of the alleged injury (noneconomic damages). To be compensated through the legal system for medical malpractice, a breach in the appropriate standard of care, compensable injury to the patient, and a causal connection between the provider's negligence and the patient's injury must be established (5).

In many malpractice claims there is a considerable time lag between treatment and the recognition of an injury due to alleged negligence. Data from the nation's largest professional liability insurer, the St. Paul Companies, indicate that on average, approximately 30% of claims have been filed in the year of treatment, 30% in the year after treatment, 25% in the third year, 7% in the fourth year, and 8% in the fifth year or later (6). For providers and insurers this pattern often has resulted in a "long tail" of exposure to unfiled malpractice claims. Traditionally, most health care providers have been insured for medical malpractice with policies written on an occurrence basis. This type of policy provides insurance for claims resulting from treatment delivered during the coverage period, regardless of when the claim is filed. Occurrence-based policies create considerable uncertainty for insurance companies who must determine appropriate premiums and reserve levels to cover future claims.

The 1970s Crisis

Liability insurance received little attention by physicians or hospital administrators until the mid-1960s because coverage could be obtained at low rates that remained fairly constant. Contractions in availability and escalations in premium costs in the late 1960s and early 1970s led to the identification of professional liability as a major national problem.

In one of the first detailed studies of this issue, the national Commission on Medical Malpractice examined information from approximately 15,000 claims closed during 1970. On the basis of this analysis, as well as on other commissioned studies, they concluded in 1973 that the mounting costs of malpractice liability insurance, the dramatic increases in claims frequency, and a perceived growing tendency of physicians to practice "defensive medicine," had all profoundly affected medical care practice, the delivery of health services, and the overall cost of health care (7).

In the next few years an explosive growth in claims frequency was seen. The St. Paul Companies experienced an average 20% increase in claims filed each year between 1970 and 1976 (6). During this period four times the number of malpractice claims were filed nationally as in the preceeding 35 years combined (6). Claim severity — the average amount in settlement or award for claims closed with payment to the claimant — also increased at an accelerating rate.

These large increases in claims and claim costs are thought to have resulted from several factors (3,6,8). First, widely publicized technologic advances in many areas of medicine contributed to heightened — and sometimes unrealistic — expectations of beneficial outcomes by both providers and consumers. These technologies also fueled rapid growth in the number of medical procedures performed, many of which were invasive with some potential for harm. Along with these changes were trends toward the depersonalization of physician-patient interactions; a more litigious climate in general; increasing numbers of attorneys experienced in health law and physicians willing to serve as expert witnesses; and in many states, pro-plaintiff changes in the legal system that increased access to the courts and eased the burden of proof.

Although increases in claims frequency and severity occurred nationally, there was significant variation from state to state. In California, for example, the number of claims closed in 1976 per 100 physicians was 8.81, whereas in Maine the rate was 0.47 (9). Danzon (9) studied factors associated with state variation in claims frequency and severity during this period. She found that the number of physicians per capita was a significant determinant of claim frequency, but not claim severity. In contrast, number of attorneys per capita had little effect on claim frequency after controlling for other factors such as availability of physicians, but did have a significant effect on claim severity. The single most powerful predictor of both claim frequency and severity, however, was state variation in degree of urbanization.

Analysis results also indicated that pro-plaintiff changes in common law doctrines contributed to the rapid growth of both claim frequency and severity during the early 1970s. The study compared states that had abolished the locality rule* and charitable immunity and that had adopted *respondeat superior*† and informed consent, with states that recognized none of these legal doctrines. Findings indicated that states with these pro-plaintiff doctrines by 1970 averaged 53% higher claim frequency per capita and 28% higher claim severity; by 1976 they also had averaged 86% higher total claim costs per capita. Danzon (9) concluded that the extension of these pro-plaintiff doctrines to other states was one factor narrowing the gap between the most and least litigious states by the late 1970s.

By the mid 1970s, many states were experiencing twofold and threefold increases in liability insurance rates, followed by the withdrawal of some carriers from the malpractice insurance market. Many companies that remained refused to take on new risks, prompting strong reaction among the medical community, including refusal by physicians in California to provide any care other than emergency services.

---

*Under the locality rule the standard of care in a given instance is measured solely by the practice patterns of other physicians in the same locality. Pro-plaintiff changes include various approaches to broadening the scope of appropriate standards of care.

†Under this doctrine liability is based on the principle of holding the superior, including an organization, responsible for the negligence of his or her agents or employees.

Among the major causes of this situation were the substantial increases in frequency and severity of malpractice claims when many of the liability insurers had both inadequate financial reserves and lower than anticipated investment income due to stock market fluctuations. To some degree these problems also resulted from the inability of insurers to predict risk due to the "long tail" of exposure characteristic of malpractice claims, the absence of adequate data describing the nature of these risks, and the relatively small number of physicians who provided a base across which these risks could be spread (3,6,8,10).

State Responses to the 1970s Crisis

In response to the alarming increases in malpractice insurance rates during the mid-1970s, most state legislatures passed new statutes to stabilize insurance markets, modify traditional tort laws, or introduce new procedures for resolving medical malpractice disputes. Virtually every state legislature in some way changed traditional civil practice laws by placing limits on provider liability, restructuring the circumstances under which individuals could bring suit, codifying how provider negligence could be established, or altering usual practices in civil action proceedings that were thought to promote large settlements and awards (10,11).

One of the most common changes in tort laws governing medical malpractice cases — instituted in about half the states — involved placing a statute of limitations on how long after the injury a claim could be filed. More than half the states prohibited plaintiffs from stating in their initial pleadings the amount of monetary damages and other relief being requested. This portion of the claim, known as the *ad damnum* clause, was thought to promote larger awards. In about one third of the states, changes were legislated that placed limits on either the total amount of an award or on particular types of damages — typically noneconomic losses. Other changes allowed for the periodic payment of damages over the lifetime of the plaintiff or during the period of disability; defined the issues to be considered in legally establishing departure from a standard of care; and permitted defendants to introduce evidence of collateral sources of payment to the plaintiff.* Various other reforms were instituted less commonly, including tightening the qualifications required of expert witnesses and various approaches to attorney fee regulation. In addition, about half the states introduced new procedures, such as binding arbitration or pretrial screening panels, for the resolution of medical malpractice disputes.

---

*Traditionally, the collateral source rule in tort cases prohibits introducing into evidence at trial indication that the plaintiff has received compensation for the injury from any source other than the defendant (for example, reimbursement from health insurance for medical expenses incurred as a result of the injury). Changes in the rule usually either allowed consideration of a collateral payment to be considered in establishing the amount of award, or required that such payments be deducted from malpractice awards (10).

Other changes were intended to help stabilize liability insurance markets. Some states, for example, created joint underwriting associations to provide increased professional liability protection to physicians and hospitals. Many large health care organizations and consortia established self-insurance programs. In about 30 states, physician groups — usually the state medical society — created not-for-profit insurance companies. Throughout the medical liability insurance industry, companies attempted to reduce their own risk and uncertainty by moving from occurrence-based to claims-made policies that insure providers only for incidents in which claims are filed within the year of coverage.

Trends in Claim Frequency, Claim Severity, and Premium Costs

After a large increase in the number of claims filed during the first half of the 1970s, frequency declined from 1975 through 1978. It is estimated that nationally the annual number of claims filed decreased from 24,240 in 1975 to 17,238 in 1978 (6). Annual decreases up to 30% were seen during this period even in states that initially were hardest hit by the professional liability problem. What caused the decline in frequency is unclear. There is no evidence that tort reforms enacted during the mid-1970s had a direct effect on the decline in claims filed. It is possible, however, that publicity about the professional liability situation, uncertainties generated by rapid changes in the malpractice insurance industry, and questions concerning the constitutionality of many of the legislative reforms either discouraged or delayed the filing of claims (6).

Whatever the causes of the 1975 to 1978 decline, by 1979 the number of claims again began to increase rapidly. Most estimates indicate that claims at least doubled by the early 1980s. The National Association of Insurance Commissioners, for example, found that the average incidence was 3.3 claims per 100 physicians before 1978, and 8.0 claims per 100 physicians during the late 1970s and early 1980s (6). Physician surveys conducted by the American Medical Association (AMA) indicate an increase from an average of 3.3 claims per 100 physicians in the late 1970s to 10.1 claims per 100 physicians in 1985 (3). The St. Paul Companies reported an increase from 7.9 to 17.9 claims per 100 physicians from 1976 to 1985 (3).

Malpractice awards and settlements did not show a decline in severity comparable to the decline in claims frequency during 1975 to 1978. Instead, there was first a steady increase, and then a dramatic upswing in both the average size of paid claims and in awards over $1 million (6,12). The St. Paul Companies, for example, experienced an increase from $17,600 to $70,200 in the average paid claim against physicians during 1976 to 1985 (3). The most recent data available indicate a 264% increase in the total amount of medical malpractice claims paid by U.S. insurers from 1980 to 1987 (13).

Until recently, growth in average malpractice premium costs was much slower than growth in the frequency and severity of claims, or than increases in the Medical Care Price Index. Although average physician premium expenses grew by 51% between 1976 and 1983, this percentage increase was slower than the average growth in physician income. As a result, average malpractice premium expenses were 4.4% of physician gross income in 1976, but had declined to 3.7% of gross income by 1983 (6,11).

During this period, total medical malpractice insurance losses increased by 145% (from $817 million to approximately $2 billion), whereas insurance premiums for the total medical professional liability industry increased by only 31% (from $1.2 billion to $1.57 billion) (6). Return on investments at high interest rates still permitted overall profit-making during the late 1970s and early 1980s among companies writing malpractice insurance. By 1984, however, *Best's Insurance Management Reports* concluded that "medical malpractice is reaching the point of no return in terms of producing investment income from loss reserves that exceeds the underwriting loss" (6).

Insurance companies responded with substantial increases in medical malpractice premiums, with an average growth rate of about 30% per year (13,14). It is important to note, however, the enormous variation by state, degree of urbanization, and specialty: St. Paul's rates in 1985, for example, varied from $1,369 for a relatively low-risk general practitioner in Arkansas to $92,570 for a Miami, Florida neurosurgeon with the same coverage (15).

More recently, rates have begun to moderate as malpractice insurers have accumulated greater reserves (13,14). In addition, several states have experienced a leveling off or decrease in number of claims. This does not yet appear to signal a nationwide trend, however, and there has been no change in the rate of increase for claim severity. For 1989, St. Paul has announced it will lower rates by 1% to 14% in 8 of the states where it offers medical malpractice coverage; an overall increase of 5.5% (ranging up to approximately 25%) is projected, however, for the remaining 34 states it serves (14).

The Impact of Tort Reforms

There is general consensus that the legislative reforms and insurance initiatives of the 1970s were effective in ensuring the availability of medical malpractice coverage; the subsequent effects of these changes on claim frequency and severity, or on the price of liability insurance are less clear (11). In a major national study of claims closed from 1975 to 1984, Danzon (16) concluded that although the frequency and severity of claims continued to climb steadily during this period, tort reforms tended to slow the rate of increase.

More specifically, Danzon found that states with statutes of limitations and laws that permitted or mandated the reduction of awards in the presence of collateral benefits had a slower increase in claim frequency. States that allowed or mandated the consideration of collateral benefits also had a slower rate of growth in claim severity, as did states that had placed limits on the size of awards. Danzon also found that arbitration statutes tended to increase claim frequency but reduce the average size of settlements or awards; neither screening panels nor limits on attorney contingency fees appeared to have any systematic effect on either claim frequency or severity. Other major influences on both frequency and severity included the degree of urbanization and the rate of surgery, or ratio of surgeons to medical specialists, in the state.

Several states have recently passed or are currently debating additional tort reform legislation. Among the changes frequently proposed have been various approaches to health claims arbitration, limits on punitive damages, and caps on awards for pain and suffering. No-fault liability coverage for birth-related severe neurologic injuries — a class of cases that traditionally has generated the largest awards — recently has been approved by two state legislatures (Virginia and Florida) and is being discussed in several other states (17).

At the same time, many proponents of tort reform have expressed growing dissatisfaction with the relatively small magnitude and apparent unevenness of its impact (13). A 1986 General Accounting Office (GAO) study of six states that instituted reforms in the mid-1970s is cited frequently. Despite these legislative changes, the study concluded that "insurance costs for many physicians and hospitals increased dramatically, as did the number of malpractice claims and the average amounts paid" (18). The growing number of courts that have declared tort reform legislation to be unconstitutional is also of significant concern. Court decisions in Kansas, Wyoming, Florida, Virginia, Texas, and Oklahoma, as well as constitutional challenges in many other states, have been part of a growing trend toward "tort deform" that has created considerable uncertainty about how to find solutions to the medical malpractice problem (13).

The Search for Other Strategies

One focus of increasing interest has been on the potential of risk management activities designed both to decrease the number of iatrogenic injuries that may result in claims, as well as to more effectively resolve claims that do emerge. The impetus for increased risk management efforts has come from several sources. First, many of the malpractice insurance alternatives that developed after the mid-1970s crisis, as well as traditional commercial carriers that continued to offer liability insurance, began to require formal risk management programs as a condition of coverage (2). Second, a series of court decisions starting in the late 1950s had extended the legal responsibilities of hospitals for ensuring the clinical competence and performance of both employees and all practitioners granted clinical privileges (19-21). As the malpractice crisis deepened, many hospitals — particularly those participating in some type of self-insurance arrangement — became more concerned about managing and preventing claims due to their own increased exposure.

More recently several national groups, including the GAO (22), the Department of Health and Human Services' Task Force on Medical Liability and Malpractice (5), and the American Hospital Association's Medical

Malpractice Task Force (4) have advocated the strengthening and expansion of hospital risk management programs. New standards that became effective in 1989 require all hospitals seeking accreditation from the Joint Commission on Accreditation of Healthcare Organizations (JCAHO) to have programs linking quality assurance and patient care to clinical risk management (23). In addition, nine states now mandate some form of risk management activities as a condition of hospital licensure (24).

State legislators and federal policymakers increasingly have come to view risk management, medical discipline, and quality control activities as an important complement to tort reforms that may limit provider liability and patient recovery of damages. An ongoing debate at both the state and federal levels concerns the extent to which public policy in this area should focus on controlling the costs of malpractice claims, or on finding methods for reducing the incidence of patient injuries related to medical care. Evidence regarding the estimated size and scope of this latter problem is reviewed in the next section.

PATIENT INJURIES RESULTING FROM MEDICAL CARE

Studies Based on Closed Malpractice Claims

As the malpractice insurance crisis intensified during the early 1970s, better information was needed that could be used to guide legislative activities and develop risk-reduction strategies in healthcare delivery settings. To address this need the National Association of Insurance Commissioners (NAIC) began a comprehensive study based on the claim files of all U.S. insurers that had written malpractice premiums of $1 million or more in any year since 1970 (25). The completed database included information on 71,788 claims closed by the 128 participating insurers during a 3.5-year period from July 1975 through December 1978.

Study results showed that 78% of all incidents resulting in paid claims occurred in hospitals; these claims accounted for 87% of all payments to claimants. Triggering events were most likely to occur in operating rooms (39%) and emergency departments (18%); most involved physicians. Injuries reported by claimants involved only emotional damage in 7% of claims, were of a temporary nature in 55%, created permanent disability in 21%, and resulted in death in 15%.

Approximately one third (35%) of all paid claims alleged improperly performed procedures. Of these, the most frequent incidents involved a foreign object left in an operation site with further surgery required for its removal. Other frequent events included the accidental laceration of pelvic and gastrointestinal organs during surgery, other types of surgical complications requiring additional surgery, and postoperative wound infections.

Approximately one fourth (27%) of all paid claims were related to diagnostic errors. The most frequent problems involved delay in treatment due to misdiagnosis, delay due to failure to diagnose an abnormal condition, misinterpretation of diagnostic tests or roentgenograms, inadequate physical examinations, and the improper performance of diagnostic tests. Ten percent of paid claims resulted from medication problems, 10% from patient falls, and 15% from other events or a combination of precipitating factors.

Although only 3% of all claims were generated by anesthesia injuries, these on average were the most costly, and accounted for 11% of all dollars paid in settlements and awards. Large average payments also resulted from claims involving operations on the nervous system (particularly the spinal cord) and obstetrical procedures. Secondary issues most likely to be associated with claims resulting in large payments included problems with emergency equipment, failure or delay in seeking consultation, failure to prevent an abnormal condition, malfunctioning anesthesia equipment, failure to disclose matters of concern to patients in a timely fashion, and patient abandonment.

The greatest increases in average payments over the study period were for claims alleging grave permanent injuries, particularly those involving cardiac arrest, quadraplegia, or severe brain damage resulting from anesthesia accidents, patient monitoring problems, or birth-related injuries. The average amount paid for these types of claims increased from $213,777 in 1975 to $349,203 in 1978.

Analysis of claim emergence and disposition patterns during this period indicated that claims were filed an average of 17 months after the precipitating incident, and were resolved an average of 21 months after filing. However, time required for claim emergence ranged from less than 1 month to 20 years, with even greater variation in the amount of time spent on claim resolution. Thirty-eight percent of all claims resulted in payment to the claimant. When all claims related to a single incident were consolidated, about half (49%) of all incidents were shown to result in at least one paid claim.

The percentage of claims requiring a formal court disposition for resolution increased each year from 7% of all claims in 1975 to 18% of all claims (and 21% of claims against physicians) in 1978. Although defendants won most (86%) of cases decided in court, court dispositions resulted in average payments that were 2.8 times higher than private settlements. The trend toward more litigation also resulted in greater expenses associated with claim defense: Regardless of the outcome, claims requiring a court disposition took an average of 9 months longer to resolve and averaged 2.1 times greater expenses than claims settled privately. The lowest expenses were reported for claims settled before the formal filing of a lawsuit. During the study, both payments and claim expenses increased by an average of 70%, or approximately 42% after adjusting for inflation.

More recently the GAO conducted a national study using a random sample of malpractice claims closed in 1984 by a randomly selected group of 25 liability insurance companies (26). Closed claims resulting from 1,706 incidents were included in the sample. These data were used to provide national estimates describing the 73,472 medical malpractice claims involving 103,255 health care providers that were closed by 102 insurance companies in 1984.

Although claim frequency, size of payments, and defense costs had all increased substantially between the two periods, many of the general patterns regarding claim characteristics revealed in the GAO analysis are similar to the earlier NAIC findings. For example, 80% of the claims included in the GAO study resulted from incidents that occurred in hospitals. Paid claims in the GAO analysis, like the earlier NAIC study, were most likely to allege improperly performed procedures (surgical and obstetrical) and diagnostic errors. Obstetrical claims in the GAO analysis, however, accounted for 27% of the total amount of payments — more than twice their proportion of indemnity payments during the earlier study.

Claims closed during the two periods were equally likely to include incidents resulting in death (15% of all claims), but those included in the GAO study were more likely to involve permanent disability (28% compared with 21% in the NAIC analysis) and to be closed with payment to the claimant (43% compared with 38%). Although less likely to require a formal court disposition, claims in the GAO analysis required an average of 4 months longer to resolve.

The results of the NAIC analysis, as well as more limited data from individual insurers, provided an initial information base supporting the development of both quality assurance and risk management programs targeted toward physicians in hospital settings, particularly those involved in obstetrics, other surgical specialties, and anesthesiology. The more recent GAO analysis also suggests the appropriateness of this focus. In addition, results from these studies have underscored the potential importance of timely identification and resolution of patient complaints, as well as prompt attention to and compensation for justifiable claims, in order to reduce the costs of defense and possibly the size of settlements and awards.

Detection of Adverse Occurrences Based on Medical Chart Reviews

The information derived from closed claim studies obviously is limited to patient injuries (and alleged injuries) that have resulted in demands for compensation. There is little evidence on the frequency with which patient injuries actually occur during medical care, or the extent to which these injuries are the result of provider error.

The most comprehensive investigation of these issues is the Medical Insurance Feasibility Study conducted during the mid-1970s under the sponsorship of the California Medical Association and the California Hospital Association (27). The study was prompted by a widely held belief within the health care community that most bad outcomes of medical and surgical management were litigated successfully by plaintiff attorneys regardless of whether or not they resulted from provider negligence. This perception generated considerable interest in the potential benefits of a no-fault system designed to compensate patients for adverse outcomes according to a fixed schedule of benefits without regard to provider error. It was believed that this approach could be more equitable and efficient, and less costly than the fault-based litigation system, with its high administrative costs and unpredictability.

The California study aimed to determine the cost and feasibility of a no-fault compensation system by conducting a detailed examination of the frequency, severity, and characteristics of patient disabilities resulting from health care management. The study was designed and implemented by Don Harper Mills, John Boyden, and David Rubsamen with the assistance of a team of medical consultants coordinated by Charles Jacobs of InterQual, Inc. Twenty-three hospitals were chosen to be representative of all California acute care hospitals in terms of size, region, ownership, and teaching status. From these institutions a sample of 20,864 medical records were selected to represent all California hospital discharges during 1974 with respect to age, gender, race, and payment source.

To help identify injuries related to medical care that might be compensable, 20 screening criteria were developed that denoted adverse incidents of major significance. Examples included a patient admitted for a condition suggesting potential prior failure or adverse results of medical management; death during the hospitalization; hospital-incurred trauma; adverse drug reaction; unplanned return to the operating room; or temperature of 38.5°C or greater on last full day before or day of discharge. Many of the screening criteria had specific exceptions that exempted the chart from further review. For example, a death during the index hospitalization was excluded from further analysis if the patient had been admitted for planned terminal care. Similarly, medical charts documenting hospital-incurred trauma or an adverse drug reaction were omitted from any additional review if the records indicated that the resulting problems resolved before discharge and did not require treatment extending the length of stay.

The initial screening by a staff of medical chart reviewers identified hospital admissions in which patients had experienced one or more adverse incidents as defined by the screening criteria. If specified exceptions were not present, these medical records were examined next by physicians and physician-attorneys to determine whether a potentially compensable event had occurred. Such an event was defined as an incident resulting in temporary or permanent disability most probably caused by health care management. Further, the injury sustained must either have led to the index hospitalization, prolonged hospitalization, or resulted in substantial treatment after hospitalization. Charts containing a potentially compensable event were then further evaluated to determine the likelihood of an adverse jury decision if the incident had resulted in a claim litigated to a court verdict. These judgments were made by four of the study investigators, all of whom were both physicians and attorneys, and experienced in evaluating malpractice claims. They based their analysis not only on whether in their judgment professional negligence had occurred, but also on several other factors likely to be considered in a court decision, including the type and degree of severity of the injury; why certain treatments were administered and others withheld; whether the disability could have been prevented under "ordinary" standards of care; and the state of the medical records.

The investigators concluded that 970 of 20,864 (4.65%) medical records examined contained information indicative of a patient disability caused by health care management. It was further estimated that 17% of these iatrogenic injuries (or 0.8% of the total) would probably have resulted in a jury finding of provider liability under the tort system. The remaining 83% were judged to derive from adverse events produced by the normal risk of medical treatment. These results imply, however, that 1 of every 126 patients admitted to California hospitals in 1974 experienced, either before or during hospitalization, a significant injury due to negligence (as legally defined) that was judged to be compensable if it had resulted in a malpractice claim.

A classification of all patient injuries resulting from health care management indicated that 82% were due to the adverse effects of treatment, and an additional 3% resulted from failure to prevent the problem or protect the patient. Both categories of events precipitated new abnormal conditions other than the problems for which patients had sought medical treatment. Fifteen percent of the injuries were classified as the effects of incomplete treatment or diagnosis in which expected and achievable medical care outcomes were not attained. Patients in this category had a problem that persisted, further deteriorated, or recurred, usually accompanied by progression from a less severe to a more severe stage of disease. Examples include the occurrence of cancer metastasis caused by a medical delay in diagnosing and treating the original lesion, or prolonged postoperative disability arising from the preoperative rupture of an appendix resulting either from medical delay in diagnosis or surgical delay in treatment of an otherwise uncomplicated acute appendicitis.

Primary causal events in two thirds (66%) of the cases were specific procedures, most often improperly performed. About one fifth (19%) of the injuries involved medication problems, and 5% were the direct result of diagnostic errors, including nondiagnosis (2.7%) and misdiagnosis (2.2%). Other causal events were categorized as involving defective devices (3%), problems in general medical management (3%), nursing management (2%), administration of anesthesia (2%), and nondefective devices (1%).

It is important to note that although these problems were detected in the medical charts of hospitalized patients, one third of the adverse events actually had occurred outside of the hospitals, usually in physicians' offices and clinics. The effects, however, were severe enough to result in hospitalization. Unlike inpatient events, these incidents were most likely to involve problems with medications (46%), followed by specific procedures (35%), general medical management (5%), and misdiagnosis (4%).

Due to restrictions placed on the study to safeguard confidentiality, investigators were not able to determine how many of the patients injured in adverse events actually filed malpractice claims. This number has been estimated, however, by Danzon (8), who compared the 1974 injury information with aggregate claims data for California available from the NAIC survey of claims closed during July 1975 to December 1978. Danzon restricted her analysis to adverse events in hospitals, and compared the number of claims relative to the number of injuries by age of the injured party, severity of the injury, and type of medical error.

Results from Danzon's analysis suggest that at most 1 in 10 of the patients experiencing an injury due to error actually filed a malpractice claim. Danzon notes that this proportion is likely to be an overestimate because it assumes that all injuries due to error in the California study were identified through the medical record review. Furthermore, during this period California had one of the highest frequencies of claims per physician and claims per capita in the nation. If the incidence of iatrogenic injuries due to provider error was similar throughout the country, the proportion of injuries resulting in claims was likely to be lower in most other states. Of the claims filed, only about 40% resulted in payment to the claimant, leading Danzon to conclude that at most 1 in 25 patient injuries due to negligence resulted in compensation through the medical malpractice system.

A comparison of types of injuries resulting from error with characteristics of claims filed and claims paid suggested that the likelihood of filing a claim appeared to be greater for permanent than for temporary injuries, and lowest for incidents resulting in death. Age of the injured party was a significant predictor of claim payment: The probability of an injury due to error resulting in a paid claim ranged from 1 in 55 for persons over age 65 to 1 in 18 for persons aged 20 to 44. With respect to the types of medical errors resulting in claims, the analysis indicated that errors of performance, rather than errors of judgment or diagnosis, appeared to be the primary cause of injuries and the principal allegation in claims. As Danzon and others have noted, iatrogenic injuries due to omissions in health care management may be as common, but they are harder to identify from hospital charts than problems due to commission. Similarly, injuries due to diagnostic errors, compared with procedural errors, may be harder to detect — whether by patients, plaintiff attorneys, or research investigators.

In summary, evidence suggests that the relationships among patient injuries associated with medical care, provider errors, and malpractice claims may be represented by the diagram in Figure 1. Area A represents all medical injuries among hospitalized patients, estimated on the basis of the California study as 4.65%, or about 1 in 20, of all patient admissions. Area B represents the incidence of all legal misconduct by health care providers, the extent of which is unknown.

Area C defines injuries due to provider error that would constitute negligence as defined legally. Theoretically, these are "actionable" injuries under the tort system of liability and should result in compensation if claims are filed. The overlap of area A and area C constituted 17% of area A, or 0.79% (1 per 126) of all patients admitted to acute care institutions in California in 1974. Applying the same rate to national hospital admissions figures suggested that during that year approximately 260,000 patients in the United States experienced injuries due to errors in the delivery of medical care.

More recent but much less comprehensive investigations of adverse events and provider error have found rates similar to, or greater than, those observed during the California study. An examination of the rate of iatrogenic illness among 815 consecutive patients admitted to the general medical service at a university hospital in 1979 concluded that 36% experienced some form of

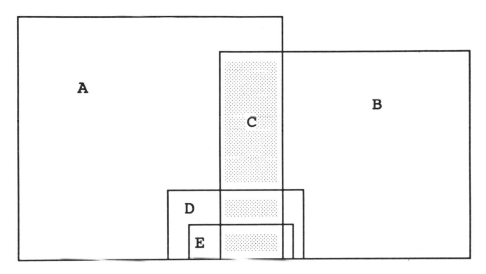

Figure 1. Relationships among patient injuries, legal fault, and malpractice claims. A = incidence of patient injuries; B = incidence of errors during medical care, C = patient injuries due to errors during medical care (shaded area); D = filed malpractice claims; and E = filed claims resulting in claimant compenation.

iatrogenic illness (28). One quarter of these events (representing 9% of all patients) were life-threatening or resulted in substantial disability. These adverse incidents were judged to have contributed to the death of 2% of the patients. The most frequent complications involved drug reactions, cardiac catheterizations, and falls. The investigators did not determine the contribution of provider error to the rate of iatrogenic problems. They concluded, however, that given the increasing number and complexity of diagnostic procedures and therapeutic agents, the careful monitoring of untoward events has become essential.

The rate of patient injury due to provider error was examined in a study of surgical mishaps due to error among 5,612 surgical admissions at Peter Bent Brigham Hospital (29). The investigation identified 36 surgical mishaps — a rate of injury due to provider error (0.64%) that is comparable to findings in the California study. The investigators emphasize the high social and economic costs of these "low-frequency events." Twenty of thirty-six patients died in the hospital, and for 11 of the patients, death was directly attributable to the error. Five of sixteen surviving patients were discharged with serious physical impairment. The average hospital stay for the 36 patients was 42 days, and the total costs of their treatment were more than $1.7 million (in 1980 dollars).

More comprehensive data that would update the California study are not available. New York state, however, has commissioned the Harvard Medical Practice Study Group to review approximately 30,000 medical records for patients hospitalized in New York during 1984. Study objectives include the determination of which patients suffered injuries in the course of their hospital treatment, and the extent to which these injuries resulted from substandard treatment (Harvard Medical Practice Study Group, "Medical care and medical injuries in the state of New York: a pilot study." Cambridge, Massachusetts, April 1987). The project includes an initial review of all medical charts using 17 screens adapted from the California study, followed by physician review of flagged records to confirm the adverse event, estimate probable causation, and assess the probability of provider negligence.

Area D in Figure 1 represents the number of malpractice claims filed. Based on Danzon's analysis, at the height of the malpractice crisis in the mid-1970s only about 10% of the injuries due to provider error resulted in filed claims. As indicated by area E, approximately 40% of these claims resulted in payment to the claimant, suggesting that during this period about 1 in 25 patients who experienced an injury due to medical care error received compensation. Even if we assume that the claim filing rate has tripled over the past decade, it seems unlikely according to Danzon's analysis, that the malpractice problem is simply due to litigious patients (8).

ALTERNATIVE STRATEGIES FOR DETECTING ADVERSE PATIENT OCCURRENCES

By the late 1970s the increasing costs of malpractice claims and liability insurance, coupled with a growing recognition that iatrogenic injuries resulting from provider errors were a large and potentially costly problem, prompted many institutions to search for methods to improve patient care and limit their own liability. The first step in such efforts involved the development of strategies to identify in a timely manner problems that had occurred and situations that posed a significant risk for patient injury. For many hospitals this need led to a major reevaluation of their traditional risk management activities.

Traditional Incident Reporting Systems

During this period most hospitals already had some type of administrative reporting system for adverse incidents involving patients or visitors. Incident reports usually involved a written description of the injury, adverse outcome, or mishap by nurses or other hospital employees (2). In most institutions the types of injuries reported did not include adverse occurrences during medical or surgical management; they usually were limited to the results of hospital employee actions or problems associated with the physical plant of the hospital.

The reporting systems were created to notify hospital risk managers, administrators, and insurers of when injuries occurred; to aid in the management of injuries in order to minimize damage; and to reduce the litigation costs associated with these injuries. These functions were performed with great variability from hospital to hospital, depending on the level of interest and cooperation of the hospital administration and insurance carrier, as well as the degree of risk management expertise.

Despite this variation, traditional incident reporting systems can be credited with identifying many important problems involving dietary and medication errors, intravenous infusion difficulties, equipment malfunctions, and patient falls. Resulting management innovations included development of wristband identification for inpatients, side rails and high-low beds, unitary medication systems, and several other improvements in ancillary services. These changes were implemented mainly by hospital nursing and administration with little medical staff awareness or involvement.

Most incident reports were of limited value to liability insurers, however, because they rarely involved injuries related to medical or surgical care — the adverse occurrences most likely to result in significant legal actions. Therefore, claims representatives in many companies usually waited for legal notice (a formal letter of intent or notice of law suit) before opening a claim file, investigating, or assigning the matter to a defense attorney.

These insurer perceptions were supported by results from the California study that concluded that traditional incident reporting as practiced during the early 1970s identified at most 10% of all potentially compensable events (27). A study of incident reporting systems during the late 1970s in Ohio hospitals found that although incident reports had been filed for about 70% of claims resulting from injuries that occurred in patient rooms, they served as advance notice for only 30% of claims arising from incidents in treatment locations such as the emergency department (30).

The reasons traditional incident reporting systems failed to serve as an effective risk management tool have been summarized by Orlikoff and Vanagunas (2). First, within most hospitals there was no clear definition of an "incident," resulting in confusion regarding what kind of occurrences should be reported. These systems were widely regarded as a nursing activity oriented toward the hospital's safety committee, thus discouraging participation by physicians and other health care providers.

Incident reports also were considered by many as possible admissions of negligence that could increase exposure to legal actions. Consequently, reports were seldom filed on major occurrences. In addition, the follow-up of incident reports for individual cases often was too slow to initiate corrective action before claim emergence; whereas the absence in most hospitals of a system to analyze incident report data and identify trends hindered the development of strategies to reduce preventable adverse occurrences.

The most important problem, however, was the failure of incident reporting to capture significant clinical adverse events. Occurrence screening and occurrence reporting are two data-gathering strategies designed during the late 1970s to overcome this deficiency. Most systems using these approaches are based on criteria developed and knowledge gained by investigators during the California study.

Occurrence Screening

During the California study it became apparent that the generic screening criteria and methodology could be adapted for hospital medical staff self-evaluation and risk control (27). It was believed a data collection and analysis system based on this approach would have obvious advantages from a risk management perspective over the traditional system for incident reporting, because the purpose of screening was to identify occurrences that would ultimately result in legal actions.

Screening for adverse occurrences, with subsequent review to detect the possible contribution of provider error, also was perceived as potentially superior to quality assessment activities based on medical chart audits. The audit approach, used by most hospitals and advocated by the Joint Commission on Accreditation of Hospitals, usually involved the development of criteria regarding the medical care process for a specific diagnosis, problem, or procedure. Medical charts were then reviewed for the limited number of patients to whom the audit criteria might apply to determine if the care received was appropriate or optimal.

By the late 1970s this approach was widely faulted for using unvalidated criteria and for failing to detect important problems in medical care (31). Physicians tended to view the audits as "tedious, costly, and nonproductive" requirements characterized by a heavy emphasis on data collection and few results that could be used for follow-up activities (32). It was hoped by its developers that, in contrast, the occurrence screening approach would identify more serious problems for a much more comprehensive sample of patients, as well as potentially provide more timely information on adverse outcomes that could be used to initiate corrective action and prevent claims emergence.

One example of the generic occurrence screening approach is the Medical Management Analysis (MMA) system designed by Joyce Craddick, MD (33). The system uses a set of screening criteria adapted from those developed during the California study in which Craddick was a participant. In approximately 200 hospitals where the system is in use, these screens are used by trained data retrieval personnel to review all patient records within 48 to 72 hours after admission, every 3 to 4 days during the hospital stay, and approximately 2 weeks after discharge. Occurrences perceived as serious are reported immediately for further review and possible action. For every admission, summary abstracts are prepared by the hospital quality assurance program. Medical charts with an adverse occurrence flagged by this screening process undergo peer review for an assessment of the clinical care provided. In addition, information on adverse occurrences is aggregated to identify possible trends.

Increasingly, regulators and accrediting bodies also are developing and implementing adverse incident detection methods that rely on the occurrence screening approach. At the national level, the JCAHO is developing clinical indicators for use by hospitals in screening cases for quality problems. It is anticipated that use of clinical indicators as quality screens eventually will be required as part of the hospital accreditation process.

The Health Care Financing Administration (HCFA) currently mandates the use of "generic quality screens" in reviews of the hospital care received by Medicare patients. Utilization and quality control peer review organizations (PROs) have been required since July 1986 to apply the generic screens to every case they review, or approximately one quarter of all Medicare hospital discharges (34). Medical records that fail the quality screens are referred by nurse reviewers to physician advisors for further analysis. Quality problems identified through this process may lead to corrective actions ranging from education and intensified review to sanctions. HCFA also has developed criteria for detecting quality problems that will be used to screen patient records in hospital outpatient departments, home health agencies, and skilled nursing facilities. Starting in 1989 these screens will be used to review ambulatory services received by Medicare beneficiaries. The U.S. Department of Defense also uses process and outcome clinical criteria to screen medical records for about 10% of all discharges from its 167 hospitals, with physician review of cases failing to meet these screens.

Virtually all adaptations of occurrence screening use this two-step approach in which explicit screening criteria are used in an initial review by trained personnel, followed by physician peer review of flagged cases with unanticipated and undesirable outcomes. This strategy is regarded by many as an effective and valid method of identifying adverse occurrences, as well as potentially compensable events resulting from substandard care. It also is seen as costly and inefficient, however, due to the large number of "false positives" identified during the initial review (34). Several approaches have been developed in efforts to address this problem.

Focused Occurrence Screens.   One strategy has been to augment (and sometimes replace) the generic hospital-wide outcome criteria with more focused screens developed specifically for departments or locations perceived to be at high risk for adverse events. The MMA system, for example, has developed several specialty-specific screens. Within this system, screens also can be added that incorporate JCAHO and utilization review requirements so that all medical record reviews can be conducted in one coordinated process (33). In addition to its hospital-wide quality indicators, JCAHO is developing focused screens, beginning with indicators for medical record reviews of obstetric and anesthesia services. Several studies (35,36) have examined the rate of agreement among trained data retrieval personnel in the detection of adverse events. Results suggest much higher levels of agreement (inter-rater reliability) for an approach in which the medical charts of patients with selected problems or diagnoses are reviewed using focused occurrence screens than for a more general review of all patients using generic screens.

Adjusting for the Risk of Adverse Occurrences.   Several recent efforts to provide more efficient and useful occurrence-screening tools examine adverse occurrences within the context of patient risk factors. The Adverse Patient Occurrences (APO) Inventory, for example, is a generic screening instrument developed by Schumacher and associates (36). It incorporates 11 items from the California study and the original MMA System with 6 new items, and produces a ratio for each patient chart reviewed that incorporates both information on adverse occurrences and patient risk for adverse events. A second example is the JCAHO quality indicators effort in which information is collected not only on adverse events, but also on patient risk factors and other information (or covariates) that may influence outcomes.

"High-Yield Screens."   The general objective of many groups who rely on occurrence screening has been to develop an abbreviated list of "high-yield" screens for which strong inter-rater agreement can be obtained. This process often requires a fairly lengthy period of experimentation with screening criteria and their definitions to determine within the particular practice setting or organization the screens that: permit high levels of agreement during the initial screening phase regarding the presence or absence of an adverse event; and identify significant patient problems or potential malpractice claims when submitted for physician review.

A good example of this process is a recent Kellogg-sponsored demonstration project undertaken by the Sisters of Mercy Health Corporation, in which location-specific occurrence screens were developed with extensive physician input (37). However, after using the screens to review 2,082 surgical charts and 743 obstetric records it was still found that "imprecise definitions of five of the (surgical and obstetric) criteria made them overly sensitive, causing many events to be erroneously identified as adverse occurrences." Three of the screens, including "neurologic deficit not present on admission," "maternal injury," and "infant abnormality and/or injury" were in retrospect not defined rigorously enough to be useful. Other screens, including "transfer from the operating room to a special care unit or bed" and "return to surgery on this admission" were found to be overly sensitive because they identified routine transfers and planned returns to surgery as well as adverse incidents. The project implemented suggestions for sharpening definitions to correct the problem. Other projects also have reported difficulties in defining and using certain screens. The presence of nosocomial infection, for example, has been particularly troublesome both for HCFA and others who have attempted to standardize definitions for use by data retrieval personnel (34).

The Sisters of Mercy project also found four screens to have a particularly "high yield" in that they flagged adverse occurrences in 10% or more of the records in several divisions, and they often were judged to indicate significant problems during subsequent physician review. These screens included the postoperative transfer from a general care bed to a special care unit or bed; unplanned removal, injury, or repair of an organ or structure during surgery; postanesthesia recovery time longer than 2 hours for patients having an abdominal or pelvic operation; and infant transferred to operating room or neonatal intensive care unit (ICU).

Occurrence Reporting

Occurrence reporting is another strategy for identifying clinically significant adverse events that grew out of efforts to improve the efficiency of occurrence screening. In recognition of the high costs associated with the two-stage approach used in the California study, Mills and colleagues (27) in the late 1970s extracted a set of criteria from the generic screens that could be used as "reportable" adverse clinical events in an improved incident reporting system. This approach to the identification of adverse occurrences subsequently was adopted by more than 300 hospitals in California and Nevada.

An example of this strategy is a list of 40 adverse events that must be reported at the time of their occurrence that has been designed by the New England Medical Center Hospitals in Boston. Occurrence reporting criteria, like screening approaches, also can be focused on specific departments, services, or locations. Examples include the lists of reportable occurrences developed by the Chicago Hospital Risk Pooling Program for high-risk areas, including operating and recovery rooms, emergency departments, labor and delivery suites, and ICUs. These criteria, developed with extensive physician consultation, are used in addition to their general system for incident reporting (2,4).

Several states now require the reporting of certain adverse events to the state department of health or the state medical board (34). New York requires hospitals to report within 24 hours of the occurrence incidents involving patient death or impairment "other than those related to the natural course of illness, disease, or proper treatment in accordance with generally accepted medical standards." Since 1987 Massachusetts has required hospitals, clinics, and health maintenance organizations to submit quarterly incident reports to the state medical board. Detailed information — including identification of the provider, a brief description of the incident, and patient characteristics — must be submitted for four types of major adverse events: maternal death related to delivery; fetal death (excluding abortion); death in the course of or resulting from ambulatory surgical care; and a chronic vegetative state resulting from medical intervention. The definition of this latter event currently is being refined at the request of the medical profession.

Early Warning Systems

The potential ability of focused occurrence screening and occurrence reporting to serve as an early warning of possible claims activity has been examined in several studies. In the Sisters of Mercy Health Corporation "Patient Care Assessment" project, surgical and obstetric screens were used to review the records of 40 surgical and 37 obstetrics patients who had filed malpractice claims or who had been involved in known potentially compensable events (37). The objective of the analysis was to determine whether these incidents could have been identified close to the time they occurred if staff had used the screening criteria to review care during or directly after hospitalization.

Of the 37 obstetric cases, 24 involved patients admitted for vaginal deliveries. Review of these records against the obstetric screens resulted in the identification of one or more adverse occurrences in 19 (79%) of the cases. The most frequently noted occurrences were identified by the screens for "infant's Apgar score six or less at five minutes"; "infant abnormality and/or injury"; and "infant transferred to operating room or neonatal intensive care unit." Most of the adverse occurrences not identified by the screens that resulted in claims alleged that failure to perform a timely caesarean section or failure to respond appropriately to fetal distress had led to mental retardation or other subsequent problems.

The remaining 13 obstetric cases involved caesarean sections, and therefore were reviewed using both the obstetric and surgical screens. Adverse occurrences were identified for all 13 patients. Thus, the screening criteria, if applied during or directly after hospitalization, would have flagged 32 of 37 (86%) cases as representing an adverse event. Notification of the occurrences by attorneys, patients, or others was actually received, however, less than 1 month after the event in 8 of the cases, between 1 month and 1 year later for 9 cases, 1 to 3 years later for 10 cases, and more than 3 years after the incident for 10 cases.

For the surgical cases, 32 of 40 (80%) charts contained one or more adverse occurrences identifiable through chart review using surgical screens supplemented with criteria developed for anesthesia review. Notification of these events had occurred within 1 month of the incident for 11 cases, between 1 month and 1 year later for 14 cases, and more than 1 year later for the remainder. Based on these analyses, it was concluded that if the screening criteria had been in use when the adverse events occurred, there would have been better documentation of the occurrences and the surrounding circumstances, and the Sisters of Mercy Health Corporation might have been in a more favorable position for legal defense. As a consequence of the project, the corporation adopted occurrence-screening for both risk management and quality assurance functions. They also revised their traditional incident reporting system to include a check list of reportable adverse clinical occurrences.

A recent study by the Chicago Hospital Risk Pooling Program examined 7 years of malpractice claims experience to analyze relationships between types of claims filed against member hospitals and the lists of reportable events used in their risk management system (38). Of the 1,121 claims filed, 46% were related to occurrences in one of four high-risk areas for which reportable adverse event check lists had been developed. For claims related to high-risk areas, 79% of the 77 labor and delivery claims, 60% of the 10 ICU claims, and 54% of both the 238 operating room and recovery room, and the 196 emergency department claims involved reportable adverse occurrences. (The analysis did not examine, however, the percentage of adverse events that actually were reported by physicians or hospital staff members close to the time of their occurrence.)

The study also determined which criteria on the lists were associated most often with a filed claim, as well as the characteristics of occurrences frequently resulting in claims that did not correspond to any of the reportable events. For example, emergency room criteria that appeared most frequently in claim files included return to the emergency room within 7 days of hospital discharge or previous emergency room visit; emergency room interpretation of roentgenogram that differed from radiologist's reading; patient or family complaint about treatment; and treatment or procedure error. Forty-six percent of the emergency room claims could not have been flagged by criteria used to determine reportable events. Of these, most (62%) alleged failure to diagnose a fracture, illness, or foreign body.

As a result of the study, reportable criteria for adverse events in three of the high-risk areas have been revised. In addition, occurrence reporting for ICU events is no longer recommended because that area accounted for only 2% of the claims from high-risk locations, and it was determined that the most important data would appear in standard mortality reviews.

Strategies To Detect Adverse Patient Occurrences

In summary, we are in a period of experimentation in which health delivery settings are developing and adapting various approaches to detect adverse patient outcomes. Several of these strategies seem promising, but none appears capable of serving as the sole data collection method for activities designed to detect and prevent adverse events. A combination of complementary approaches, tailored to the needs and specific problems of the organization, is recommended most frequently. Regardless of the methods selected, several fundamental issues must be addressed. The most important of these is securing physician support and involvement in the activities, as well as ensuring the confidentiality of information collected.

The Role of Physicians. There is widespread agreement that the most important factor promoting effective quality assurance and risk management is physician support and involvement in key activities (39,40). Physicians must be participants because, as emphasized previously, the most significant problems in health care settings — including events most likely to generate substantial malpractice claims — usually involve medical staff members and require physician participation to resolve problems. As medically related events become the major focus of risk management efforts, physicians must become involved in establishing the criteria used in screening and reporting systems to identify adverse patient occurrences.

They also must be primarily responsible for the evaluation of events selected for more intensive analysis. For each case reviewed, physicians must render opinions concerning the appropriate standard of care, factors contributing to the event, the extent of patient injury, and possible treatment or rehabilitation strategies if appropriate.

In addition, many health care settings place a high priority on facilitating physician reporting of significant clinical adverse events. A common approach is to supplement ongoing clinical reporting and screening activities with a 24-hour "hot line" for the verbal communication of incidents that may require immediate action by risk management staff. It is important to emphasize, however, that for any of these reporting strategies to be successful, physicians and staff members must be assured that adequate precautions have been taken to safeguard the confidentiality of such reports.

Confidentiality of Risk Management Activities. A common reason for failure to report adverse clinical events is fear of increased liability exposure if such reports are "discoverable" by plaintiff attorneys. Two methods most frequently considered for protecting the confidentiality of reports are "cloaking them under attorney-client privilege," or including them under peer review or other quality assurance activities protected by state statute if one exists (2). The method chosen will determine appropriate information flow and review procedures. If attorney-client privilege is used, analysis procedures must include attorney review. If protection is sought under a state statute, then an appropriate quality assurance or medical staff peer review committee must be included in the review of event reports.

Confidentiality is afforded to medical staff review of adverse occurrence information and other peer review functions in most states by statute. As of 1988 all but a few states had enacted laws protecting the minutes of such peer review committees from discovery or admissability in a malpractice suit (exceptions were North Carolina and Utah). It should be noted, however, that applicable laws often are interpreted literally by the courts. Details such as where files are kept, who is and is not copied, and the expressed purpose of communications can affect whether or not confidentiality protections apply. The committee and departmental structures and lines of communication created for peer review and risk management by the health care organization's bylaws and procedures must be carefully tailored so that the specific state statutes are applicable.

Regardless of the method of protection used, as Orlikoff and Vanagunas (2) emphasize, "the most effective means for combating fear is to ensure that incident reports are completed in a factual manner, reflecting the occurrence as it happened and not making value judgments or 'laying blame.' " This is a particularly important message to convey in physician and staff educational efforts. It must be understood that in many adverse occurrences all the factors responsible for the event cannot be immediately determined, even by participants in the incident. Thus, judgments regarding causation usually are premature without subsequent investigation and analysis.

In addition to the importance of physician support and confidentiality precautions, several suggestions have been made for strengthening clinical adverse incident detection systems (1-3). As discussed previously, clear definitions of screens and reportable events, as well as reporting procedures that are straightforward, easy to use, and timely are critical program elements. Motivation among physicians and staff members to participate in detection activities also is enhanced when it is readily apparent through appropriate feedback that this information is used to improve malpractice claims experience and patient care activities.

USING INFORMATION ON ADVERSE PATIENT OCCURRENCES

The clinical risk management process usually is considered to have four basic components: event identification and reporting; evaluation of risk through event analysis; risk treatment, which may include clinical, patient relations, and legal aspects; and risk prevention activities (3). The previous section reviewed current approaches to the systematic identification of adverse events from a risk management perspective. Unexpected adverse patient occurrences also may be identified through ongoing activities in other areas such as quality assurance, infection control, utilization review, and patient relations. The risk management benefits of adverse patient outcome detection through these activities, however, depend on the timeliness of event identification and promptness of reporting.

Malpractice Claim Management and Prevention

Event Analysis and Risk Evaluation.   Once identified, adverse occurrences must be analyzed to determine the extent of patient injury and factors precipitating or contributing to the event. Potentially serious cases may trigger investigation, including review of the medical record and other documentation as well as interviews with individuals involved in or witnessing the occurrence. Physician review is critical, particularly with regard to the nature and extent of injury, probable causes, and appropriateness of care received. It is likely that these judgments will increasingly need to consider guidelines and standards that have been developed for assuring clinical competence in specific medical procedures. The American College of Physicians, for example, has developed guidelines for clinical competence with regard to eight procedures in gastroenterology and nephrology (41). As part of a major patient safety and risk management effort, the Department of Anesthesia at the Harvard Medical School has developed specific, detailed, and mandatory standards for minimal patient monitoring during anesthesia at its nine component teaching hospitals (42). Although the movement is not without controversy, other specialties and organized groups of medical practitioners also are vigorously debating guidelines and standards for practice, and it is likely that these efforts will be used increasingly in peer review activities.

There must be some type of organizational mechanism — such as a standing committee — that can be immediately activated to coordinate these investigative and review functions. When iatrogenic injuries are identified, this group also must have the authority to initiate appropriate clinical and managerial activities to reduce the consequences of the adverse event for the patient and to decrease the likelihood of a malpractice claim.

Reducing the Consequences of Adverse Events.   Reducing the consequences of an adverse patient event may involve developing a plan for clinical treatment to respond to the patient's injury. Decisions should be made promptly about what information should be communicated to the patient regarding the event, as well as who should bear financial responsibility for any increased charges. Nursing management should be made aware of the adverse occurrence and subsequent decisions (3).

The importance of timely and appropriate communication with the patient (and possibly family members or significant others) after an unexpected adverse occurrence is frequently emphasized (2,3). As the previous discussion has indicated, most adverse patient events (83% according to the California study) are likely to occur as part of the "normal risk" of medical treatment rather than provider error. In these cases, good patient-provider communication regarding factors contributing to the event is critical. If it has been determined or is strongly suspected that the injury is due to provider error, the patient (or family member) should be informed as rapidly as possible of treatment plans, as well as the waiver of charges and financial restitution if considered appropriate.

Orlikoff and Vanagunas (2) argue that improved patient communication should be viewed as an important risk management tool that can provide a much-needed avenue for patients and families to express dissatisfaction with physicians and the hospital apart from litigation; lessen the probability that patients will file claims if injuries or incidents do occur; aid in predicting which patients will file malpractice claims; and increase the odds of obtaining timely, reasonable settlements if legal action is threatened.

Analysis of the event also must be conducted from a legal perspective, a process that is likely to involve recommendations by reviewing physicians regarding whether the case should be settled or defended in the event of legal action, as well as guidance by legal staff, insurer representatives, and defense counsel as appropriate.

Strengthening Peer Review Activities

Adverse event information may help strengthen peer review activities, but this is unlikely without the support and involvement of key members of the medical staff, particularly clinical chiefs of service in high-risk areas such as surgery, obstetrics, and emergency services (40,43). Fifer and Patton (44), for example, stress the important role clinical chiefs can play in using clinical incident reports or occurrence screening data in medical staff performance reviews. Serious events can receive immediate follow-up, whereas all clinical incidents or occurrences can be "trended," and reviewed in aggregate form by appropriate committees and clinical chiefs.

It is important to emphasize that the clinical chief or peer review committee has several options available for using information on adverse incidents or occurrences. These reports can be used informally as a basis for discussion with the physician involved, or as a grounds for closer observation of clinical performance or analysis of relevant medical records. More formally, on the basis of a particularly serious event or pattern of incidents, the recommendation may include remedial education, proctoring, or in the most extreme cases, a limitation or revocation of privileges (44).

Medical Staff Privileging and Credentialing. Increasingly, information on adverse occurrences and incidents also is being used in hospital reappointment and credentialing decisions. Traditionally in many hospitals, renewal of privileges and recredentialing were characterized by the "empty file syndrome." Information on most medical staff members was limited to the original application for privileges, and perhaps a list of continuing medical education courses attended (44). It is becoming more common, however, to view a primary objective of effective quality assurance and risk management programs as linking findings from monitoring activities with decisions on privileging and credentialing. As evidence has accumulated regarding an association between volume of procedures performed and better quality outcomes (45), it is becoming more commonplace in credentialing decisions for peer review committees to consider whether the volume of a specific procedure or other service provided by the medical staff member is sufficient for the maintenance of clinical competence.

In many institutions increased scrutiny also is being given to new applicants for medical staff positions, particularly with respect to verification of applicant-provided information, careful checking of references, and requests for information regarding malpractice claims experience and disciplinary actions (41,46). New accreditation standards from the JCAHO effective on January 1, 1989 require hospitals seeking accreditation to have ongoing risk management activities designed to identify, evaluate, and reduce the risks for patient injury associated with care. More rigorous investigations of physicians applying for new or renewed privileges are also mandated (23). These new standards, for example, require physicians under review to report any voluntary relinquishment or reduction of privileges or licenses — a long-standing "loophole" in many states that has allowed some physicians to avoid formal actions through voluntary resignations.

The new JCAHO standards indicate that each applicant for medical staff membership must complete an application form that asks for information specified in the medical staff bylaws. Such information must include previously successful or currently pending challenges to any licensure or registration or their voluntary relinquishment, as well as the voluntary or involuntary termination of medical staff membership, or limitation, reduction, or loss of clinical privileges at another hospital. In addition, the medical staff bylaws and rules and regulations must specify the circumstances under which an applicant is to report involvement in a professional liability action. At a minimum, final judgments or settlements involving the individual applicant are to be reported.

Reappointment, renewal, or revision of clinical privileges must be based on a reassessment of the criteria outlined above, as well as information concerning the physician's current licensure, health status, professional performance, judgment, and clinical or technical skills, *as indicated in part by the results of quality assurance activities.* (Some states, however, may have additional requirements.) The new standards also specify that the medical staff must actively participate, as appropriate, in risk management activities related to the clinical aspects of patient care and safety, including the identification of general areas of potential risk, correction of identified problems, and design of programs to reduce risk.

Independent confirmation of information on disciplinary actions and liability claims experience for physicians seeking new or renewed privileges may soon be available from the National Practitioner Data Bank (47,48). The data repository, which was authorized by federal legislation passed in 1986, is scheduled to begin during the fall of 1989. It will collect information regarding any final malpractice action, including out-of-court settlements against any licensed health care provider; disciplinary actions by state medical and dental boards; final professional review actions by hospitals, health maintenance organizations, or other medical facilities that have a peer review system; as well as any adverse actions by professional societies against members as a result of a formal peer review procedure.

The data system is to be established under a 5-year, $15.9 million contract between the U.S. Department of Health and Human Services and Unisys, a Pennsylvania information systems company. Once it is operational, all U.S. hospitals will be required to consult the data bank when a physician or dentist applies for clinical privileges, as well as every 2 years regarding reappointment and credentialing decisions.

Hospital privileging and credentialing, as well as other physician peer review activities, are also of increasing concern to state legislatures. Within the past year legislatures in more than half the states have enacted measures to regulate the quality of medical care by strengthening the monitoring of physician behavior. According to a recent Intergovernmental Health Policy Project report, states hope to reduce poor quality care and malpractice problems by expanding the powers of state medical boards, increasing physician licensure requirements, adding legal protections for peer reviewers, and mandating stricter requirements for hospital reporting of adverse actions against physicians (49).

Monitoring and Improving Patient Care

An important objective of most systems for the detection of adverse events is to accumulate and analyze reliable information in a manner that facilitates the identification of trends and possible problem areas (2,3). Such information can provide a focus for quality assurance efforts, as well as a means of measuring their impact. It also can be used by governing boards as one approach to monitoring the quality of patient care. To be most useful for these purposes, the number of adverse events should be analyzed, and trends over time displayed, according to the type of occurrence, location of the event, severity of the injury, time of day, shift on which the incident occurred, and relevant characteristics of patients and staff involved.

As more organizations begin to collect this information, it may become possible to identify particular problem areas through comparisons with peer institutions. Currently there is substantial variability among systems for identifying adverse events. In addition, there is little standardization of data elements collected or data collection procedures (34). This situation may change due to the screening and clinical incident reporting activities by regulators and accrediting and licensing bodies that have been discussed previously.

In addition, there are substantial efforts among hospitals and multihospital systems to develop comparable adverse event information that will allow meaningful comparisons and better data interpretation. The Maryland Hospital Association, for example, has undertaken a project with funding from the Robert Wood Johnson Foundation to develop a limited number of "clinical indicators" that can be commonly defined and that will permit meaningful comparisons among hospitals with similar characteristics (50). The major objective is to provide governing boards with a tool for monitoring the quality of care provided by their institutions. After a 3-year period of development and pilot testing, the indicators presently being used include surgical wound infections, autopsy rates, newborn deaths, perioperative deaths, cesarean sections, hospital readmissions, unplanned admissions after ambulatory surgery, intensive care unit readmissions, and unscheduled returns to the operating room. Currently approximately 250 hospitals are participating in the demonstration (Summer SJ. Personal communication).

Risk Management Activities and Malpractice Claims Experience

There is little empirical evidence regarding the degree to which hospital risk management activities result in a more positive malpractice claims experience. This relationship is difficult to assess because the length of time between an incident and the emergence of a formal claim often is considerable. In addition, a substantial amount of time may be required before the final outcome is apparent regarding the claims resolution process. These factors necessitate a longitudinal study design that permits examination of claims emergence and resolution for events or incidents that may have occurred during the period when risk management program activities were in place.

A recent study of 40 Maryland community hospitals attempted to take these factors into consideration in an analysis of risk management activities and subsequent claims experience (Morlock LL, Malitz FE. Do hospital risk management programs make a difference? Final report to the National Center for Health Services Research and Health Care Technology Assessment, 1988). The study used the earliest systematic information available on hospital risk management activities — a 1980 survey of all hospitals in the state conducted by the Maryland Hospital Education Institute. Survey responses included information on the role of the governing board in risk management activities, risk management program components, hospital policies for handling adverse medical incidents, and educational programs offered by the hospital in quality assurance and risk management. The professional liability experience of each hospital was assessed through data on claims resulting from hospital-based incidents (whether or not the hospital was a defendant) that occurred during 1980 to 1982, and that were resolved by the end of 1987. Claims experience was adjusted for hospital differences in exposure by including information in the analysis on hospital bedsize, and the volume of services performed in high-risk locations, including surgical and obstetrical suites and emergency departments.

Analysis results indicate that after adjusting for differences in exposure to claim risk, the total number of claims was lower in institutions that had implemented in-hospital programs regarding physician and nurse responsibilities in quality assurance and risk management. The number of claims in which defendants were found liable and total dollars awarded in damages were significantly less in hospitals that by 1980 had established a governing board oversight committee for quality assurance and risk management, that included risk management information in regular reports sent to the governing board, and that had a formal policy indicating that clinical chiefs must be notified of adverse medical incidents. In addition, the number of claims in which defendants were found liable was significantly lower for hospitals that had formal policies indicating whether patients or families should be informed of medical errors, and specifying who had responsibility for communicating such information. Hospitals with these characteristics did not have higher rates of private settlements.

This study included a relatively small number of hospitals in a single state that should be considered "early adopters" of risk management activities. Findings provide some of the first evidence available, however, for several key tenets in the clinical risk management literature, including the importance of educating clinicians regarding their role in risk management efforts; formalizing channels of communication that can facilitate early intervention if needed with patients and families after adverse medical events; and establishing a strong organizational structure for using information on unanticipated adverse occurrences.

EMERGING ISSUES IN CLINICAL RISK MANAGEMENT

Currently we are in a period of experimentation, characterized by various approaches to the detection of adverse patient occurrences, as well as considerable variation in strategies for the use of such information. There is relatively little empirical evidence regarding the efficacy of alternative approaches, either as mechanisms for the "early warning" of claims activity or in terms of their usefulness for improving the quality of patient care.

An on-going Robert Wood Johnson funded project by Mills, Lindgren, and Christensen is examining the effectiveness of various "early warning systems" for malpractice claims management and prevention implemented by the Professional Risk Management Group and others in inpatient health care settings in California. Among the issues being addressed are the relative advantages of "broad-based" clinical incident reporting, focused reporting, and occurrence screening approaches to adverse event detection; as well as how improvements can be made in the utilization of information available through these strategies for malpractice claim management and prevention. Research also is needed on these issues in other types of settings.

An area of intense controversy within the medical profession has been whether the development of guidelines or standards for clinical performance will result in decreased or increased malpractice claims activity. This issue is being examined by Bunker and colleagues with respect to anesthesia-related claims. Clearly it merits investigation in other areas as well.

The use of malpractice claims information in the medical staff privileging and credentialing process is now mandated by the JCAHO. If plans are realized for the National Practitioner Data Bank, reliable data on claims experience will become increasingly available. Little is known, however, regarding how such information can be most effectively used in peer review activities.

Future Trends

In the past few years sweeping changes in health care delivery have been seen. One trend has been an increasing amount of services delivered outside of the hospital setting. Most approaches to adverse event detection and other risk management strategies have been hospital-based efforts. One exception is the HCFA-sponsored projects to develop occurrence screens for ambulatory settings that have been discussed in previous sections. Some efforts also are underway to design and implement programs tailored to the liability problems and risk management opportunities specific to each type of delivery setting. An excellent example is the risk management model program developed for hospital-sponsored home health care by the Institute on Quality of Care and Patterns of Practice at the Hospital Research and Educational Trust (2). The development, implementation, and evaluation of similar efforts in primary care and long-term care settings should receive high priority.

Other significant trends have resulted in greater cost containment pressures imposed by utilization review requirements, more emphasis on managed care alternatives, and in many settings, new roles for physicians as gatekeepers who must weigh the potential benefits and costs of each additional health care service (51,52). It is reasonable to speculate that in the past most incentives provided by third party reimbursement and the predominant forms of health care delivery encouraged the provision of additional procedures and other services. Under these circumstances adverse events and provider errors probably were most likely to result from "acts of commission." Current risk management tools have been designed to reflect this assumption.

The 1990s, however, are likely to be characterized by the rationing of health care services through various organizational and payment mechanisms. These constraints, in the absence of countervailing forces, will almost certainly produce a higher rate of "errors of omission." The design of appropriate risk management and quality assurance strategies to detect and address problems created by these pressures is perhaps our greatest challenge.

References

1. Bader & Associates, Inc. *Patient Safety Manual: A Guide for Hospitals and Physicians to a Systematic Approach to Quality Assurance and Risk Management*. 2nd ed. Chicago:American College of Surgeons;1985.

2. Orlikoff JE, Vanagunas AM. *Malpractice Prevention and Liability Control for Hospitals*. 2nd ed. Chicago:American Hospital Publishing, Inc.;1988.

3. Kilduff R. *Clinical Risk Management — A Practical Approach*. Chicago:InterQual, Inc.;1985.

4. American Hospital Association. *Medical Malpractice Task Force Report on Tort Reform and Compendium of Professional Liability Early Warning Systems for Health Care Providers*. Chicago: American Hospital Association;1986.

5. Department of Health and Human Services. *Report of the Task Force on Medical Liability and Malpractice*. Washington, DC:DHHS;1987.

6. American Medical Association Special Task Force on Professional Liability and Insurance. *Professional Liability in the '80s. Report I*. Chicago:American Medical Association;1984.

7. Department of Health, Education and Welfare. *Report of the Secretary's Commission on Medical Malpractice*. Publication No. (OS) 73-88. Washington, DC: U.S. Government Printing Office; 1973.

8. Danzon PM. *Medical Malpractice: Theory, Evidence and Public Policy*. Cambridge:Harvard University Press;1985.

9. Danzon PM. *The Frequency and Severity of Medical Malpractice Claims*. Santa Monica, California: The Rand Corporation; 1983.

10. American Medical Association Special Task Force on Professional Liability and Insurance. *Professional Liability in the '80s. Report 2*. Chicago:American Medical Association;1984.

11. Pierce R. What legislators need to know about medical malpractice. Denver: National Conference of State Legislatures; 1985.

12. Jury Verdict Research. *Current Award Trends*. Solon, Ohio:Jury Verdict Research;1985.

13. Holthaus D. After tort reform: what's next? *Hospitals*. 1988;**62**:48-53.

14. Lund DS. Oregon malpractice rates to fall in '89 — many other states, however, will see a predictable increase in premiums. *HealthWeek*. 1988;**2**:13-4.

15. Williams S, ed. *Medical Malpractice Resurfacing as Issue for States*. Washington, DC:Alpha Centerpiece;1985.

16. Danzon PM. The frequency and severity of medical malpractice claims: new evidence. *Law Contem Prob*. 1986;**49**: 57-84.

17. Fisher RS. Physician discipline emerges as a state priority. State Health Notes, The George Washington University, 1988.

18. United States General Accounting Office. *Medical Malpractice: Six State Case Studies Show Claims and Insurance Costs Still Rise Despite Reforms*. Washington, DC:GAO;1986.

19. Southwick AF. Hospital liability; two theories have been merged. *J Legal Med*. 1982;**4**:1-50.

20. Curran WJ. A further solution to the malpractice problem: corporate liability and risk management in hospitals. *N Engl J Med*. 1984;**310**:704-5.

21. Jessee WF. *Quality of Care Issues for the Hospital Trustee: A Practical Guide to Fulfilling Trustee Responsibilities*. Chicago:The Hospital Research and Educational Trust;1984.

22. United States General Accounting Office. *Medical Malpractice: A Framework for Action*. Washington, DC: GAO;1987.

23. Joint Commission on Accreditation of Healthcare Organizations. *AMH/89: Accreditation Manual for Hospitals*. Chicago:JCAHO;1988.

24. Nelson S. States adopt risk-management regs. *Hospitals*. 1988;**62**:56.

25. National Association of Insurance Commissioners. *Malpractice Claims: Medical Malpractice Closed Claims, 1975-1978*. Brookfield, Wisconsin:National Association of Insurance Commissioners;1980.

26. United States General Accounting Office. *Medical Malpractice: Characteristics of Claims Closed in 1984*. Washington, DC:GAO;1987.

27. Mills DH, ed. *California Medical Association and California Hospital Association. Report on the Medical Insurance Feasibility Study*. San Francisco:Sutter Publications;1977.

28. Steel K, Gertman PM, Crescenzi C, Anderson J. Iatrogenic illness on a general medical service at a university hospital. *N Engl J Med*. 1981;**304**:638-42.

29. Couch NP, Tilney NL, Rayner AA, Moore FD. The high cost of low-frequency events — the anatomy and economics of surgical mishaps. *N Engl J Med*. 1981;**304**:634-7.

30. Duran G. Positive use of incident reports. *Hospitals*. 1979;**53**:60-8.

31. Sanazaro PJ. Medical audits, continuing education and quality assurance. *West J Med*. 1976;**121**:241-52.

32. Affeldt JE, Walezak RM. The role of JCAH in assuring quality care. In: Pina JT, Haffner AN, Rosen B, Light DW, eds. *Hospital Quality Assurance: Risk Management and Program Evaluation*. Rockville, Maryland: Aspen Publications; 1984

33. Craddick JW. *Medical Management Analysis Series, Vol. II: Improving Quality and Resource Management Through Medical Management Analysis*. Rockville, Maryland: Medical Management Analysis International, Inc.; 1987.

34. U.S. Congress, Office of Technology Assessment. *The Quality of Medical Care: Information for Consumers.* Washington, DC: U.S. Government Printing Office; 1988.

35. Panniers TJ, Newlander J. The adverse patient occurrences inventory: validity, reliability, and implications. *QRB.* 1986:**12**:311-5.

36. Schumacher DN, Parker B, Kofie V, Munns JM. Severity of illness index and the adverse patient occurrence index. *Med Care.* 1987;**25**:695-704.

37. Sicher CM, Sisters of Mercy Health Corporation. *Approaches to Patient Care Assessment in a Multihospital System.* Chicago:JCAHO;1987.

38. Vanagunas A, Halleen N. CHRPP completes study of concurrent monitoring. *Occurrence.* 1986;**1**:1-5.

39. Fifer WR. Risk management and medical malpractice. *QRB.* 1979;**5**:9-13.

40. Craddick JW. Medical management analysis in 1986. In: Chapman-Cliburn G, ed. *Risk Management and Quality Assurance: Issues and Interactions.* Chicago:JCAH;1986.

41. Roberts JS, Radany MH, Nash DB. Privilege delineation in a demanding new environment. *Ann Intern Med.* 1988;**108**:880-6.

42. Eichhorn JH, Cooper JB, Cullen DJ, Maier WR, Philip JH, Seeman RG. Standards for patient monitoring during anesthesia at Harvard Medical School. *JAMA.* 1986;**256**:1017-20.

43. Troyer GT, Salman SL. *Handbook of Health Care Risk Management.* Rockville, Maryland:Aspen Systems Corporation;1986.

44. Maryland Hospital Education Institute. Reference file no. 11: application of occurrence screening to performance-based credentialing. In: *Compendium of Professional Liability Early Warning Systems for Health Care Providers.* Chicago:American Hospital Association;1986.

45. Luft HS, Hunt SS. Evaluating individual hospital quality through outcome statistics. *JAMA.* 1986;**255**:2780-4.

46. Burda D. Liability reshapes hospital/physician relationships. *Hospitals.* 1987;**61**:56-60.

47. Wilson MA. National practitioner data bank. *Bull Fed State Boards Med Exam.* 1988:163-72.

48. U.S. to establish system tracking doctors, dentists. *The Baltimore Sun.* December 31, 1988.

49. Fisher RS. Physician discipline emerges as a state priority. *State Health Notes.* 1988;**84**:1-6.

50. Summer SJ. Maryland's experiment with quality measures. *Bus Health.* 1987;**5**:14-6.

51. Winkenwerder W, Nash DB. Corporately managed health care and the new role of physicians. *Cancer Invest.* 1988;**6**:209-17.

52. Reagan MD. Physicians as gatekeepers: a complex challenge. *N Engl J Med.* 1987;**317**:1731-4.

COMMENTARY

The risk management article by Morlock and associates summarizes a very complex topic. It also finally brings the area of risk management into the quality of care measurement family. Traditionally the two have been separate and distinct disciplines with professionals in one area not familiar with the latest developments in the other. This chapter goes a long way to rectifying this situation, and it is hoped that increased communication and cooperation between the disciplines will result. Readers of this book will certainly see the parallels and ties in the two research fields; adverse patient occurrences in risk management as compared to outcomes (*see* chapter by Dubois) measurement in quality of care; and the potential importance of measuring patient satisfaction (*see* chapter by Kaplan and Ware) for both early feedback on potential risk management problems and designing strategies after an incident has occurred. Finally, as in quality of care measurement, there is no magic bullet that can accurately and, at low cost, pinpoint risk management problems. Both risk management and quality of care measurement are multidimensional. Morlock and associates recommend "a combination of complementary approaches, tailored to the needs and specific problems of the organization."

The editors have tried to demonstrate throughout this book the importance of structuring quality into the very marrow of the health care institution. Morlock and associates clearly document how important this is in the area of risk management. This is true for traditional indemnity and managed care situations, in the hospital, and in the physician's private office.

The whole structure of the risk management process beginning with incident reporting, moving on to malpractice claim management, and closing the loop with feedback to the entire organization (not just the affected individual) fits in perfectly with the Deming approach to incorporating quality into the entire management process (*see* chapter by Batalden and Buchanan). Historically, unfortunately, risk management activities have not had the necessary visibility at the executive level to permit the diffusion of results (the feedback loop) of risk management investigation throughout the organization. With the increased risk that skyrocketing malpractice settlements have posed to the financial health of an institution has come an increased executive attention to the role of risk management in the entire management process.

With respect to the hospital, the locus of the lion's share of risk management activity, Morlock and associates appropriately highlight the credentialing process. Credentialing can become a more rigorous and objective structural component of the quality management process. In the managed care situation, credentialing and its follow-up can be tied in innovative ways to the compensation process. At a minimum, the incident reporting process should be tied to the credentialing mechanisms. The current continuing education routine where a physician needs to take a certain amount of course work in any area he or she wants needs to be changed in favor of a system wherein continuing medical education is tied into specific skill improvements needed for the individual physician. This approach again is more amenable to the managed care situation.

The legal implications of risk management activities pose a potential cooperation barrier between quality assurance and risk management. Morlock and associates have appropriately emphasized the need to protect risk management activity from legal disclosure. Quality of care measurement has no similar legal protection. Although the editors have been blending the line between risk management and quality assurance activities, a separate and distinct separation will be necessary for plaintiff attorneys.

The line probably lies, and needs to be clearly specified, at adverse patient occurrences that transpire at the individual patient level.

It is very interesting from a quality management point of view to read Morlock and associates' summary of the literature pertaining to incident reporting and occurrence screening. Who should fill out incident reports? The more specific the information and the closer the author of the report is to the event (preferably the physician involved, if such was the case), the more accurate and relevant is the report. With respect to occurrence screening, we are struck by the parallels to the quality of care measurement literature. Though more research needs to be done to document this finding, focused occurrence screening, a process measure, is more valuable when it is tied to specific diagnostic screens. A similar trend can be seen in process measures for ambulatory care (*see* chapter by Greenfield).

After all is said and done, many physicians will ask if quality assurance and risk management activities make any difference? Do they result in lower malpractice claims? Morlock and associates have thoroughly documented how this is a difficult hypothesis to prove. As physicians in malpractice themselves painfully realize, one can get sued years after an incident has occurred. Despite these methodologic problems, in separate studies, Morlock has shown that "the total number of claims experienced was lower in institutions that had implemented in-hospital programs regarding physician and nurse responsibilities in quality assurance and risk management." This bottom line impact on both the financial and quality of care vigor of a health care institution clearly demonstrates the need to tie these disciplines together and to infuse the information throughout the organization. The achievement of this twin goal cannot be accomplished without the leadership of both the local and national physician community. (The Editors)